齊仲甫《女科百問》

CHANNELING THE MOON
A TRANSLATION AND DISCUSSION OF QÍ ZHÒNGFǓ'S
HUNDRED QUESTIONS ON GYNECOLOGY

———◆———

PART TWO · QUESTIONS 15–50

齊仲甫《女科百問》

CHANNELING THE MOON

A Translation and Discussion of Qí Zhòngfǔ's
Hundred Questions on Gynecology

PART TWO ⌒ QUESTIONS 15–50

SABINE WILMS, PHD

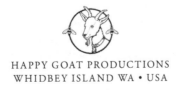

HAPPY GOAT PRODUCTIONS
WHIDBEY ISLAND WA • USA

Published by Happy Goat Productions
Whidbey Island, WA · USA
www.HappyGoatProductions.com

Published in the United States of America

First published in 2020

ISBN 978-1-7321571-4-9

ADDITIONAL COMMENTARY
Sharon Weizenbaum, LAc · whitepinehealingarts.org
Genevieve LeGoff · www.betweenheavenandearth.org

Photos © Linda Schwarz · www.whidbeyartists.com/schwarz
Cover photo *Ebey's Dusk* · Inset photo *Blue Moon*

Book design by Barbara Tada · www.pixelgardendesign.com

Education in Traditional Chinese Medicine
www.HappyGoatProductions.com
Online · Books · Teaching

DEDICATION

This book is dedicated to my parents, Ute and Klaus Wilms, both physicians and my first teachers of medicine. Through their lived example, I learned from the moment I entered this world what it means to dedicate yourself to your profession and Golden Path. And even though it took me more than a dozen years after high school to find my way back to this profession and I don't practice clinical medicine or work in the biomedical system that my parents, sister, uncles, and grandparents practiced in, maybe it gives me a little old-fashioned legitimacy to cite the old Chinese saying:

醫不三世，不服其藥。

When a physician does not come from three generations
[of doctors], don't take their medicine!

Of course this book is also dedicated to my daughter, my favorite peach dumpling and shining light, and to my old dog Nilson who has made sure I stay sane and healthy by insisting on beach walks. He keeps my feet and heart warm under my desk while I write, and always waits patiently by the shore when I find bliss and wash away the effects of a long day at the computer in the icy salty waters of the Puget Sound.

...And to my deepest teacher the sea,
     great mother of us all and ultimate embodiment of Yīn...

Contents

LIST OF PHOTOGRAPHS

Acknowledgments

IN MY DECADES OF WORKING WITH BOOKS AS AN AUTHOR, EDITOR, reviewer, reader, and publisher, this is the most important thing that I have learned: It truly does "take a village", in this case a passionate dedicated community of experts, to "raise a child" or bring a book to fruition. Once again I have been so fortunate to receive this kind of support in the process of shepherding this newest creation of mine from the state of a raw translation to the beautiful finished book you are holding in your hand. Innumerable colleagues, both academic and clinical, have generously shared their time and expertise to help me shed some light on a world far removed from our own in time, geography, and language, and yet, I believe, with important messages for our modern world. Please know that the following list, no matter how long I could make it, would always be incomplete. As it is, it represents just the tiny cherry on the top of a delicious pile of whipping cream, in the form of countless colleagues, students, friends, and family members, who have all given so generously in service of this powerful medicine.

To begin with, I thank my esteemed clinical colleagues Genevieve LeGoff, Brenda Hood, Sharon Weizenbaum, Zhou Guangying, Z'ev Rosenberg, Long Rihui, and Debra Betts, for their insights into gynecology in the tradition of Chinese medicine. Their teachings have informed my own, and their clinical work in this field has made a huge difference in the increasing recognition of traditional Chinese gynecology as a highly effective medical paradigm for the treatment of women's conditions. Very slowly, the standard of education in this key subject is rising in Chinese medicine schools and continuing education programs, as students are starting to demand and receive full semester- or year-long classes in genuine Chinese gynecology (as opposed to the "biomedicine light" version sold as "integrative" TCM in simplistic weekend workshops). Word is also getting around among inquisitive and demanding patients that medical care can be more advanced than the prescription of pain relief or birth control pills for menstrual pain, or a hysterectomy to treat endometriosis or fibroids. I am so grateful for the inspiring work of the leading clinicians in this important field as teachers and practitioners!

I also want to thank the medical historians whose research in the historical and cultural context of traditional Chinese gynecology has proven invaluable for this translation project. Among many others, Charlotte Furth, Yi-Li Wu, Francesca Bray, and Jen-der Lee have produced contributions that I believe to be essential reading for practitioners interested in the history of traditional Chinese gynecology.

As with all my work, I want to thank Nigel Wiseman for his accomplishment in laying the foundations for the translation, and accurate transmission, of Chinese medical literature into Western languages by creating a professional, historically accurate, yet clinically useful technical terminology of Chinese medicine in English. While translators may or may not choose to adapt his specific term choices, his and Feng Ye's *Practical Dictionary of Chinese Medicine* continues to be the single most important publication and reference work on the topic of translating Chinese medicine into Western languages.

A number of people were directly involved in the production of this book. I deeply treasure the content of the Chinese texts that I translate in my books, and it is such a privilege to have developed a team of expert professionals at Happy Goat Productions who share my respect for this wisdom and my dedication to creating books that aim to reflect the value of these texts. Once again, Barbara Tada has worked her magic in creating the perfect layout to present the complex combination of textual layers in a reader-friendly and beautiful format. As in the past, it has been such a pleasure and honor to witness the evolution of her design of the cover to represent my hard work inside. As the perfect compliment to Barbara's design work, I am so very grateful to the talented artist, and new friend, Linda Schwarz for permitting us to use her gorgeous artwork for the cover and inside illustrations. All of her photographs in this book were taken within a few miles of my home, right here on beautiful Whidbey Island. The soft, watery, "yīn" quality of Linda's art immediately struck me as the perfect addition to this book on gynecology, when I first came across it in a local gallery. Leo Lok, Eugene Anderson, Sharon Weizenbaum, and Genevieve LeGoff generously agreed to read my manuscript patiently and critically, and helped me to straighten out a number of potential or real confusions and misunderstandings. I cannot thank them enough, but of course take full responsibility for all mistakes that are still inside these pages! Chris Flanagan, copy editor extraordinaire, has once more taken a giant load off my back by editing my writing with her skilled hawk eyes. How lucky I am to have found an editor who combines professional English editing skills with clinical expertise in Chinese medicine as well as a knowledge of Chinese! She is truly a unique asset to our profession. For any writer, but for perfectionists like myself in particular, it is a huge relief to have this level of support!

As in the first volume of *Channeling the Moon*, Sharon Weizenbaum has again increased the clinical value of the information in this book immeasurably by adding her pearls of wisdom as clinical commentary throughout the book. It has been one of my favorite parts of the process of producing this book to receive her insights and feedback on my own work and see what she would do with this information.

I am so happy to acknowledge my wise friend and advisor Lillian Pearl Bridges who continuously sets me straight, keeps me on my "Golden Path," feeds me delicious meals cooked with love, reminds me of the magic of 靈 *líng*, and helps me make sense of, or at least function in, a world that often feels like a very foreign planet. This book would not exist without her friendship and love, belief in the relevance of my work, and professional and spiritual encouragement!

Last but definitely not least, I continue to be infinitely grateful for the enthusiasm, interest, and support expressed by my students and readers all over the world who have convinced me of the need to take on and persevere in this challenging translation project. I will never stop appreciating my extraordinary good fortune as a historian and scholar to receive such personal feedback and to know that my work is making a real difference in the lives of my readers', and students', and colleagues' patients! It is a privilege and honor to work in this field, which I consider the crown jewel of the treasure trove of Chinese medicine.

INTRODUCTION

THE PRESENT BOOK, TITLED *CHANNELING THE MOON, PART TWO*, contains my translation and discussion of Questions 15 to 50 of Qí Zhòngfǔ's *Hundred Questions on Gynecology*. After discussing the theoretical foundations of women's physiology and then addressing conditions related to menstruation in Questions 1–14 (published as *Channeling the Moon, Part One* by Happy Goat Productions, 2019), Qí Zhòngfǔ next concerns himself with women's miscellaneous conditions, or in other words, with any conditions that he saw as related specifically to the female body. The reasons for their inclusion in this book are varied, fascinating, and not always obvious. Therefore they have much to teach us modern humans about the way Qí Zhòngfǔ and his contemporaries viewed gender, reproduction, health and illness, sexuality, women's social and natural environment, medicine as a whole, and many other topics. Perhaps more than the other three volumes in what will be a series of four volumes, this particular one provides insight into what it meant in Sòng dynasty China to inhabit a female body beyond the obviously female experiences of menstruation (volume one), pregnancy (volume three), and childbirth and postpartum recovery (volume four).

We live in a fascinating time and world of rapid medical, social, and cultural change when it comes to defining and delineating the fluid boundaries of maleness and femaleness, masculinity and femininity, sex and gender. Obviously, the meaning of the words "man" and "woman," and the territory of fertile borderland between these two, was radically different in Sòng dynasty China from what it is in modern America, where, to name just one factor, the clinical treatment with hormonal and surgical therapy provides new options for people whose gender differs from the sex assigned to them at birth. I raise this issue here with some hesitation because our language and culture are evolving so rapidly that my ruminations, as a proud member of the "wrinklies" living a fairly reclusive writer's life with my head in ancient Chinese texts, are bound to offend some critical readers. Please bear with me, however, because of the point I am hoping to make, not about contemporary America but about the way in which we need to look at information from a far distant culture and society.

We are so used to thinking of Sòng dynasty China as a backwards time of patriarchy and misogyny, characterized by foot-binding, concubinage, women's physical and social isolation within the confines of the home, and their lack of access to political power and public expression. But what do we really know about the embodied experience of women's daily lives in the thirteenth century? How did men and women, parents and children, rulers and subjects, even experience hierarchy in a Confucian society built on the dual foundations of 義 *yì* ("justice" or "righteousness") and 仁 *rén* ("humaneness" or "compassion") in the spirit of two-directional family relations of love, caring, and obligation? How did not only the male medical authors but also their readers and female patients experience, express, and interpret women's emotional and physical distress? What were the key vulnerabilities and etiological factors that they saw as affecting the healthy functioning of female bodies, including but perhaps most interestingly not limited to menstruation and reproduction? And ultimately, what was considered "healthy" or "normal," and what was considered "pathological" or "irregular" during this time? For so many reasons, these are not questions whose answers we can take for granted on the basis of our modern experience. Our current gender fluidity is only one, if perhaps the most obvious, change that should make us pause before we take our basic assumptions about the female body, however we want to define it, for granted. Beyond offering useful clinical treatment options for common gynecological conditions, the text that you are about to read presents new perspectives and angles from which to look at situations that you may never have considered before in the contexts of either a specifically female body or of a pathology that can be influenced positively in treatment. More than anything, I ask you to approach this information with an open mind and critically assess your own preconceptions as you join me in exploring the "Hundred Questions on Gynecology" posed by Qí Zhòngfǔ and the answers he presented. In particular, you may want to watch out for questions and answers that strike you as unusual or initially as only of historical value. Rather than dismissing them, why not contemplate how you might translate Qí Zhòngfǔ's ideas into the modern clinical context?

For far too long, the supposed "backwardness" and misogyny of traditional China has allowed contemporary practitioners of the TCM version of Chinese medicine in the West to flippantly dismiss the wealth of historical knowledge on gynecology (婦科 fùkē, literally "specialization in women") in China. As Qí Zhòngfǔ's and other texts of the Sòng period show, however, gynecology in thirteenth-century China was a dynamic and blossoming field of new inquiry with an abundance of ideas sprouting in the deep and fertile topsoil of the Hàn and Táng classical foundations. For the sake of your female patients and all of our efforts to improve women's lives in general, I ask you to take this material seriously and look beyond the mainstream Western view of traditional China as misogynistic and therefore incapable of producing information on women's health that can benefit and enlighten us today.

There are many possible reasons why the high standard of gynecological care throughout the history of Chinese medicine is rarely reflected in the current practice of TCM in the West. Depending on your background and personal experience, you may want to blame this unfortunate fact on any or all of the following: the misogynistic history of Western biomedicine, which is regrettably still the dominant and unquestioned medical paradigm for too many Western practitioners of Chinese medicine; the institutional limitations of TCM education in the West; political and economic factors affecting both providers of healthcare and their patients; ignorance and lack of exposure among practitioners and/or patients to Chinese knowledge and clinical practice on this topic; lack of access to primary sources and their transmission; and/or the popularity in the West of acupuncture over medicinal therapy, which forms the core of traditional gynecology in China but is still in its infancy in the West. What I hope to demonstrate with this book series, however, is that you can no longer blame traditional Chinese gynecology for the lack of training, resources, and clinical efficacy with which far too many Western practitioners of Chinese medicine still approach the female body.

Qí Zhòngfǔ's answers to his "Hundred Questions" are drawn from a wide range of sources that span the preceding millennium and present a panoply of etiological, pathological, diagnostic, and therapeutic pearls. The thirty-six questions discussed in the present volume address conditions that were seen as associated with the female body beyond the immediate effects and processes of menstruation and reproduction. They include standard conditions still treated in TCM gynecology and directly related to female physiology centered around blood and physiological factors like the breasts, vagina, and uterus: abnormal bleeding anywhere in the body, abdominal distention and masses, vaginal discharge, spotting and hemorrhaging, etc. Interestingly enough, there is no mention of what could be read as the traditional precursors of the modern condition of breast cancer.

In addition to the obviously female-specific conditions mentioned above, we see discussions of issues related to the emotions and the Shén, like panic, cravings, weeping and less joy and more anger, mental instability and delirious behavior especially at night, and "having intercourse with ghosts at night." There are questions that address women's conditions caused by their greater susceptibility to external invasions of wind and cold in particular, resulting in blackout vision, seizures, and mania, and congestion, pain, and lack of flow, respectively. And then we have discussions for such standard conditions as jaundice, lumbar or arm pain, plum-pit Qì, eczema, or Dissipation Thirst, which are included in this book because the manifestation of these conditions in the female body can be explained from and therefore also treated by a specifically female angle.

There are three separate but obviously related and mutually reinforcing etiological factors in the formation of gynecological conditions that appear consistently throughout this volume: vacuity, openness, and taxation. All of these are due to women's reproductive processes, namely the monthly discharge of menstrual blood when healthy and not pregnant, the formation and nurturing of the fetus during pregnancy, the often traumatic and extremely draining process of childbirth, and then the further burden on the female body from breastfeeding. As a result, the formation, management, and replenishing of blood and fluids is of utmost importance in the vast majority of these conditions. It certainly rings true after reading this book that "women are ruled by Blood"! As Qí Zhòngfǔ points out in Question Forty-Four:

> 若血氣調和，不生虛實痛証。

> If the blood and Qì are harmoniously attuned, they do not engender vacuity or repletion pain patterns.

Looking at the material in this volume from the perspective of physiology rather than pathology, Qí Zhòngfǔ's writings reflect an image of the healthy female body as a fertile landscape dominated by fluid: In its most basic form as blood, it flows freely and swiftly in rivers and channels, sweeping away blockages and bringing life and sustenance to the most distant reaches of the body. It pools in fertile marshes and backs up in swamps and reservoirs that drain on a regular basis in alignment with the ebb and flow of cosmic forces, rinsing away impurity and staleness. In the form of *yíng* Provisioning, it seeps and soaks into the surrounding tissue as vital nourishment. And ultimately it gathers and comes to rest in the Chōngmài as the limitless

"Sea of Blood." As Question Thirty-Five explains in the context of "heat entering the Blood Chamber" as the cause for women speaking deliriously at night:

何以明之？室者，屋室也，謂可以停止之處。人身之血室者，
營血停止之所，經脈留會之處，即衝脈也。

衝為血海，王冰云「陰靜海滿而去血」，內經云「任脈通，
太衝脈盛，月事以時下」者，是也。

How do we know this? Chamber means a house, referring to a place where you can stop moving and stay. The Blood Chamber in the human body is the place where *yíng* Provisioning and blood stop and where the channels come together. Thus, it is precisely the Chōngmài.

The Chōngmài is the Sea of Blood. This is what Wáng Bīng's statement, "when Yīn is still and the Sea is filled, the [menstrual] blood leaves," and the *Nèijīng* statement, "the flow in the Rènmài goes through, the flow in the Great Chōngmài is exuberant, and the monthly period therefore descends in time," are talking about.

A healthy human body obviously depends on all *zàngfǔ* organs functioning harmoniously and fully. Nevertheless, the importance of blood in the female body means that two organs are of particular importance, due to their role in blood physiology: the heart, which governs the flow of blood in the vessels, and the liver, which stores the blood. In addition, the spleen and stomach provide and manage moisture, and the kidney, due to its role in reproduction, is also intimately involved, especially in the context of being threatened by exhaustion. Question Forty-Eight, states:

常觀血之流行，起自於心，聚之於脾，藏之於肝。此三經者，
皆心血所系之處也。

> According to the standard view, the flow of blood starts in the heart, gathers in the spleen, and is stored in the liver. These three channels are all places linked to heart blood.

When the delicate dynamic equilibrium between Qì and blood is disturbed and this flow is mismanaged or out of control, however, pathology manifests in natural metaphors of water being out of place. Results range from Landslide Collapse and flooding to spilling over, draining, leaking, and spotting, or the opposite, namely the lack of flow, which causes desiccation and congealing to form masses, blockages, and obstructions. Lastly, related to this central importance of fluids and water in the female body, another potential pathogenic factor is fire, or heat. This "evil" threatens to dry up the fluids in the body and, through its Five Dynamic Agents association, disorders the heart in particular, when it rises up from the womb along the Chōngmài. In this context, we must pay special attention to the womb, or the "Blood Chamber" in a narrower sense, as the entryway through which pathogenic factors manage to sneak into a vacuous and exhausted female body, especially during menstruation and childbirth or its immediate aftermath.

We can see from this constellation of vulnerabilities, weaknesses, and potential pathologies why women's conditions were already in the Hàn dynasty referred to as *dài xià* 帶下 "below the belt." A modern TCM practitioner may be tempted to read this expression as referring to the Dàimài in the sense of "the area located below the Dàimài," but it must be noted that early gynecology texts do not yet emphasize the role of this vessel in their etiologies. Thus, the term must have originally referred not to the vessel in this location, but to the location of "below the belt" itself. In the Hàn period text *Jīnguì yàolüè* 《金匱要略》 (Essentials from the Golden Cabinet) by Zhāng Zhòngjǐng 張仲景, women's conditions are referred to as the "thirty-six diseases of women" (婦人三十六病 *fùrén sānshíliù bìng*) in the introduction. In Chapter Twenty-Two on women's miscellaneous conditions, these are explained as "all being located below the belt" and summarized in this way:

婦人之病，因虛，積冷，結氣，為諸經水斷絕，至有歷年，血寒積結，胞門寒傷，經絡凝堅。。。

此皆帶下，非有鬼神。久則羸瘦，脈虛多寒；三十六病，千變萬端；審脈陰陽，虛實緊弦；行其針藥，治危得安；其雖同病，脈各異源，子當辨記，勿謂不然。

Women's diseases are due to vacuity, accumulated cold, and bound Qì, causing all the various interruptions in the flow of the menstrual fluids. If this continues for a number of years, blood and cold accumulate and bind, there is cold damage in the entrance to the womb, and the channels and network vessels become congealed and hard...

These are all "below the belt" [diseases], and not due to the presence of ghosts and spirits. Over time, they result in marked emaciation, vacuity in the vessels, and a preponderance of cold. These "thirty-six diseases" have a thousand alterations and ten-thousand variations. Examine the pulse for being Yīn or Yáng, vacuous or replete, and for being tight and string-like. Carry out your needling or medicinal therapy, to manage crises and obtain peace. Even though these conditions may be an identical disease, the pulse may each have a different source. You must differentiate and take note of this! Do not contradict this statement!

In its most comprehensive meaning at this early period, Charlotte Furth has suggested in her outstanding book on the history of Chinese gynecology *A Flourishing Yin* that the term *dàixià* referred to "women's reproductive malfunctions in terms of an energy field holding the womb in place and regulating the flow of fluid discharges from the vagina." It is significant here that the primary symptom of female pathology was, already at this early stage in the development of gynecology, identified as interrupted menstruation, a condition with much broader consequences and connotations than a mere inability to reproduce.

After the *Jīnguì yàolüè*, the next transmitted text in the history of Chinese medicine to attempt a categorization of women's symptoms by applying the structure of these so-called "thirty-six diseases of *dàixià*" is Cháo Yuánfāng's 巢元方 *Zhūbìng yuánhòu lùn* 《諸病源候論》 (Discourse on the Origins and Signs of the Various Diseases) from 610 CE. Here, the entries on menstrual disorders immediately precede those on conditions of vaginal discharge, which are referred to, in what is for a modern reader a slightly confusing terminology, in the narrower sense of the term as *dàixià*. These are followed by sections on vaginal leaking, Landslide Collapse (a life-threatening condition associated with profuse vaginal discharge or hemorrhaging), and various types of abdominal masses, concluding with an essay on the "thirty-six diseases of *dàixià*." The pathologies of menstrual inhibition and vaginal discharge are explained with almost identical etiologies: In both cases, the condition is ultimately caused by taxation damage to Qì and blood, leading to physical vacuity and an invasion by wind and cold, in terms that will sound familiar to readers of Part One of *Channeling the Moon*, which discussed menstrual conditions. This wind-cold lodges in the uterus and damages the channels, in partic- ular the Hand Shàoyīn Heart Channel and the Hand Tàiyáng Small Intestine Channel, which are responsible for the descent of blood as menstrual fluid. Excessive cold causes the blood to congeal instead of flowing freely and being discharged as menstrual fluid (or turn- ing into breast milk after childbirth or providing nurturance for the fetus during pregnancy). When Qì is depleted and therefore unable to constrain and control blood, this pathology can easily turn into vaginal discharge in the various colors when "the blood in the chan- nels is injured and therefore mixed with filthy fluids, forming vaginal discharge." The color of the discharge gives an etiological clue about which of the five *zàng* organs is primarily affected according to the

Five-Phases association of *zàng* organs and colors: green pointing to the liver, yellow to the spleen, red to the heart, white to the lungs, and black to the kidneys. In the entry following the five entries on vaginal discharge in each of the five colors, an alternative etiological explanation links white discharge to the presence of excessive cold and red discharge to the presence of excessive heat.

The next entry, which introduces the pathological category of abdominal lumps, states that they are caused by an accumulation of cold Qì and by a failure to disperse food and drink, causing them to lodge below the rib-sides instead. Several entries on specific types of accumulations repeatedly relate all of them to reproduction and menstruation, either because they are caused by childbirth-related depletion and weakness, or because they cause menstrual stoppage and interrupt women's ability to bear children. The *Zhūbìng yuánhòu lùn* then cites a list of "thirty-six diseases of *dàixià*," which is almost identical to Sūn Sīmiǎo's 孫思邈 slightly later list in his *Bèijí qiānjīn yàofāng* 《備急千金要方》 (Essential Formulas Worth a Thousand in Gold to Prepare for Emergencies, 652 CE). The entry concludes with a reference to Zhāng Zhòngjǐng: "The thirty-six types of diseases mentioned by Zhāng Zhòngjǐng are all due to cold and heat and taxation damage in the uterus, causing [a woman] to suffer from vaginal discharge, arising inside the genitals...."

Finally, supporting Furth's link of vaginal discharge, menstrual irregularities, and reproductive malfunctions, Cháo Yuánfāng concludes this volume with an essay on infertility. This is again related to taxation damage to Qì and blood and an imbalance of heat and cold, causing wind-cold lodging in the uterus, blocked menstruation, Landslide Collapse, or vaginal discharge. Faced with this confusion of categories based on symptoms related to menstruation, vaginal discharge, abdominal masses, and infertility, we might agree with Alfred North Whitehead that "classification is a halfway house between the immediate concreteness of the individual thing and the complete abstraction of mathematical notions... Classification is necessary. But unless you can progress from classification to mathematics, your reasoning will not take you very far."[1]

There is a striking difference between the minimal and often over-lapping or even identical explanations for the various conditions of gynecology that we find in the early gynecological literature and the sophisticated theoretical explanations and formula treatments offered by Qí Zhòngfǔ. His illustrious colleague Chén Zìmíng 陳自明, the author of the voluminous and slightly later *Fùrén dàquán liángfāng*《婦人大全良方》(Compendium of Excellent Formulas for Women, composed in 1237 CE), spelled out the pivotal role of blood in women's physiology and pathology in the very introduction to his text, paraphrasing Qí Zhòngfǔ's discussion of the *tiānguǐ* in Question Four without giving him credit:

> 岐伯曰：女子七歲腎氣盛，齒更髮長；二七而天癸至，任脈通，太沖脈盛，月事以時下。天，謂天真之氣降；癸，謂壬癸，水名，故云天癸也。
>
> 然沖為血海，任主胞胎，腎氣全盛，二脈流通，經血漸盈，應時而下。所以謂之月事者，平和之氣，常以三旬一見，以像月盈則虧也。
>
> 若遇經脈行時，最宜謹於將理。將理失宜，似產後一般受病，輕為宿疾，重可死矣。蓋被驚則血氣錯亂，經脈斬然不行，逆於身則為血分、癆瘵等疾。若其時勞力，則生虛熱，變為疼痛之根。若恚怒則氣逆，氣逆則血逆，逆於腰腿，則遇經行時腰腿痛重，過期即安也。逆於頭、腹、心、肺、背、脅、手足之間，則遇經行時，其證亦然。若怒極則傷肝，而有眼暈、脅痛、嘔血、瘰癧、癰瘡之病，加之經血滲漏於其間，遂成竅穴，淋瀝無有已也。
>
> 凡此之時，中風則病風，感冷則病冷，久而不愈，變證百出，不可言者。所謂犯時微若秋毫，感病重如山嶽，可不畏哉！

---

1 *Science and the Modern World*, p. 28.

Qí Bó said: "When girls reach the seventh year of life, their kidney Qì is exuberant, their adult teeth come in, and the hair on the head grows long. At two times seven, the *tiāngui* arrives, the flow in the Rènmài goes through, and the flow in the Great Chōngmài is exuberant. The monthly period descends on time." Heaven refers to the descent of the Qì of heavenly perfection; *gui* refers to *réngui*, which is the name of water. Thus we call it *tiāngui*.

This being so, the Chōngmài is the Sea of Blood, while the Rènmài is in charge of the womb. When kidney Qì has reached its peak, the two vessels stream and flow through. The menstrual blood gradually builds up and descends in response to its proper timing. The reason why we call it "monthly affair" is that it normally appears once every three ten-day cycles, just like the moon's waxing and waning.

At the time when the menses flow, you must be most circumspect in regard to healthcare and recuperation from illness. When these are not carried out properly, it is like contracting an illness after childbirth: A mild illness will become a chronic condition, while a severe illness will result in death! If the woman is exposed to panic, the blood and Qì become chaotic, and the movement in the channels is abruptly cut off. Counter-current movement in the body then leads to the formation of illness in the blood aspect and conditions like consumption. If the woman taxes her physical energy during this time, this engenders vacuity heat, which transforms into the root of pain. Rage and anger result in Qì moving counter-current, which in turn results in blood moving counter-current. Counter-current movement in the lumbus and legs results in severe pain there at the time of the menstrual flow, which eases off when the period is over. Counter-current movement in the head, abdomen, heart, lungs, back, rib-sides, and hands and feet results in the same kind of sign at the time of the menstrual flow. If the rage is extreme, it damages the liver, and you have the diseases of dizziness, rib-side pain, retching blood, scrofula, and welling-abscesses with sores. When this is complicated by menstrual blood oozing and leaking into these spaces, it subsequently forms openings and cavities, and dribbling that has no end.

Any time this situation occurs, being struck by wind results in falling ill with wind disease, and contracting cold results in falling ill with cold disease. When this persists for a long time with no cure, it will transform into a hundred patterns to emerge in unspeakable variety. How could you not dread this situation that is described as "tiny like autumn down feathers at the time of the violation but more serious than the highest mountain peaks when the disease breaks out"!

A few lines further down, Chén continues by citing a truism that should still be memorized by every Chinese medicine student in their first year of education:

大率治病，先論其所主。男子調其氣，女子調其血。氣血，人之神也，不可不謹調護。

然婦人以血為基本，氣血宣行，其神自清。所謂血室，不蓄則氣和；血凝結，則水火相刑。

As a general guideline for the treatment of any condition, first you discuss what the patient is governed by. In men, you attune their Qì; in women, you attune their blood. Qì and blood! These are the spirit of the human, and you must never fail to protect them with great care!

> This being so, women have blood as their foundation, and when Qì and blood flow freely, their spirit is naturally clear. What we refer to as the Blood Chamber, if nothing is hoarded there, the Qì is harmonious. But if the blood congeals and binds [there], then water and fire torture each other.

The results of this condition are obvious to any practitioner who sees women in their clinical practice. In other words, blood is the key aspect in female physiology and pathology to which we must pay attention. In terms of determining the origins of a condition, it is especially the time during the menstrual period and the even more dangerous stage of childbirth and the recovery period thereafter that are the most likely moments when external and internal pathogens are able to penetrate and wreak havoc in the female body. In the often-repeated warning, these conditions may be "tiny like autumn down feathers at the time of the violation but more serious than the highest mountain peaks when the disease breaks out"! The resulting signs and symptoms show up in myriad variations, but all tend to return to this specifically female constellation of: openness during menstruation and birth, causing increased vulnerability; compounded by exhaustion and vacuity directly and/or indirectly related to reproductive processes; allowing external factors, but especially heat, cold, or wind, to enter; resulting in pathology in the movement of fluids and of blood in particular, whether as uncontrolled flow in the wrong places or, more commonly, as lack of flow; causing problems associated with fluid accumulations and masses, but perhaps first and foremost the pain that comes from a lack of healthy movement.

So here you have it in a nutshell. This is what traditional Chinese gynecology has to say about pre-, peri-, post-, or any other kind of menstrual and even menopausal pain, and really almost any other pain that is not the immediate and direct result of an external factor like a fall or injury: It is not "normal," but a sign of serious imbalances in the female body between Qì and blood, which you can treat by attuning the menses and restoring women's physiological monthly flow of blood in resonance with the waxing and waning of the moon and her internal cycles of fertility. It is my sincere hope that the thirty-six questions on gynecology translated and discussed in the following pages may help you with the diagnosis and treatment of conditions that affect the female body so that we can allow the full strength, power, elegance, and beauty of traditional Chinese medicine to shine forth in the West, for the benefit of your patients and all women suffering from less than perfect health...

Langley, Whidbey Island,
on the eve of the Year of the Metal Rat
January 24, 2020

Notes on Reading This Book

THIS SECTION OFFERS SOME GENERAL INFORMATION AND MY explanations of a few simple stylistic guidelines that I have developed to make it easier for you to appreciate and potentially apply the information in the main section of this book in your clinical practice. I encourage you to read the following paragraphs carefully and refer back to them as the first place to look for answers if anything in this book does not make sense to you, from clinical concepts to capitalization.

First off, if you are unfamiliar with the basic theories and historical context of gynecology in premodern China, please read the "Introduction" in pages 1–66 of *Channeling the Moon: Part One*. Specifically, that chapter introduces the early history of Chinese gynecology and the most important texts up to the Sòng period, which you will find constantly referenced in both Qí Zhòngfǔ's explanations and in my discussions in the following pages. The information contained in this second volume assumes that you are familiar with the content of the first volume and therefore builds on it rather than repeating it. With this approach, I follow the manner in which the original author of the *Hundred Questions on Gynecology* would have presumably wanted his Hundred Questions read consecutively, one after the other, at least as the first exposure for readers who were not already experts in premodern Chinese gynecology themselves. Of particular importance for appreciating the explanations offered by

Qí Zhòngfǔ in the present book are his discussions in Part One on female bleeding, *tiānguǐ*, the difference between male and female bodies, and the processes involved in physiological and pathological processes of menstruation. After a first read-through, it is my hope that you will find a spot for this series of books on your clinic's bookshelf for important reference works, and consult these volumes often for ideas on etiology, diagnostic differentiation, and treatment options when your standard TCM training leaves you asking for more and different answers.

The following sections are adapted from *Channeling the Moon: Part One* as a reminder and for easy reference.

Defining "Woman" and the "Female Body" in a Non-Binary World

Before we delve into the following English translation of a thirteenth-century Chinese text on gynecology, a word on definitions is necessary to bring this book into the twenty-first century. About a decade ago, I was challenged in the middle of an introductory lecture of a semester-long course on Chinese gynecology when my students refused to accept my naïve definition that a woman is a human with a uterus who in a healthy state is able to reproduce and menstruates regularly between menarche and menopause, when not pregnant, breast-feeding, or ill. I owe a debt of gratitude to my patient, understanding, well-meaning students who have gently guided me into the twenty-first century and attempted to educate me on the contemporary meaning of "woman." Any sensitive contemporary practitioner, teacher, or writer on gynecology must recognize that not all people who menstruate are women and that not all women menstruate (given the conditions above). The meaning of such seemingly innocuous words as "female" and "male" or "man" and "woman," which used to assume a binary gender, has changed dramatically in an age of sex and gender fluidity.

While I would have liked to honor and express this fluidity in the following pages, we must recognize that gender is a social construct and that our modern understanding of gender and sexuality differs greatly from that of China in the thirteenth century. In this book I have therefore chosen to translate 女 nǚ consistently as "woman" or "female" and 男 nán as "man" or "male," because the context is a Sòng dynasty text on gynecology, in which any person who menstruated was by definition female and in which a woman was indeed implicitly defined as a person capable of reproducing, had a uterus, and menstruated, carried a fetus, or lactated between the times of menarche and menopause unless she was ill. Similarly, the term "sexual intercourse" alone does not in itself imply anything about the sexuality or gender of the participants, whether in the modern English or in the traditional Chinese version. But the specific medical context should make it clear in any particular instance whether the implication is one that is limited to heterosexual intercourse, such as when an exchange of Yīn and Yáng Essences or the potential for pregnancy and procreation are involved. As you translate the ideas expressed in the following pages into your modern practice, you may have to modify my translation, such as, for example, by replacing the term "woman" with "person who menstruates," because the act of menstruation is not limited to women in clinical practice. For the sake of historical accuracy, however, I have chosen to retain a literal translation style and trust that the reader can make these adjustments on their own. I sincerely hope that this choice will not cause offense and always appreciate mutually respectful constructive criticism and feedback if you disagree with my approach.

Formatting Conventions and Terminology

As in *Channeling the Moon: Part One*, the following rules should help to make sense of most instances of italicization, capitalization, hyphenation, and spacing that you might notice in this book.

With all of my books, I generally follow the technical terminology presented so comprehensively in Nigel Wiseman and Feng Ye's *Practical Dictionary of Chinese Medicine* and note any divergences from this terminology in the "Discussion" sections. I am hoping that this will make it easy for the educated reader to recognize quotations from classical literature and notice both similarities to other texts and subtle but potentially significant differences. It also enables the reader to look up the often-extensive explanations for many technical terms that are found in the *Practical Dictionary*. Instances where I deviate from this terminology are usually due to the specific needs of a thirteenth-century text on gynecology or my extensive experience in working with texts that tend to be considerably earlier than the literature that Wiseman and Feng were focusing on.

In addition, however, technical terminology in contemporary and clinically applied Chinese medicine in the West has been evolving, like any living language, but much more rapidly over the last decade or two, along with the profession as a whole. This evolution has generally been in a positive direction towards greater accuracy and refinement. I have thus taken the liberty to update Wiseman and Feng's terminology on the basis of what have become accepted Pīnyīn terms in the profession, like the extraordinary vessels or medicinals. My reason for these changes is that this book is primarily aimed at contemporary practitioners in the English-speaking world who are by now more familiar with the Pīnyīn terms for medicinals, for example, than with their Latin or common English identifications. Following current practice in many Chinese medicine educational programs in the US, I render terms for which no direct English equivalents exist in italicized Pīnyīn, from disease names like *bì* Impediment to such untranslatable concepts as *tiānguǐ*, the *zàng* and *fǔ* organs, and the *hún* and *pò* souls. For better clarity, I have tried to pair the Pīnyīn term, whenever possible and helpful, with an English equivalent or explanatory term, such as *yíng* Provisioning and *wèi* Defense. Any terms that I translate differently from Wiseman and Feng's terminology, as found in their *Practical Dictionary of Chinese Medicine*, are listed in the Glossary in the appendix of this book.

Unfortunately, most acupuncturists continue to use "excess" and "deficiency" instead of the more accurate "repletion" and "vacuity," or even "fullness" and "emptiness," as translations for the Chinese concepts of 實 *shí* and 虛 *xū*. Given that these terms do not always carry negative implications in Chinese, even in a medical context, but are originally value-free (note especially that the character for "excess" consists of a treasure under the roof!), I simply cannot make myself translate them into what I consider incorrect terms, as "excess" and "deficiency." As a translator who is producing a book for a professional audience in the field of Chinese medicine, I see it as my role to offer an accurate transmission of the original meaning of the text that is as literal and faithful to the original as possible. Of course your needs as a clinical practitioner in communicating with your patients are different from this, and you may choose more common English terms to express your diagnostic findings. In a similar vein, I just cannot make myself translate the term 五行 *wǔ xíng* as "five elements" but insist on sticking with the far less elegant "five dynamic agents." In both cases, I hope that the profession might eventually catch up with me or that we might simply adopt the pinyin terms here, just like we no longer feel the need to translate Qì into the very different and grossly misleading English concept of "energy" but have simply accepted that it needs to stand on its own and remain in Pīnyīn. I do sincerely apologize for any discomfort this may cause some of my readers.

In terms of handling Chinese terms and issues of translation, I have tried to strike a balance that makes this book useful, accessible, and enjoyable to as many readers as possible since I strongly believe in the importance of the material contained in the following pages. Thus, I have avoided the temptation to create an overly technical and highly annotated academic tome that will only appeal to readers with years of academic training in literary Chinese and clinical practice. At the same time, Sòng dynasty gynecology is too complex to be presented in a simplistic rendering that brushes over cultural, linguistic, and medical differences or biomedicalizes the material, to give the reader a false sense of familiarity. I have included Chinese characters in discussions of etymology to open up a window into Chinese medicine to readers unfamiliar with the written language. I have also added the Chinese source text to most quotations from medical classics, so that readers who are literate in these texts can form their own opinion instead of having to rely on my translation. As with all my work, it is my sincere hope that this book will inspire some practitioners to start learning even a little bit of classical medical Chinese in order to gain a more accurate understanding of this ancient medicine through its abundant literature treasure trove.

In general, Pīnyīn terms are written in lower case and in italics, with the exception of a number of terms that I treat as having become part of the English vocabulary at this point and therefore capitalize as proper nouns. These exceptions include Qì 氣, Yīn 陰 and Yáng 陽, Dào 道, Sānjiāo 三焦, and Shén 神. Reflecting standard practice among US practitioners at this point in time, medicinal names are treated like Western herb names and are therefore not italicized or capitalized but given in Pīnyīn pronunciation in a single word, such as gāncǎo or rénshén. In contrast, channel names (Chōngmài, Rènmài, Yángmíng, etc.) are capitalized as proper nouns and spelled in one word. Likewise, formula names are treated as proper nouns and therefore capitalized, not italicized, and broken up by word, not by character and syllable. Thus, for example I write Dāngguī Sì Nì Tāng. The same holds true for point names, which are also treated as proper nouns and therefore capitalized, not italicized, and spelled in a single word, such as Láogōng. Personal names and place names are treated in the same way. To allow them to stand out from other technical Pīnyīn terms, text titles are capitalized, intoned, broken up into words, and italicized (like English titles) in accordance with standard Pīnyīn spelling rules for titles, such as *Huángdì nèijīng*. In addition, they are accompanied by the Chinese characters in Chinese title brackets, such as 《黃帝內經》, and followed by the English translation in parentheses (Yellow Emperor's Inner Classic) at their first occurrence. In subsequent citations, I merely give the Pīnyīn title. You can always look any cited text up by Pīnyīn title in the "Primary Sources" section of the Bibliography. Technical terms can be found by consulting the Reference Tables for Formulas and for Medicinals, and the relevant sections on "Actions for Medicinal and Formula Preparation," "Other Terms Related to Medicinals and Formulas," "Gynecology and Pathology," and "Other Technical Terms" in the Glossary in the back of this book.

Lastly, I have resisted the temptation to make my translation appear more directly clinically applicable by adding metric measurements to the text itself. The reader is advised to consult the table below but use caution since the equivalents between traditional Chinese and contemporary metric units changed from one dynasty to the next and formulas were often copied from much older texts without updating or changing the measurements. As you will see from my often inconclusive detective work in the following translation, it can be impossible to know how old the original formula is or even when it was first recorded in writing. It is therefore wiser to read formulas in terms of proportional rather than absolute measurements. This is a thorny subject, and readers must rely on their clinical experience and specialized training rather than blindly applying any formulas translated below.

TABLE OF MEASUREMENTS DURING THE SÒNG PERIOD

Unit of Measurement	Equal to Smaller Unit	Metric Equivalent	English
1 斗 dǒu	10 升 shēng	6700 mL	"peck"
1 升 shéng	10 合 gě	670 mL	"pint"
1 合 gě		67 mL	"gill"
1 斤 jīn	16 兩 liǎng	633 g	"catty"
1 兩 liǎng	10 錢 qián	40 g	"tael"
1 錢 qián	10 分 fēn	4 g	"cash" or "mace"
1 分 fēn		0.4 g	"candareen"

齊仲甫《女科百問》

Qí Zhòngfǔ · *Hundred Questions on Gynecology*

QUESTIONS 15 – 50

第十五問

婦人多驚者，何也？

答曰：婦人者眾陰之所集，而以血為之主。夫心主行血，脾主裹血，肝主藏血。因產蓐過傷，或因喜怒攻損，是致營血虧耗。

內經云：「血氣者人之神，」血既不足，神亦不定，所以驚怖。

巢氏有風驚悸候云：「心藏神，為諸臟之主。若血氣調和，則心神安定，若虧損，則心神怯弱，故風邪乘虛干之，防以驚悸。若久不止，則變為恍惚也。」

QUESTION FIFTEEN

What is the Reason for Women's Propensity to Panic?

ANSWER: Women are characterized by the accumulation of multitudes of Yīn, and they are ruled by blood. Now the heart rules moving the blood, the spleen rules swathing the blood, and the liver rules storing the blood. Whether because of excessive damage during childbirth or the postpartum period or because of injuries sustained from elation and anger, the result is that the *yíng* Provisioning blood is consumed and exhausted.

As the *Nèijīng* states, "The blood and Qì are the Shén of humans," and when the blood is insufficient, the Shén is also unsettled. This in turn causes panic and terror.

In an essay on Wind Panic Palpitations, Master Cháo states: "The heart stores the Shén and is the ruler of all the other *zàng* organs. If the blood and Qì are harmonious, the Shén in the heart is at ease and settled. If they are debilitated, the Shén in the heart is timid and weak. Therefore, wind evil exploits the vacuity and interferes with it. Guard against panic palpitations! If they occur over a long time without stopping, the condition will transform into severe mental confusion."

Discussion

The term 主 *zhǔ* deserves an explanation to shed additional light on the oft-cited saying that "women are ruled by blood while men are ruled by Qì." Tracing this saying back to its purported origin, the *Fùrén dàquán liángfāng* in the third entry of the first volume cites the preface to a lost ninth-century text called "Treasure Formulas for Childbirth" (《產寶方》 *Chǎnbǎo fāng*):

> 大率治病，先論其所主。男子調其氣，女子調其血。氣血，人之也，不可不謹調護。然婦人以血為基本，氣血宣行，其神自清。所謂血室，不蓄則氣和；血凝結，則水火相刑。

As a general guideline, in the treatment of disease we first discuss that by which [a patient] is ruled. In men, you attune their Qì, and in women, you attune their blood. Qì and blood are the Shén of humans. In all circumstances, you must attune and protect these with great caution. This being so, women take blood as their foundation, and when Qì and blood move smoothly, their Shén is naturally clear. When nothing is retained in the so-called Blood Chamber, the Qì is harmonious. When blood congeals and binds, water and fire torment each other.

As the text explains, the clinical significance of this term "rule" here is that the physician needs to "attune and protect" the specific ruling aspect as the foundation of the gendered body. In the case of the female body, health manifests specifically in the free and uninhibited flow of blood, with no blood being retained in the "blood chamber." Therefore the consistent goal that any medical treatment of a female body should carefully attend to is to ensure such a state.

So far, there should be no surprises for any reader with even a cursory understanding of traditional Chinese gynecology. But maybe we can dig a little deeper by looking at the etymology of the character 主: While the modern character simply looks like the character for "king" (王 *wáng*) with a dot on the top, its origin suggests a slightly different meaning. The original form 主 depicts an oil lamp consisting of a stand and a bowl-shaped container for lamp oil, which holds a large flame in the middle.

As the commentary to the second-century character dictionary *Shuōwén jiězì* explains, the top is what holds the lard or oil, and the fire is that which is being "ruled," or perhaps better "contained." It has a very small physical form and yet lights up a whole room. These associations might explain why the character means not only "to rule" or "dominate" in all its grammatical variations, but also "host," in the sense of the container that "hosts" the flame or of course a person who "hosts" a visitor. In addition and even more closely related to its technical meaning in formula and materia medica literature, it can mean "to indicate," in the sense of serving as a sign that augurs or portends a turn of events like good or bad luck or a certain weather event. In the medical context, it is used to link a single ingredient or medicinal formula or point prescription to the particular pathology or constellation of symptoms that it "rules," "hosts," or "is indicated for." If we refrain from seeing it as derived here from the meaning "to rule" in the sense of a formula that rules over a condition by overpowering it, how does the meaning of this connection between medicine and physiological effect change when we think of the medicine as the small container that holds the flame that brightly illuminates the entire room? For example, what does it mean that rénshēn is described in the *Shénnóng běncǎo jīng* as follows?

主補五臟，安精神，定魂魄，止驚悸，除邪氣，明目，開心益智。

Indicated for supplementing the five *zàng* organs, calming the Jīngshén and settling the *hún* and *pò* souls, stopping panic palpitations, expelling evil Qì, brightening the eyes, and opening up the heart and boosting wisdom.

Returning to the passage above, how might our thinking now change about the saying that women "are ruled by" blood? Most directly, the phrase obviously takes on far greater significance for diagnosis when we recall the meaning of 主 as "to augur," so that blood is thus the single most important characteristic by which a skilled physician determines the health and harmony of the female body. On an even deeper level, could we even think about blood in the female body (and Qì in the male body) as something like the container that holds, or "hosts," the flame that illuminates the entire room? Here blood is far from the ruler that dominates the female body but should rather be envisioned as the subtle yet far-reaching protective life force that holds the entire body together and makes it shine. Most Chinese medicine practitioners are probably more accustomed to seeing Qì in this role. Of course, blood and Qì always operate as an interdependent pair, and male and female are merely the names for the two extreme poles along a continuum of the human body that we should be careful not to see in the absolute gendered terms that we are used to from a biomedical perspective. T important role of blood in female physiology and diagnosis strikes me as the single most valuable contribution that traditional Chinese gynecology makes to our understanding of the human body.

In this context, it behooves us to once again consider the effect of cultural attitudes and biomedical hormonal birth control measures on menstruation from a Chinese medicine perspective. Besides being a "Chinese medicine nerd," I am also a closet medical anthropologist and a devoted mother who raised a girl to an adult woman in contemporary US culture. In that role, I spent a precious year in my daughter's middle school classroom leading a weekly session for only the female students on "Girls' Talk," as a safe space for them to explore their changing bodies and ease their initial experiences with menstruation. In later years, I offered our female-only home and my presence, when invited, as a non-judgmental resource or sounding board for discussions on birth control. The sharp contrast between traditional Chinese medical ideas and mainstream American attitudes towards menstruation among modern girls and young women is a topic of great interest to me and also, I believe, of great clinical significance and potential. In the traditional Chinese gynecology texts, the monthly flow of blood is an "indicator" (主 zhǔ) of health, balance, and abundance in the female body. From this perspective, what does it mean that most young women in the US greet the arrival of their period with dread and shame and the anticipation of pain, or as an inconvenience or detriment to academic and athletic performance, and that they actively attempt to hide or even avoid it through medical intervention? Making matters worse, this attitude is reinforced by advertising, popular culture, and most parents, doctors, teachers, and coaches. In sharp contrast, my background in Chinese medicine has taught me to experience my monthly periods as welcome opportunities to check in with my body and to honor the obvious signals it offers me on my body's needs, from cold and heat to emotional states, stress, and physical resources like diet, exercise and rest, and sleep. These signals then allow me to actively make changes, as much as I can in any given month, to address any signs of imbalance and improve my health, or I pay the price down the road.

In our modern Western version of Chinese medicine, we have become masters at reading the state of Qì in our patients' bodies, but what about the blood? Are we not missing out on one half of the diagnostic toolbox, at least in menstruating bodies, if we ignore the messages presented each month by the female blood flow? Worse yet, what happens to this excess of blood in female bodies that are deprived of this important opportunity to "get rid of the old and bring in the new" (推陳出新 *tuīchén chūxīn*)? The connection between the etiology of impeded blood flow and the pathology of blood binding into all sorts of abdominal masses like Accumulations and Gatherings and Concretions and Conglomerations is logical and its importance in Chinese gynecology can hardly be overstated. Obviously, one eventual outcome is often infertility, which brings more and more patients to Chinese medicine practitioners. It is wonderful that word is getting out about the clinical potential of Chinese medicine in fertility disorders, but wouldn't it be even better if we could address these issues, in the spirit of the classics, when the problem is as tiny as autumn down feathers instead of waiting until it has grown to the size of a giant mountain? This reminds me of the famous rhetorical question from *Sùwèn* Chapter Two:

夫病已成而後藥之，亂已成而後治之，譬猶渴而穿井，鬭而鑄錐，不亦晚乎。

Now to have an illness that has already formed and only afterwards treat it with medication, to have chaos that has already formed and only afterwards put it in order, this is just like being thirsty and then digging a well, or like being in the middle of combat and then forging sharp weapons. Isn't it too late indeed at this point?

Returning to the Qí Zhòngfǔ's answer to Question Fifteen on Women's Propensity to Panic, the citation from the *Nèijīng* comes from *Sùwèn* Chapter Twenty-Six. The citation by "Master Cháo" is an almost literal quotation of the entire entry on Wind Evil Panic Palpitations in Volume Thirty-Seven in the gynecological section of Cháo Yuánfāng's *Zhūbìng yuánhòu lùn*. The major difference is that the term that I have translated as "severe mental confusion" above, namely 恍惚 *huǎnghū* (rendered by Wiseman as "abstraction" and defined as "inattention to present objects or surroundings, or low powers of mental concentration. It is a sign of heart disease.") is followed by a second sign: worry and apprehension (憂懼 *yōujù*) in Cháo's original text.

The message to take away from this question and answer is that clearly panic is a key factor to take into consideration when treating women. On the one hand, panic has the potential, as an etiological factor, to scatter the Shén, upset the Qì dynamic by interfering with the physiological downward flow, and throw off menstruation, with all the dreadful consequences that these situations entail. The emphasis here though is that panic is additionally important as a pathology that women are particularly prone to contract because of their affinity with blood and the depletion of blood through the physiological processes of menstruation, childbirth, and breastfeeding, and through the etiological factor of vacuity taxation in particular.

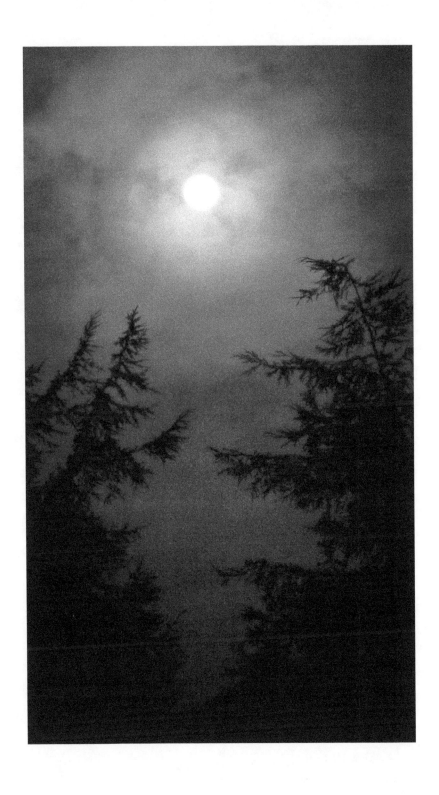

經濟丹

治婦人血氣不足，營衛俱虛，心氣不定，夜臥驚怖，夢寐不祥，心虛自汗，乏力倦怠，飲食減少，咳嗽痰實。

常服補心養血，安神定志，令人血壯氣實。極有神效。

白茯苓	
白茯神	
白芍藥	各一兩
遠志(去心)	一兩
乳香(別研)	半兩
當歸(酒浸)	一兩
酸棗仁(去殼，炒)	半兩
人參	一兩
沒藥(研)	一兩
朱砂(別研)	半兩
石菖蒲(真者)	一兩

只用棗仁丸亦得。

上十味為末，煉蜜為丸桐子大，將朱砂為衣，每服三十丸，加至五十丸。棗湯參湯食前任下，飲後亦可。

Jīng Jì Dān
(Fording the River Elixir)

A treatment for women's insufficiency of Qì and blood, dual vacuity of both *yíng* Provisioning and *wèi* Defense, unsettled heart Qì, panic and terror when sleeping at night, ominous dreams, heart vacuity with spontaneous sweating, lack of strength and fatigue, reduced appetite for food and drink, and coughing with plentiful phlegm.

Taken consistently, it supplements the heart and nurtures the blood, puts the Shén at ease and settles the will, and makes the person's heart strong and Qì replete. It possesses utmost divine efficacy.

báifúlíng	
báifúshén	
báisháoyào	1 *liǎng* each
yuǎnzhì (remove the cores)	1 *liǎng*
rǔxiāng (grind separately)	0.5 *liǎng*
dāngguī (steep in rice wine)	1 *liǎng*
suānzǎorén (remove the shells and mix-fry)	0.5 *liǎng*
rénshēn	1 *liǎng*
mòyào (grind)	1 *liǎng*
zhūshā (grind separately)	0.5 *liǎng*
shíchāngpú (the genuine variety)	1 *liǎng*

You may also just use Zǎorén Wán (Jujupe Pit Pill).

Process the ten ingredients above into a powder, use refined honey to make pills the size of *wútóng* seeds, and coat them with the zhūshā. Take 30 pills per dose, increasing the dosage to up to 50 pills. Ingest them as you wish before meals by downing them with jujube or ginseng tea. It is also permissible to take them after drinking alcohol.

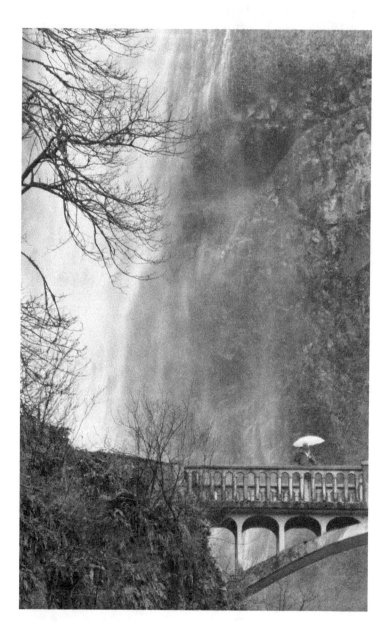

Formula Note

Translating the name for this formula into English is challenging indeed, and to a certain extent impossible, especially when we read it in the context of this question and the following formula. Originally and before working on the following formula, I had chosen the perhaps more elegant English title "Rule and Rescue Elixir" as a translation of 經濟丹. To arrive at this English name, I chose to read the two characters 經 *jīng* and 濟 *jì* as a fairly common compound that in the received literature has the meaning of "to govern the country and rescue the population," safely ignoring the modern meaning of the compound as "economics." Nevertheless, as an individual character, 經 has the two meanings of "channel" and "to pass through, to experience," while 濟 on its own originally means "to ford a river," and from there by extension "to rescue, to assist," all of which is relevant here. Hence the formula name can also be rendered, with some grammatical discomfort, as "Channel Rescue Elixir" or, as my final choice, "(Going through) Fording the River Elixir," suggesting perhaps the sense that this elixir is intended for the stage where one is in the middle of fording. The significance of 濟 as "fording the river" is particularly relevant in light of the name for the following formula, which consist of a combination of the two *Yìjīng* trigrams Water (坎 kǎn) and Fire (離 lí). Placing the trigram for Water ☵ on top of Fire ☲ creates hexagram sixty-three ䷾, which is called 既濟 *jì jì*, meaning "having forded across" or "Consummation," as opposed to hexagram sixty-four, with Fire over Water ䷿, which is called 未濟 "not yet forded across." At this point, I hope it is obvious that it is impossible to find an English equivalent to express all these connotations. The closest approximation in English to this literal sense of 經濟 would be something like "passing through the stage of fording a river," which is unfortunately not an acceptable formula name. For this reason, I have chosen the more elegant and brief "Fording the River Elixir." All of these connotations would have been familiar and significant to any educated reader in the Sòng period, adding important information on the indications and intended actions of both this formula and the next one.

坎離丹

既濟水火，補心滋腎，白濁夢遺。

辰砂(另研)	一兩
酸棗仁(酒浸去殼研淨)	一兩
附子(去皮臍)	一個
乳香(令隔水乳缽細研入)	半兩

上先用附子碾細羅末，次入三味和勻，煉蜜丸如雞頭大。每服一粒溫酒下，空心一服。須是臘月合，瓷器盛之。

Kǎn Lí Dān
(Fire and Water Elixir)

"Having forded the river" (*Yìjīng* hexagram sixty-three), this is Water and Fire. Supplementing the heart and saturating the kidney, it is indicated for white turbidity and dream emissions.

chénshā (grind separately	1 *liǎng*
suānzǎorén (steep in rice wine, remove hulls, grind, and clean)	1 *liǎng*
fùzǐ (remove the skin and bottom)	1 piece
rǔxiāng (let the water separate out and grind it finely in a mortar before adding it)	0.5 *liǎng*

Of the ingredients above, first take the fùzǐ, crush it finely with a roller, and sift it into a powder. Next add the remaining three ingredients and blend everything evenly. Form pills with refined honey that are the size of a chicken's head. For each dose, drink down one pill in warm rice wine, a single dose on an empty stomach. This [medicine] must be compounded during the twelfth lunar month and stored in a porcelain container.

石斛散

治虛勞羸瘦，乏力，少食，倦怠，多驚畏。

石斛(去根，淨洗，銼，酒炒)	四錢
牛膝(酒浸)	
柏子仁(去皮，研)	
五味子	
遠志(炒)	
杏仁(去皮尖，炒)	
木香	
肉蓯蓉(酒浸，焙乾)	各三錢
訶子肉(炮)	
青橘皮	
柴胡	
人參	
熟地(蒸)	
白茯苓	四錢
甘草(炙)	二錢
乾薑(炮)	一錢半
神曲(研炒)	
麥	各六錢

上為細末，每服二錢。米飲調下，食前日二三服。

Shíhú Sǎn
(Dendrobium Powder)

A treatment for vacuity taxation with marked emaciation, lack of strength, reduced eating, fatigue, and increased panic and fear.

shíhú (remove the roots, wash clean, grate, and stir-fry in rice wine)	4 *qián*
niúxī (steep in rice wine)	3 *qián* each
bǎizǐrén (remove the skin and grind)	
wǔwèizǐ	
yuǎnzhì (stir-fry)	
xìngrén (remove the skin and tips and stir-fry)	
mùxiāng	
ròucōngróng (steep in rice wine and roast until dry)	
hēzǐròu (blast-fry)	
qīngjúpí	
cháihú	
rénshēn	
shúdì (steam)	
báifúlíng	4 *qián*
gāncǎo (mix-fry)	2 *qián*
gānjiāng (blast-fry)	1.5 *qián*
shénqǔ (grind and stir-fry)	5 *qián* each
mài	

Process the ingredients above into a fine powder and take 2 *qián* per dose. Down it mixed into thin rice gruel. Take 2 to 3 doses per day before meals.

第十六問

婦人多因風冷而生諸疾者，何也？

答曰：風乃陽邪也，冷乃寒氣也。風隨虛入，冷由勞傷。夫人將攝順理，則血氣調和，風寒暑濕不能為害。若勞傷血氣，便致虛損，則風冷乘虛而干之。

或客於經絡，則氣血凝澀，不能溫養於肌膚；或入於腹內，則沖氣虛虛，不能消化於飲食。大腸虛則多利，子臟寒則不生。或為斷絕，或為不通者，隨所傷而成病，皆不逃乎風冷之氣也。

Question Sixteen

What is the Reason for Women's Propensity to Generate All Sorts of Conditions as the Result of Wind Cold?

Answer: Wind is surely a Yáng evil, and cold is surely the Qì of winter-cold. Wind follows vacuity to enter, while cold is caused by taxation damage. If people rest and nurture their health in accordance with cosmic principles, the blood and Qì are harmonious, and wind, winter-cold, summer-heat, and dampness are not able to cause harm. If taxation damages the blood and Qì and then causes vacuity detriment, however, wind and cold exploit this vacuity and interfere.

Perhaps they intrude into the channels and network vessels, congealing and impeding the smooth flow of Qì and blood so that they are unable to warm and nourish the skin. Or they enter the inside of the abdomen, resulting in depletion of the Chōng Qì and inability to digest food and drink. Vacuity in the large intestine results in propensity to diarrhea. Cold in the uterus results in failure to bear children. Whether it is a matter of interrupted flow or of a failure to flow through, illness is formed in response to the nature of the damage, which in all of these cases does not deviate from the Qì of wind and cold.

DISCUSSION

The expression 沖氣 *chōng qì* has a number of connotations that are all relevant in the present context. First, we can read it literally as "thrusting Qì," not negatively but rather as Qì that moves dynamically and forcefully, instead of stagnating and congealing. In addition, since the Chōngmài is the Sea of Blood (see Question Seven, translated in *Channeling the Moon, Part One*), it makes sense to read 沖 here as implying the Chōngmài or "Thoroughfare Vessel," since 沖 is often used interchangeably with 衝, and both characters are used to refer to the Chōngmài in medical texts. However, to complicate matters further, we must not ignore a third dimension: Even though when dealing with a medical text we should always prioritize the technical meaning, the expression 沖氣 has another, non-medical meaning that is based on a famous line from the *Dàodéjīng* 《道德經》 (Classic of the Way and its Virtue-Power):

道生一，一生二，二生三，三生萬物。萬物負陰而抱陽，沖氣以為和。

The Dào engenders the One, the One engenders the Two, the Two engender the Three, and the Three engender the Ten Thousand Things. The Ten Thousand Things carry Yīn on their shoulders and wrap their arms around Yáng. Through this process, thrusting Qì becomes harmonized.

This literary significance would not have been lost on any educated member of Sòng society. In this passage, 沖 describes the ideal of dynamic yet harmonious movement of Qì that facilitates the generative flow between the poles of Yīn and Yáng, heaven and earth, with humanity in the middle. Lastly, the character 沖 can also be used as a substitute for the character 中 *zhōng* ("middle"), so 沖氣 also implies the notion of "central Qì." To summarize, this expression 沖氣 here should be understood to have implications of dynamically moving Qì, of Qì in the Chōngmài, and of the Qì that flows in the center of the body like a "thoroughfare." It is impossible to express all these connotations in a single English term, so we must step back, on encountering polysemous expressions like this, and explore their significance in the original language rather than choosing a single English translation for the sake of elegance and ease of reading.

The last sentence of the essay on women's propensity to wind-cold pathologies above contains two words for flow that might strike an English reader as more or less identical. The intentional specificity in the original source, though, is emphasized clearly here by the repetition of the sentence particle 或 *huò*, meaning "whether... or...," indicating that the text is describing two alternative scenarios, rather than just giving rhetorical alternatives. As such, the author emphasizes here that an "interruption" (斷絕 *duànjué*) is not the same as a "failure to flow through" (不通 *bù tōng*), but that in both cases, the grave consequence of developing pathologies related to wind-cold is unavoidable. What exactly the substance is whose flow is either impeded temporarily or prevented from flowing through remains unsaid. While we ordinarily assume that a medical author speaks of Qì when discussing flow, the gynecological context suggests that Qí Zhòngfǔ meant both Qì and blood, if not primarily blood. This short sentence here shows that gynecological authors in the Sòng period did indeed place importance not just on the symptom of a stopped menstrual flow but on the precise timing, nature, and duration of this stoppage, and viewed a temporary disruption differently from the much more serious situation of "failure to flow through." While this latter expression might strike the modern English reader as awkward, I translate it consistently as not just "stopped" or "blocked" menstruation. Similarly, I render its counterpart 通 ("to flow through" or "promote through-flow"), which frequently occurs in formula names and descriptions of formula effects or healthy physiology, not just as "free flow" or "restoring flow" or "opening up," but always incorporate the notion of flowing THROUGH, of penetrating all the way to the end. Admittedly this makes for less elegant passages in English, but it is essential to me to preserve the seriousness of the condition, and the implication that something that should be getting discharged and reaching an important target is getting blocked and consequently forced to either exit elsewhere from the body or bind into masses. The dire long-term consequences of this pathology should be obvious to anybody who has seen floodwaters break through a dam or an avalanche roll down a mountain.

補陰丸

治婦人百疾，或經不調，或崩中漏不止，腰腿沉重，臍腹作痛，潮熱往來，虛煩自汗，中滿氣短，嘔噦不時，肢體煩疼，不思飲食，日漸瘦弱。

此藥順肌體，悅顏色，調營衛，逐風寒，進飲食，化痰涎。

藥材	用量
熟地	各七兩
生地	
白朮	五兩
蒼朮(泔浸一宿)	五兩半
藁本(去土)	四味各十兩
牡丹皮	
當歸	
秦艽	
細辛	七兩
肉桂(去皮)	八兩
甘草(炙)	六兩半
蠶蛻布(燒存性)	七兩
大豆黃卷(炒煙去)	六兩半
枳殼(麩炒)	六兩
陳皮(去白)	六兩
乾薑(炮)	各五兩
羌活	
白芷	六兩
白茯苓	六兩
糯米(炒黑色，火煙出)	三升

上為細末，蜜丸，每一兩作十九。每服一丸，溫酒化下，醋湯亦得，食前。

Bǔ Yīn Wán
(Yīn-Supplementing Pill)

Treats the hundred illnesses of women, perhaps with unattuned menses or with Landslide Collapse of the center and spotting that will not stop, heaviness in the lumbus and legs, pain in the navel and abdomen, intermittent tidal heat, vacuity vexation and spontaneous sweating, fullness in the center and shortness of breath, randomly occurring retching, vexing aches in the limbs, no interest in food and drink, and daily progressing frailty.

This medicine smooths out the flesh, makes the complexion pleasing, attunes *yíng* Provisioning and *wèi* Defense, expels wind cold, promotes eating and drinking, and transforms phlegm and drool.

shúdì	7 *liǎng* each
shēngdì	
báizhú	5 *liǎng*
cāngzhú (steep in rice rinsing water overnight)	5.5 *liǎng*
gǎoběn (remove soil)	10 *liǎng* for each of these four ingredients
mǔdānpí	
dāngguī	
qínjiāo	
xìxīn	7 *liǎng*
ròuguì (remove the skin)	8 *liǎng*
gāncǎo (mix-fry)	6.5 *liǎng*
cántuìbù (i.e. cántuìzhǐ. Burn [carefully] to preserve its nature)	7 *liǎng*
dàdòuhuángjuǎn (stir-fry until the smoke is gone)	6.5 *liǎng*

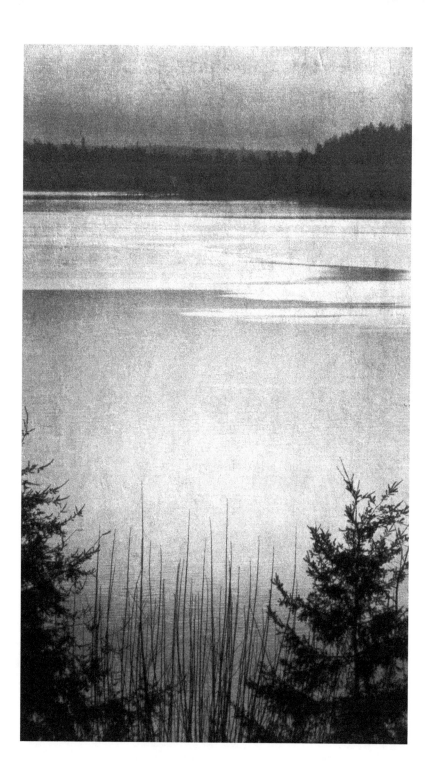

zhǐké (bran-fry)	6 liǎng
chénpí (remove the white parts)	6 liǎng
gānjiāng (blast-fry)	5 liǎng each
qiānghuó	
báizhǐ	6 liǎng
báifúlíng	6 liǎng
nuòmǐ (stir-fry until black and smoking)	3 shēng

Process the ingredients above into a fine powder and form into honey pills, making 10 pills with every 1 *liǎng*. Take 1 pill per dose, downing it dissolved into warm rice wine, or possibly also in vinegar or hot water, before meals.

丹鉛丹

治一切虛寒冷病。

鹿茸	
靈砂	
白龍骨	
川椒	
陽起石	
牡蠣粉	
肉桂	
肉蓯蓉	
石斛	
川巴戟	
木賊	
澤瀉	
天雄(酒浸,炮)	
沉香	
菟絲子(酒浸)	
膃肭臍	各一兩
磁石(醋淬)	
麝香	各半兩

上為細末,煉蜜為丸,梧桐子大。每服一百丸,溫酒或鹽湯下。

Dān Qiān Dān
(Cinnabar and Lead Elixir)

Treats all conditions of vacuity cold.

lùróng	
língshā	
báilónggǔ	
chuānjiāo	
yángqǐshí	
mǔlìfěn	
ròuguì	
ròucōngróng	
shíhú	
chuānbājǐ	
mùzéi	
zéxiè	
tiānxióng (steep in rice wine and blast-fry)	
chénxiāng	
tùsīzǐ (steep in rice wine)	
wànàqí	1 *liǎng* each
císhí (quench in vinegar)	
shèxiāng	1.5 *liǎng* each

Process the ingredients above into a fine powder and mix with refined honey into pills the size of *wútóng* seeds. Take 100 pills per dose by downing them in warm rice wine or hot salty water.

FORMULA NOTE

It is easy to read through this formula quickly and overlook a curious ingredient that is just innocently tucked in among all the others: 膃肭臍 wànàqí, a.k.a. seal penis and testicles. The reader only interested in directly clinically applicable information is invited to skip over the following discussion. Nevertheless, my love of seals, based on my interactions with these curious, personable, graceful creatures when I swim in the Puget Sound north of Seattle, induces me to indulge in a small detour. What is the significance of this rarely-used ingredient in a formula for vacuity cold in a book that otherwise almost exclusively contains herbal medicinals with only a few minerals in alchemically oriented formulas here and there? Obviously, lùróng (velvet deerhorn), báilónggǔ (dragon bone), mǔlì (oyster shell), and shèxiāng (musk) are also substances derived from animals, albeit much more commonly used ones.

So what is this mysterious ingredient, wànàqí, which, I have to admit, I had never before come across? Also called 海狗腎 hǎigǒushèn ("sea dog kidney"), it is clear that its historical meaning and continued traditional use refers to the penis and testes of male seals, and not to the kidney. Of course the kidney is closely related to the reproductive organs in Chinese medicine, the original character in the Chinese name (臍 qí) actually means "navel," and the penis and testes are sometimes referred to as the external kidney anyway. According to the Zhōngyào dàcídiǎn 中藥大辭典 (Great Dictionary of Chinese Materia Medica), the substance is salty and hot, enters the liver and kidney channels, and is used to "warm the kidney, strengthen Yáng, boost Essence, and supplement the marrow. It treats vacuity detriment and taxation damage, Yáng wilting and debilitation of Essence, and weakness in the lumbus and kidney." In Volume Fifty-One of the Běncǎo gāngmù from 1596, it is described as follows:

"Its Qì and flavor are salty, greatly hot, and non-toxic. It is indicated for demonic Qì and corpse influx, dreams of intercourse with ghosts, demons, goblins and fox spirits, heart and abdominal pain, malignity strike with evil Qì, abiding blood binding into clots, Strings and Aggregations, and marked emaciation. In men, it treats abiding Concretions and Qì lumps, accumulating cold and taxation Qì, kidney Essence weakness, taxation caused by too much sexual activity, and haggard emaciation. It supplements the center and boosts kidney Qì, warms the lumbus and knees, assists Yáng Qì, breaks Concretions and bindings, and cures panic, *kuáng* mania, and seizures. It is most excellent for the five taxations and seven damages, Yīn wilting and lack of strength, kidney vacuity, taxation oppression in the back and shoulders, and black face and cold Essence.

One of the most outstanding characteristics of seals, which as an avid open-water swimmer myself in the cold Pacific Northwest I envy them greatly for, is that they frolic comfortably in very cold water because of their large amount of insulating blubber. It thus makes intuitive sense that they would be a good substance for the treatment of cold. The spectacular mating behavior of male seals, from the powerful and aggressive establishment of their rookeries to the subsequent defense of their large harems, is easily observed since it occurs on land. Additionally, penises in general are a potent Yáng-supplementing medicinal in Chinese medicine, whether derived from dogs, stallions, or seals, since they combine the concentrated power of the male "jade stalk" with the inherently Yīn nature of all reproductive organs as associated with the kidney and the innermost aspect of the body. Seal testicles are thus a widely used tonic for sexual functions. Even though they are not a common medicinal in gynecological formulas, we can see how their greatly heating and Yáng-supplementing quality makes them a perfect ingredient for a condition of vacuity cold. It is even possible that this formula was originally not gendered but used for male cases of vacuity cold as well. Unfortunately, I have not been able to trace it back to an earlier source.

第十七問

婦人多頭眩而冒者，何也？

答曰：眩者，暈也，謂轉運之運，世之為頭運者是也。冒者冒蒙之冒，世為昏冒者是也。《明理論》曰：「眊，非毛而見其毛；眩，非玄而見其玄。」眊謂眼花也，眩謂眼黑也。

《針經》云：「上虛則眩，下虛則厥。」眩雖為虛，蓋風家亦有之者，風主運動故也。婦人頭運，挾痰多嘔吐者，狀若醉頭風也。

QUESTION SEVENTEEN

What is the Reason for Women's Propensity to Blackout Vision and Veiling?

ANSWER: Blackout vision means dizziness. This is a reference to a rotating motion, popularly known as head spinning. Veiling means clouded. This is popularly known as fainting. According to the *Mínglǐ lùn*, "Blurred vision means that there is no hair and yet one sees hair. Blackout vision means that there is no blackness and yet one sees blackness." Blurred vision means flowers in the eyes, while blackout vision means blackness in the eyes.

According to the *Zhēnjīng*, "Vacuity above results in blackout vision; vacuity below results in Reversal." Even though blackout vision is [there identified as] a [state of] vacuity, it is also something that affects patients with [pathological] wind. The reason for this is that wind rules movement. Women's condition of head spinning complicated by copious phlegm and retching and vomiting resembles the condition of alcoholic head wind.

Discussion

This answer is difficult to adequately put into English because the Chinese text uses certain characters to explain other characters based on similarity in sound and etymology, in a way that is impossible to recreate literally in English. For example, the character運, meaning "motion," is pronounced *yùn*, which is almost exactly the same as the pronunciation of the character 暈 for "dizziness," pronounced *yūn*. In other words, the Chinese text explains blackout vision by equating it first with *yùn* and then equating that with *yūn* to explain that blackout vision has to do with spinning. The explanation quoted from the *Mínglǐ lùn*, which is an abbreviation for *Shānghán mínglǐ lùn* 《傷寒明理論》 (Discourse on Elucidating Principles of Cold Damage, composed by Chéng Wújǐ 成无己, 1156), can only be fully appreciated when we look at the etymology of the characters for "blurred vision" and "blackout vision": In both cases, the radical of the character is 目 ("eye"), which is then combined with the character for hair 毛 and blackness 玄, respectively. In both cases, the character thus refers to a vision problem that involves seeing things that are not there, in the case of blurred vision, hair, and in the case of blackout vision, blackness. Isn't Chinese brilliant?

The next quotation is identified as coming from the *Zhēnjīng* 《針經》 (Needle Classic), an alternate name for the *Língshū jīng* 《靈樞經》 (Classic of the Divine Pivot), the second half of the *Huángdì nèijīng*. The quotation is found in Chapter Fifty-Two on "*Wèi* Defense Qì." The full extent of the quotation is:

凡候此者，下虛則厥，下盛則熱；上虛則眩，上盛則熱痛。故石者，絕而止之，虛者，引而起之。

Whenever we investigate these locations, vacuity below means Reversal, exuberance below means heat. Vacuity above means blackout vision, exuberance above means heat and pain. For this reason, [treat] repletion cases by interrupting and stopping [the flow of pathogenic Qì], and [treat] vacuity cases by drawing in and raising up [the flow of physiological Qì].

The present question on "Women's Propensity to Blackout Vision and Veiling" serves to reinforce the importance of wind as a pathogenic factor in Chinese medicine in general and in women's health in particular. The meaning of wind in Chinese medicine is a topic worthy of a separate book and impossible to do justice here in a brief comment. Before we delve into the treatment of head wind with clinical formulas, however, it might be helpful to review the most basic notions about wind as they are outlined in the early classics, since they are so different from our modern biomedical conception.

To begin with, the etymology of the character for wind, 風 *fēng*, can already provide some insights. It is a depiction of a bug 虫 under a sail 凡. Some scholars explain this by the fact that the stirring of wind brings insects to life. More relevant to the nature, effects, and manifestations of wind in the human body is that wind, like bugs, invades an old house through crumbling walls and gaps in the windows and doors. Like bugs, it likes to crawl into vacant buildings and empty spaces, and has a difficult time squeezing into something that is already full. Once inside, it appears now here and now there, showing up briefly, wreaking havoc, then going underground, only to reappear unexpectedly somewhere else at an opportune moment. Anybody who has tried to eliminate ants inhabiting a kitchen in an old adobe house knows what I am talking about. Wind, like bugs, looks for the easy way in or out, and your best defense is to very carefully plug up any cracks and then maintain a tight seal. Think about standing on a wintry mountain top in a knitted sweater versus in a wind-proof jacket zipped up tight all the way from top to bottom.

In the human body, conditions associated with wind are said in Chinese medicine to move around and go underground in periods of remission, only to erupt elsewhere unexpectedly, just like the above-mentioned ants that might hide in old walls or closets and tunnel through to another room where they make an unexpected appearance, create a temporary nuisance, and then once again go into hiding, only to erupt someplace else. We see this in roaming pain, such as in joints and muscles, and with random eruptions of latent conditions. As *Sùwèn* Chapter Forty-Two states,

風者善行而數變。腠理開則洒然寒，閉則熱而悶。

> Wind loves to move and frequently transforms. When the interstices are open, it results in shivering and [feeling] cold. When they are closed, it results in [feeling] hot and oppression.

The body is described in terms of a fortress that needs to be tightly sealed and carefully guarded against outside invasion. Thus the "Discourse on Heavenly Truth in the Ancient Past" 上古天真論 (*Sùwèn*, Chapter One) explains:

夫上古聖人之教下也，皆謂之虛邪賊風，避之有時，恬惔虛无，真氣從之，精神內守，病安從來。

> In the ancient past, the sages taught those below them always by framing it in terms of vacuity evil bandit wind, which must be avoided at the [necessary] times. In a state of tranquility and ease, of emptiness and absence [of desires and external stimulation], the genuine Qì follows along. Safeguarding the Jīngshén inside, where could disease possibly come from?

Wind as a pathology is discussed in great detail in the *Nèijīng*, with an entire chapter dedicated to it in both the *Sùwèn* and the *Língshū*. It is often paired with the term "bandit" as 賊風 *zéifēng*, implying that wind, like bandits, sneaks into a house that is not carefully guarded and then stealthily removes the person's health or wealth. This attack tends to be sudden and take the victim by surprise, just like a "wind strike" pathology causes rapidly developing and unexpected symptoms like fainting, seizures, or paralysis. And like the constant movement of wind, wind conditions in the body tend to be associated with trembling, shaking, dizziness, twitching, and similar symptoms. As emphasized in *Sùwèn* Chapter Five, "when wind prevails, movement results" (風勝則動). Given the affinity of wind with bugs in terms of their behavior (stealthy, unpredictable and with no fixed location, suddenly appearing and suddenly disappearing again, etc.), it should come as no surprise that bugs are common ingredients in formulas to get rid of wind, since they are able to track the pathogen down into the tiniest nooks and crannies and forcefully expel it outward. For just one example from this text, see the formula for Shèxiāng Wán (Musk Pill) below, which contains scorpion and earthworm to treat joint running pain. Moreover, wind is a condition that is associated with Yáng and with a movement upward and outward, and which primarily affects the upper part of the body. As Sùwèn Chapter Twenty-Eight states, "Damage by wind means that the upper body receives it first" (傷於風者，上先受之). Its nature is to open and drain and it therefore intrudes first into the head and fleshy exterior, manifesting as headache, sweating, aversion to wind, etc., and with a superficial pulse.

Again and again, as in the passage above, it is also associated with vacuity, to drive home the message that the carefully guarded, well-maintained, balanced human body will not fall ill because disease is unable to invade it. This is surely one reason why it is such a threat for women in particular during the extremely vulnerable postpartum period, when new mothers are thoroughly exhausted from pregnancy, labor, and delivery and have lost a large amount of Qì, blood, and fluids. For this reason, it is essential to protect new mothers from wind (and cold) during the period of "sitting out the month" (坐月子 zuò yuèzi) as still practiced by traditional women in China and beyond. The most dreaded result of wind invasion right after childbirth is therefore the condition of arched-back rigidity, (角弓反張 jiǎogōng fǎnzhāng). We will return to postpartum care in the later part of this book.

The grave danger of wind is emphasized again and again in the classics, most famously perhaps in the "Discourse on Wind" 風論 in Sùwèn Chapter Forty-Two:

故風者，百病之長也。至其變化，乃為他病也。無常方，然致有風氣也。

Wind! It is the leader of the hundred diseases. Arriving at its transformations, it causes other diseases. It has no constant direction [from which it comes] and yet it is all caused by the presence of wind Qì.

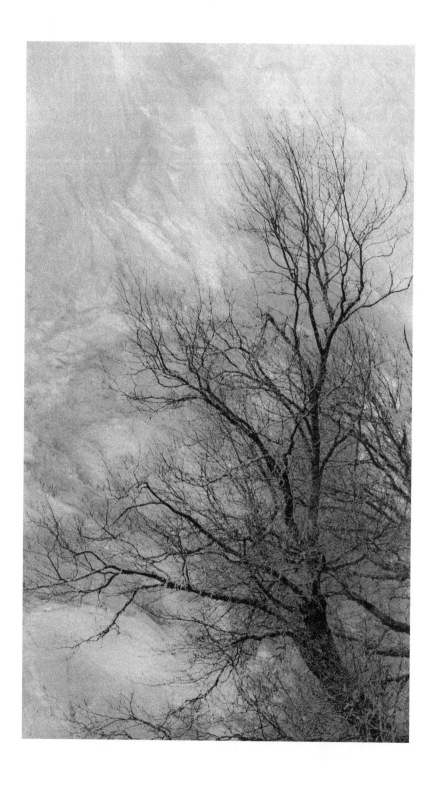

In that particular chapter, wind refers mostly to wind that invades from the outside as one, if not THE, primary factor among the six climatic Qì (wind, cold, summer-heat, dampness, dryness, and fire) that cause disease in the body. In this role, it is often paired with the other pathogenic factors, as in wind-cold, wind-heat, wind-damp, etc. There is, however, also another type of wind that is generated or located inside the body. This type of internal wind is associated with blood vacuity, with heat extreme, or with an overly active liver, since "the various forms of wind twitching and black-out vision are all associated with the liver" (諸風掉眩，皆屬於肝). (from the famous "Nineteen Lines," *Sùwèn* Chapter Seventy-Four).

芎羌散

治婦人患頭風者十居其半，每發必掉眩如在車上。蓋因血虛，肝有風邪襲之耳。

《素問》云：「徇蒙招尤，目瞑耳聾，下實上虛，過在足少陽厥陰甚則入肝。」蓋謂此也。方比他藥捷而效速。

川芎	一兩	藁本	
當歸	三錢	荊芥穗	
羌活		半夏	
旋復花		防風	各半兩
細辛	各半兩	熟地	
蔓荊子		甘草(炙)	
石膏(生)			

上為粗末，每服二錢。水一大盞薑五片，煎至七分，去滓溫服。不拘時候。氣虛者，此藥送養正丹五七十粒。

Xiōng Qiāng Sǎn
(Chuānxiōng and Notopterygium Powder)

A treatment for women suffering from Head Wind of which half invariably exhibit trembling and vertigo like motion sickness during each episode. This is caused by blood vacuity and the presence of wind evil that has assailed the liver.

When the *Sùwèn* states: "Rapid dizziness and extreme shaking, blurred vision and deafness means repletion below and vacuity above. The trespass is in the Foot Shàoyáng and Juéyīn vessels, and in serious cases it enters the liver," this is the condition described here. Compared to other medicines, the present formula is nimble, and its effect is rapid.

chuānxiōng	1 *liǎng*	gǎoběn	
dāngguī	3 *qián*	jīngjièsuì	
qiānghuó		bànxià	0.5 *liǎng* each
xuánfùhuā		fángfēng	
xìxīn	0.5 *liǎng* each	shúdì	
mànjīngzǐ		gāncǎo (mix-fry)	
shígāo (raw)			

Process the ingredients above into a coarse powder and take 2 *qián* per dose. Simmer in a large cup of water with five slices of ginger until reduced to 70 percent, remove the dregs, and take warm. Do not restrict the timing. For Qì vacuity, pair this medicine with 50-70 pellets of Yǎng Zhèng Dān (Nurturing the Upright Elixir).

FORMULA NOTE

There is no formula for Yǎng Zhèng Dān in Qí Zhòngfǔ's text. However, we find a formula with this name in Volume Five of the *Tàipíng Huìmín Hé jìjú fāng* 《太平惠民和劑局方》 (Tàipíng Formulary from the Imperial Grace Pharmacy), an imperially sponsored and widely known formula collection from 1078. Here is the full text of the indications for that formula:

卻邪輔正，助陽接真。治元氣陰邪交蕩，正氣乖常，上盛下虛，氣不
升降，呼吸不足，頭旋氣短，心神怯弱，夢寐遍體盜汗，腹痛腰疼，
或虛煩狂言，口乾上喘，翻胃吐食，霍亂轉筋，咳逆不定，又涎潮，
不省人事，陽氣欲脫，四肢厥冷。如傷寒陰盛，自汗唇青脈沉，最
宜服之。及後，血氣身熱，月候不均，帶下腹痛，悉能治療。常服濟
心火，強腎水，進飲食。

[A formula] to drive back evil and assist the upright and to help Yáng and link up with the genuine. It treats entanglement of original Qì with Yīn evil, upright Qì deviating from the norm, exuberance above and vacuity below, Qì failing to upbear and downbear, insufficient inhalation and exhalation, spinning head with shortness of breath, timidity and frailty of the heart Shén, night sweating all over the body when dreaming, and abdominal pain and aching lumbus; or vacuity vexation with manic speech, dry mouth and panting, nausea and vomiting, Sudden Turmoil (i.e., simultaneous vomiting and diarrhea with severe abdominal cramps) with cramping, and counter-current cough that will not settle; as well as drooling, loss of consciousness, impending desertion of Yáng Qì, and Reversal cold in the limbs. If there is Yīn exuberance in cold damage conditions with spontaneous sweating, green-blue lips, and a sunken pulse, it is most appropriate to take this formula. And then you are thoroughly able to treat generalized heat in the blood and Qì, irregular menstruation, vaginal discharge, and abdominal pain. Taking this formula consistently rescues heart fire and strengthens kidney water, and also promotes appetite for food and drink.

The formula itself consists of a concoction of mercury, sulfur, cinnabar, and galenite, melted, doused with vinegar, and processed with glutinous rice flour into bean-sized pills, to be taken as 20-30 pills per dose by drinking them down on an empty stomach before meals in warm salty water. It is said to have divine efficacy that is indescribable.

An almost identical formula is also found in Chén Zìmíng's 陳自明 *Fùrén dàquán liángfāng* 《婦人大全良方》 (Compendium of Excellent Formulas for Women), which was composed slightly later in 1237. Here it is listed under the section for "vacuity wind with dizzy head and vision and blackout," which begins with the following introduction:

夫婦人風眩，是體虛受風，風入於腦也。諸臟腑之精，皆上注於目，其血氣與脈並上屬於腦也。循脈引於目系，目系急，故令眩也。其眩不止，風邪甚者，變成癲疾也。

Women's wind blackout vision is a condition of generalized vacuity and contraction of wind, which then enters the brain. The Essence of all the *zàng* and *fǔ* organs streams upward into the eyes and their blood and Qì join together in the vessels to rise up into the brain. The encircling vessels pull on the ties of the eyes and when these are tight, this causes blackout vision. When this blackout vision does not stop and the wind evil is severe, it transforms into the illness of *diān* insanity.

Following this introduction is the formula for Yǎng Zhèng Dān, which is here described as "indicated for vacuity wind with blackout vision and incessant drool. This medicine upbears and downbears Yīn and Yáng, supplements and links to the genuine Qì, and is not simply a treatment for stopping spinning in the head."

玉真丸

治腎氣不足，氣逆上行，頭痛不可忍，謂之腎厥。
其脈舉之弦，按之石堅。(一本作不堅)

硫黃	二兩
石膏(硬者不研)	各一兩
半夏(湯洗七次)	
硝石(研)	一分

上為細末，研和生薑汁糊為丸，如桐子大。陰乾，
每服三十丸。生薑湯米飲湯下。更灸關元穴百壯。
《良方》中硫黃丸亦佳。

Yù Zhēn Wán
(Jade Immortal Pill)

Treats insufficiency of kidney Qì and counter-current
upward movement of Qì, with unbearable headache. This
is referred to as kidney Reversal. The patient's pulse will be
stringlike when lifted and stone solid when pushed (another
edition has "not solid" instead).

liúhuáng	2 liǎng
shígāo (firm, do not grind)	1 liǎng each
bànxià (wash in hot water 7 times)	
xiāoshí (grind)	1 fēn

Process the ingredients above into a fine powder. Grind with
fresh ginger juice into a paste and form into pills the size
of wútóng seeds. Dry in the shade. Take 30 pills per dose,
drinking them down in fresh ginger decoction or thin rice
gruel. Furthermore burn 100 cones of moxa on the point
Guānyuán (REN-4). The formula for Liúhuáng Wán in the
Fùrén dàquán liángfāng is also outstanding.

FORMULA NOTE

It might strike the attentive reader as a bit strange that the text here refers to another gynecology text, Chén Zìmíng's *Fùrén dàquán liángfāng*, that was actually published in 1237, or seventeen years later than Qí Zhòngfǔ's work. Given the size of both of these works, however, it is not at all surprising that these writers were aware of each other's books and that the manuscripts might have been passed back and forth, or even that both quoted earlier formula collections that are no longer preserved. Alternatively, this reference to Chén's work could have been added by a later editor of Qí Zhòngfǔ's text. In the present case, Chén Zìmíng presents the formula for Liúhuáng Wán directly after the one for Yù Zhēn Wán, so it is obvious that this is the formula referred to by Qí Zhòngfǔ as well. Why Qí chose not to list the formula himself is unclear to me.

Here is the complete text for that formula:

硫黄丸

治頭痛不可忍，或頭風年深、暴患，無所不治，服此除根。
硝石（一兩）　硫黄（二兩）
上研令極細，滴水丸如指頭大，空心，蠟茶清嚼下。

Liúhuáng Wán (Sulphur Pill)

A treatment for unbearable headache, possibly wind in the head that has deepened over years and is causing fulminant suffering. There is no condition that this formula will fail to treat, since taking this formula eliminates the root of the condition.

Ingredients: 1 *liǎng* of xiāoshí and 2 *liǎng* of liúhuáng

Grind the ingredients above until they are extremely fine. Drip water on them until you can form pills the size of a fingertip, and on an empty stomach take [a pill] by chewing it with pure early spring tea.

醉頭風餅兒

僵蠶（去絲嘴）

天南星

上件各等分細末，生薑自然汁和作餅，如折二錢
大，濃五分。陰乾，每服一餅。同平胃散四味者三
錢重，水三大盞，薑五片，棗二個，先煎平胃散一
沸，次下餅子。捶碎入，同煎一二沸，通口服。

Zuì Tóu Fēng Bǐngr
(Alcoholic Head Wind Cake)

jiāngcán (remove silk and mouths)

tiānnánxīng

Take equal amounts of the ingredients above and process
them into a fine powder. Combine with the natural juice of
fresh ginger and shape into cakes about the size of a *zhé-èr*
coin, equal halves in concentration. Dry them in the shade
and take one cake per dose. Combine it with [an amount of]
Píng Wèi Sǎn (Stomach-Calming Powder) so that the four
ingredients [including the ginger and jujube mentioned
below] together should be a total of 3 *qián* in weight. First
simmer the Píng Wèi Sǎn in 3 large cups of water with 5
slices of ginger and 2 jujubes, bringing everything to a boil
once, then add the cake, crushed into pieces. Simmer everything together and let it come to a boil once or twice. Take
it orally.

Formula Note

Píng Wèi Sǎn is a well-known formula for settling the stomach that is described in the *Tàipíng Huìmín Héjìjú fāng*. It consists of chénpí, hòupò, cāngzhú, gāncǎo, shēngjiāng, and dàzǎo. The reference to the weight of the ingredients presumably means that one should add enough Píng Wèi Sǎn powder to a single cake and 5 slices of ginger and 2 jujubes to weigh a total of 3 *qián*.

It should be noted that "alcoholic head wind" here does not refer to a condition that occurs in a person who is addicted to alcohol, but simply to head wind that is related to the intoxication by alcohol. I briefly considered using "intoxicated" instead of "alcoholic" as a translation of 醉 *zuì* to avoid this potential misunderstanding, but that term is not specific enough. There is a huge and medically significant difference in the effect of various intoxicants on the body, and the present form of head wind is specifically related to the effect of consuming a large amount of alcohol.

桃紅散

治男子婦人氣虛，攻注頭目昏眩，偏正頭疼，夾腦風，兩太陽穴疼，眉棱骨痛。及治風痰惡心，頭運欲倒。小兒傷風鼻塞，痰涎咳嗽，並宜服之。

川烏	一兩
草烏	八錢
天南星(以上三味水洗三次)	半兩
麝香	各一錢
腦子	
朱砂(別研細)	半兩

上為細末，每服半錢。薄荷茶調下。溫酒亦得。

Táo Hóng Săn
(Peach Red Powder)

Treats Qì vacuity in men and women with invasive dizziness in the head and eyes, lateral or medial headache, brain-squeezing wind, pain in both Tàiyáng points, and superciliary arch pain. Also treats wind phlegm nausea and head spinning to the point of falling over. It is also suitable to give this to small children suffering from wind damage with nasal congestion, phlegm, and cough.

chuānwū	1 *liǎng*
cǎowū	8 *qián*
tiānnánxīng (wash the three ingredients above in water three times)	0.5 *liǎng*
shèxiāng	1 *qián* each
nǎozǐ	
zhūshā	0.5 *liǎng*

Process the ingredients above into a fine powder and take 0.5 *qián* per dose. Down it mixed into mint tea. It is also possible to take it in warm rice wine.

第十八問

身體疼痛流注不定者，何也？

答曰：身體疼者，其証不一。

太陽証表未解，法當身體疼痛，太陽中濕，一身盡痛。

若脈沉身體自利痛者，陰也。

身重背強，腹中絞痛，咽喉不利，身如被杖者，陰毒証也。

若風邪乘虛在於皮膚之間，淫淫躍躍，若刺一身盡痛，傷侵血氣，動作如蟲毒之狀者，巢氏謂之風蟲也。

QUESTION EIGHTEEN

What is the Reason for Generalized Aches and Pains Streaming All Over Without a Fixed Location?

ANSWER: Generalized aching cannot be reduced to a single pattern.

In Tàiyáng patterns when the exterior is unresolved, there should be generalized aches and pains and, when Tàiyáng is struck by dampness, pain all over the entire body.

If the pulse is sunken and the body manifests with spontaneous diarrhea and pain, this means Yīn.

Heaviness of the body and rigidity of the back, wringing pain in the middle of the abdomen, inhibition in the throat, and a body that feels as if being flogged, this is a Yīn toxin pattern.

If wind evil exploits the vacuity in the space of the skin, with a seeping and leaping [sensation] and pain as if being stung all over the entire body, if the damage has invaded the blood and Qì, and the movement feels like *gǔ* toxin, Master Cháo refers to this as wind *gǔ* toxin.

DISCUSSION

The question and initial answer start out quite vague, asking about "generalized aches and pains streaming all over without a fixed location" and emphasizing that this symptom "cannot be reduced to a single pattern." Following this introduction, however, the answer becomes increasingly narrow and concrete, starting with Tàiyáng patterns with an unresolved exterior and narrowing it down to the involvement of dampness specifically. Next, the text offers advice on differentiating a Yīn condition, and then presents further signs that allow us to identify the presence of a Yīn toxin pattern.

The last paragraph discusses a very specific condition, namely "wind gǔ toxin" and cites Cháo Yuánfāng as the authority on this subject. Based on the placement of this condition in the *Zhūbìng yuánhòu lùn*, namely as the twelfth entry in Volume Thirty-Seven on women's miscellaneous condition, we know that Cháo's view of this condition involves two aspects: the presence of pathologic wind and its manifestation as a condition characterized by discomfort in the superficial skin layer. Citing Cháo's discussion in full here, to better decode Qí Zhòngfǔ's explanation, we quickly realize, as so often in this book, that Qí's last paragraph is nothing but a slightly abbreviated paraphrase of Cháo's explanation:

風蟲者，由體虛受風，風在皮膚之間。其狀，淫淫躍躍，若蟲物刺，一身盡痛，侵傷血氣，動作如蟲毒之狀，謂之風蟲。

Wind *gǔ* toxin is caused by vacuity of the body and contraction of wind, with the wind being located in the space of the skin. Its manifestation is a seeping and leaping [sensation], as if being stung by a *gǔ* toxin substance, pain all over the entire body, invading and damaging the blood and Qì, and stirring that feels as if from *gǔ* toxin. This is what is called wind *gǔ* toxin.

For most modern readers, it is probably necessary to explain first what a "stirring that feels as if from *gǔ* toxin" might look like. The term *gǔ* 蠱 originally referred to a specific type of poisoning that was executed clandestinely by people with harmful intentions. The character is first found in Shāng oracle bone inscriptions and depicts three insects in a bowl. Attesting to its great importance in early China, the *Zhūbìng yuánhòu lùn* devotes an entire volume to it (see Volume Twenty-Five). As Cháo explains in the introduction there, *gǔ* is a toxic concoction that a person prepares intentionally by "placing several venomous insects or snakes in a container and waiting until the creatures have devoured each other. When only one creature is left alive, this is called *gǔ*." Because this poison causes all sorts of ambiguous and hard-to-pinpoint pathological changes in the victim when slipped into their food or drink, eventually leading to death, it can be used intentionally by the toxin's "ruler" for their own sinister benefit. There are different varieties of *gǔ* with different manifestations, like flying *gǔ*, snake *gǔ*, lizard *gǔ*, frog *gǔ*, or dung beetle *gǔ*, and there are a number of techniques for differentiating whether a victim is suffering from genuine, i.e. natural poisoning or from *gǔ* poisoning. For example, if you make the victim spit into water, sinking saliva is a sign of *gǔ* while floating saliva means that it is a case of natural poisoning. Alternatively, if you make a patient sleep on top of a swan skin without letting them know and this aggravates the condition, this also indicates *gǔ* poisoning. Most dreadful, perhaps, is the fact that *gǔ* poison, after successfully killing the original victim that it was intended for by its "ruler," could become "ruler-less" and randomly strike innocent people exposed to it in the wild.

In a later and more general sense, the term came to refer to dreadful chronic and deep-lying conditions of hidden causation that were therefore notoriously difficult to treat. In the contemporary clinical context, the etiological concept of *gǔ* toxin and associated formulas are employed by innovative physicians like Heiner Fruehauf in the treatment of Lyme Disease.

Let us now return to the passage above and the specific condition of gynecological "wind *gǔ* toxin" as one explanation for generalized pain with no fixed location in women. It is significant for both diagnosis and treatment that "wind *gǔ*" is not mentioned in the volume on *gǔ* toxin and thus appears not to have been a recognized non-gendered variety of *gǔ* in Cháo Yuánfāng's view. In addition, the volume on *gǔ* toxin does not emphasize skin conditions specifically, beyond the occasional reference to a feeling in the skin like insects crawling, which makes sense since the toxin is derived from insects. The second to last entry of the volume does discuss a condition called 沙蝨/虱 *shāshī*, literally "sand lice," referring to a kind of tiny parasite contracted by bathing in contaminated water or by walking through plants in wet weather. This condition does manifest with red dots on the skin and sting-like pain but strikes me as a side note by Cháo and irrelevant to our discussion of "wind *gǔ* toxin."

Based on the full description in Cháo's entry on wind *gǔ* toxin in the gynecological section of his book, I suggest that this name describes not a specific form of *gǔ* poisoning, but a condition associated with an invasion of wind that is so severe and painful that it feels like *gǔ* toxin, presumably associated with *gǔ* because of the sensation like crawling insects and perhaps also because of the severity and intractability of the condition. Obviously, this distinction has highly significant ramifications for treatment. Supporting this interpretation, Qí Zhòngfǔ also mentions wind invasion as the etiological factor, which then manifests in a sensation like being "stung all over the body," as if the patient were struck by *gǔ* poisoning. In other words, Qí merely mentions *gǔ* toxin to describe the experience of wind invasion, but does not imply anywhere that we should consider *gǔ* as a potential etiology for generalized aches and pain with no fixed location! This conclusion is also supported by the following formulas.

虎骨散

治婦人血風攻注，身體疼痛。

虎脛骨	一兩半	羌活	半兩
桂心		牛膝	
芎藭		天麻	
海桐皮	各一兩	附子	各一兩
當歸		骨碎補	

上為細末，每服一錢，空心溫酒調下。

Hǔ Gǔ Sǎn
(Tiger Bone Powder)

Treats women's blood wind assault with generalized aches and pains.

hǔjìnggǔ	1.5 *liǎng*	qiānghuó	0.5 *liǎng*
guìxīn		niúxī	
xiōngqióng		tiānmá	
hǎitóngpí	1 *liǎng* each	fùzǐ	1 *liǎng* each
dāngguī		gǔsuìbǔ	

Process the ingredients above into a fine powder. Take 1 *qián* per dose, downing it on an empty stomach mixed into warm rice wine.

透經湯

治身體疼痛。

五積散	半兩
生附子	二錢

上件用水二盞，薑七片、棗二枚，煎至八分，去滓，入麝少許，再煎三四沸。通口服，不拘時候。

Tòu Jīng Tāng
(Permeating-the-Channels Decoction)

Treats generalized aches and pains.

wǔjīsǎn	0.5 *liǎng*
shēngfùzǐ	2 *qián*

Take the ingredients above and simmer them in two cups of water with 7 slices of ginger and 2 jujubes until reduced to 80 percent. Remove the dregs, add a small amount of shèxiāng, and simmer it again, bringing it to a boil 3 or 4 times. Take it orally and do not restrict the timing.

FORMULA NOTE

The ingredient listed as Wǔjī Sǎn stands for "Five Accumulations Powder" and is a reference to a well-known formula from the *Tàipíng Huìmín Héjìjú fāng* for breaking up all kinds of Accumulations. The ingredients are 3 *liǎng* each of báizhǐ, chuānxiong, gāncǎo, fúlíng, dāngguī, ròuguì, sháoyào, and bànxià; 6 *liǎng* each of chénpí, zhǐqiào, and máhuáng; 24 *liǎng* of cángzhū; 4 *liǎng* of gānjiāng; 12 *liǎng* of jiégěng; and 4 *liǎng* of hòupò. Blast-fry all of the above except the ròuguì and zhǐqiào, which you grind separately into a coarse powder. Then process the 13 ingredients together into a coarse powder and stir-fry over a small flame until they change color, spread the mixture out to cool, add the ròuguì and zhǐqiào powder and mix it in evenly. Take 3 *qián* per dose, simmer in 1.5 cups of water with 3 slices of fresh ginger until reduced to 1 cup, remove the dregs, and ingest it slightly hot.

麝香丸

治白虎歷節，諸風疼痛，游走無定，狀如蟲嚙，晝靜夜劇，及一切手足不測疼痛。

川烏(大八角者，生)	三個
全蠍(生)	二十一個
黑豆(生)	二十一粒
地龍(生)	半兩

上為細末，入麝半字，同研，和糯米糊為丸，如綠豆大。每服七丸，甚者十丸，夜令膈空，溫酒下，微出冷汗一身，便瘥。予得此方，凡是歷節及不測疼痛，一二服便瘥。

在歙川日有一貴家婦人，遍身走注疼痛，至暮則發，如蟲嚙其肌，多作鬼邪治之。予曰：「此正歷節病也。」三服愈。（凡云一字者，二分半也。）

Shèxiāng Wán
(Musk Pill)

Treats White Tiger Joint Running; the various forms of wind pain, which roam around without a fixed location, feel like gnawing bugs, and are calm during the day but aggravated at night; and all indeterminate aches and pains in the hands and feet.

chuānwū (big ones with eight protuberances, raw)	3 roots
quánxiē (raw)	21 specimens
hēidòu (raw)	21 beans
dìlóng (raw)	0.5 *liǎng*

Process the ingredients above into a fine powder and add 0.5 *zì* of shèxiāng. Grind everything together and mix with glutinous rice flour to make pills the size of mung beans. Take 7 pills per dose, up to ten pills in serious cases. Lie down at night, make the diaphragm empty, and down them in warm rice wine. A slight discharge of cool sweat all over the body means recovery. Since I have obtained this formula, I have cured all cases of Joint Running and indeterminate aches and pains with one or two doses.

There was once a married woman in an elite household in Xīchuān who was suffering from streaming aches and pains all over the body that erupted at dusk and felt as if there were bugs gnawing her flesh. Most practitioners would consider this a ghost evil and treat it as such. I said: "This is a straight-forward case of Joint Running disease." She recovered after three doses.

EDITORIAL NOTE: It is always said that 1 *zì* equals 2.5 *fēn*.

Formula Note

White Tiger Joint Running is a subcategory of Joint Running disease, which is a painful wind condition. The reference to the white tiger suggests the severity of the pain, which can be so bad that it feels like a tiger's bite. In modern TCM it is often equated with the biomedical disease category rheumatoid arthritis and explained as a type of *bì* Impediment dominated by wind. First mentioned in Chapter Five of the *Jīnguì yàolüè* on "Pulses, Patterns, and Treatments of Wind Strike and Joint-Running Disease," White Tiger Joint Running is described there as manifesting with red swollen joints, violent pain, and inability to bend and stretch, and as caused by an invasion of wind, cold, and dampness evils due to insufficiency in the liver and kidney. Entering the joints and accumulating there over time, wind, being a Yáng evil, transforms into heat while the cold and dampness cause stagnation of Qì and blood.

The *Zhūbìng yuánhòu lùn* offers a more detailed description of the symptoms and etiology in the entry on "Joint Running Wind" that deserves to be quoted in full:

> 歷節風之狀，短氣，白汗出，歷節疼痛不可忍，屈伸不得是也。由飲酒腠理開，汗出當風所致也。亦有血氣虛，受風邪而得之者。風歷關節，與血氣相搏交攻，故疼痛。血氣虛，則汗也。風冷搏於筋，則不可屈伸，為歷節風也。

> The manifestations of Joint Running Wind are shortness of breath, discharge of white (in some editions, spontaneous 自) sweat, Joint Running pain that is unbearable, and inability to bend and stretch. It is caused by exposure to wind after drinking alcohol, which has opened the patient's interstices and caused sweating. There is also a kind [of Joint Running] that is due to contraction of wind evil as the result of a vacuity of blood and Qì. Wind runs into the joints and battles with the blood and Qì. This causes the pain. Vacuity of blood and Qì result in sweating. When wind cold assaults the joints, the patient is unable to bend and stretch. This is Joint Running Wind.

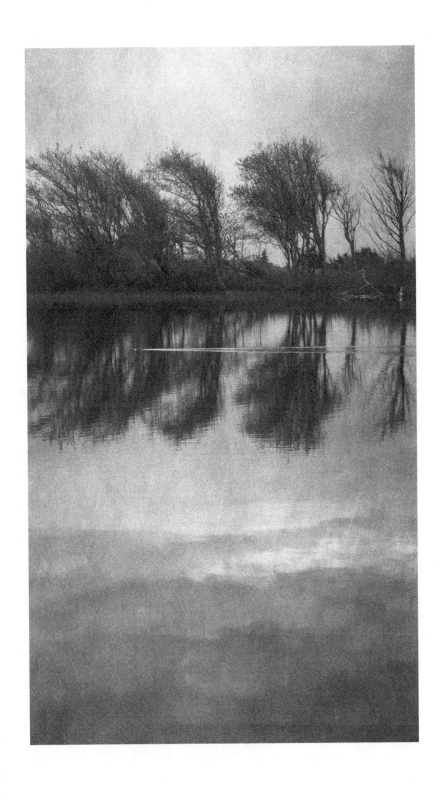

第十九問

朝食暮吐者，何也？

答曰：嘔吐之病，皆繇三焦不調，脾胃不和，清濁
相干之所致也。

大抵嘔吐本二証。嘔者，嘔而有聲，俗所謂哕是
也。吐者，吐而有物，胃中虛冷則吐。

若心下牢大如杯，或時寒熱，朝食暮吐，脈如弦
緊，則為虛寒相搏，胃氣日虧。所以不能停留水
穀，名曰胃反。

QUESTION NINETEEN

What is the Reason for Eating in the Morning and Vomiting in the Evening?

ANSWER: The disease of retching and vomiting is always caused by a lack of attunement in the Sānjiāo, disharmony in the spleen and stomach, and mutual harassment between the clear and the turbid.

Generally speaking, retching and vomiting are originally two patterns: Retching refers to heaving with a sound, while vomiting refers to ejecting a substance. When there is vacuity cold inside the stomach, vomiting results.

If there is a firm spot below the heart about the size of a cup, occasional [aversion to] cold and heat [effusion], eating in the morning and vomiting at night, and a pulse that is string-like and tight, this means that vacuity and cold are assaulting each other and that stomach Qì is diminished further with each passing day. Because the patient is unable to retain water and grain, it is called stomach reflux.

Discussion

What strikes me as most interesting about the answer to this question is the lack of any reference to a gendered dimension in this condition. Most of the previous questions in this text were concerned with menstruation, which is obviously a condition that only affects female bodies. The prior question did not specifically explain a connection to the female body, but by now any careful reader will be aware of women's affinity to Yīn, to dampness (see Question Three, quoting the famous introduction to Sūn Sīmiǎo's writings on gynecology), and to Wind (see Questions Sixteen on wind cold and Seventeen on Blackout Vision and Veiling).

In the present question, the only obvious connection to gynecology is the etiology of vacuity cold. As a Yīn evil, vacuity cold is more likely to affect women who are Yīn by nature and have a propensity to suffering from vacuity in particular during certain stages in their reproductive cycle, most notably the postpartum period. That said, vacuity cold in and of itself, as well as the present etiology of vacuity cold weakening stomach Qì, are not generally thought of as gendered conditions. A possible reason for the inclusion of this condition of retching and vomiting in a gynecological textbook is given by Cháo Yuánfāng in the entry with the very same title (*Zhūbìng yuánhòu lùn*, vol. 40):

> 胃氣逆則嘔吐。胃為水穀之海，其氣不調， 而有風冷乘之，冷搏受 於胃氣，胃氣逆則嘔吐也。

> When stomach Qì moves counter-current, this results in retching and vomiting. The stomach is the Sea of Water and Grain. When its Qì is not attuned and there is wind-cold present to exploit this, the stomach Qì is assaulted by the cold. As stomach Qì moves counter-current, retching and vomiting result.

Qí Zhòngfǔ was certainly familiar with Cháo's text and therefore with the explanation of wind-cold, as opposed to just cold, for retching and vomiting found there. And women's propensity to wind invasion is a fact that has been firmly established in previous answers by Qí Zhòngfǔ. So it is quite possible that in the mind of Qí and his contemporaries, the etiology of this condition was always associated with wind-cold instead of with just cold and that Qí did not find it necessary to state that fact here because it would have been obvious to his readers. On the other hand, it is also interesting that the very next entry in Cháo's text, which addresses "seasickness and motion sickness in women and small children," stresses the non-gendered nature of that condition, even though it is placed in the volumes on gynecology:

無問男子女人，乘車船則心悶亂，頭痛吐逆，　謂之注車、注船。特由質性自然，非關宿挾病。

No matter whether we are talking about men or women, riding in a chariot or boat results in heart oppression and disorder, headache, and vomiting, which is called "chariot flux" or "boat flux." In particular, this is due to natural disposition and is not related to any chronic illness.

Returning to the *Hundred Questions on Gynecology*, the inclusion of retching and vomiting as the result of vacuity cold debilitating stomach Qì gives us an important clue about the conception of the female body in Sòng dynasty Chinese medicine and also about the greatest threats to women's health, as perceived by Qí Zhòngfǔ and his colleagues. It should alert contemporary practitioners to pay special attention to the etiology of vacuity cold when treating women and to perhaps pass this information on to their patients for preventative care and lifestyle changes. This is especially important since this is not a concept widely shared by our contemporary culture or biomedicine.

Lastly, this association of the female body with vacuity cold has important consequences for treatment and is clearly reflected in the prevalence of warming and supplementing medicinals in the vast majority of gynecological formulas.

紫金丹

治嘔吐、心腹疼。

丁香	
木香	
蓽澄茄	
胡椒	
五靈脂(西者)	
肉豆蔻(煨)	
乾薑(炮)	
半夏末	半兩
附子(炮)	
硫黃水銀砂子(二件，如靈砂法炒青金頭角)	一兩

上為細末，半夏末薑汁打糊丸，如桐子大。每服七
十丸，空心米飲下。

Zǐ Jīn Dān
(Precious Gold Elixir)

A treatment for retching and vomiting and for pain in the heart and abdomen.

dīngxiāng	
mùxiāng	
bìchéngqié	
hújiāo	
wǔlíngzhī (from the West)	
ròudòukòu (roast over embers)	
gānjiāng (blast-fry)	
bànxià (process into a powder)	0.5 *liǎng*
fùzǐ (blast-fry)	
liúhuáng shuǐyín shāzǐ (2 pieces, stir-fry as in the method for língshā until it turns into qīngjīntóujiǎo)	1 *liǎng*

Process the ingredients above into a fine powder. With the pinellia powder and ginger juice, beat everything into a paste and form pills the size of *wútóng* seeds. Take 70 pills per dose and ingest them on an empty stomach by drinking them down in thin rice gruel.

Formula Note

Finding more information on this formula has proven challenging since there are dozens of formulas in Chinese medicine with this title that differ widely in terms of ingredients and indications. There is even a second formula with this same name listed in the next Question below, which only shares the ingredient sulfur but is otherwise unrelated.

The ingredient liúhuáng shuǐyīn shāzǐ 硫黄水銀砂子, literally "sulfur liquid-silver sand," has caused me many grey hairs. The compound shuǐyīn 水銀, literally "water/liquid silver," means quicksilver, or in other words, the pure and natural form of mercury in its liquid state at room temperature. In historical China, it was produced by extracting it from cinnabar or mercuric sulfide (HgS), which occurs naturally especially in Western China. The cinnabar is roasted until the mercury is released as vapor into the air and then condensed. Both mercury and cinnabar were common ingredients in not just alchemical but also medicinal formulas throughout the history of Chinese medicine. Obviously, mercury is a highly toxic substance that should not be used in contemporary practice regardless of its use in historical formulas. While cinnabar is less toxic than pure mercury because of its low solubility and hence low bioavailability, it is not an ingredient considered safe by most modern practitioners. Regardless of the precise meaning and end product of the alchemical refinement described here for this ingredient, this formula should therefore not be used in clinical application.

Originally, I followed the punctuation of most printed and online editions of this text, which pair shuǐ 水 ("water") with liúhuáng 硫黄 (sulfur), thus creating the ingredient "sulfur water" and treat this as a separate ingredient from yīnshāzǐ. Eventually, I ended up choosing a different punctuation in my listing of ingredients based on the following instructions, which call for powdering the medicinals before they are processed with ginger juice into a paste. It simply does not make sense to me that sulfur water would be listed among the other dry ingredients but then processed according to the following instructions, or that quicksilver, which is liquid in its natural state at room temperature, is measured as a "sand." Additionally, these editions then list the final ingredient as yīnshāzǐ 銀砂子, literally "silver sand." Yīnshā as a compound can sometimes refer to vermilion, which is the English name for the pigment that is a side-product of mercury mining, compounded by grinding powdered cinnabar (mercury sulfide). With assistance from Leo Lok, I realized that reading this string of characters as two separate ingredients is wrong and that we instead have to combine the two terms liúhuáng (sulfur) and shǔiyīn (quicksilver) into a single item, because when we mix these two substances, the end result does take the form of a rough chunky powder or "sand."

The term língshā, literally "magical sand," is a reference to the alchemical product mercuric sulfide, created by combining and heating mercury and sulfur in a particular manner. Chemically, the combination of these two substances can take two forms, red cinnabar (α-HgS) or, as the present case presumably desires, the black variety called "metacinnabar" (β-HgS), which in its natural form is characterized by a metallic luster but in the alchemically produced compound takes on a bluish grey hue. This is presumably what the term "blueish metal" (青金 qīngjīn) refers to in the final product. I gratefully acknowledge Leo Lok's assistance in alerting me to a passage in the Jiǔzhuǎn língshā dàdān 《九轉靈砂大丹》 (Eightfold Transformation Magical Sand Great Elixir), by an unknown author from the Táng to Sòng periods, that equates the two terms língshā 靈砂 and qīngjīntóumò 青金頭末. This text describes a complicated procedure that involves two people sitting across from each other stir-frying the mixture of sulfur and mercury in an iron wok coated with wax with an iron shovel-like implement until it smokes, then dousing the mixture with rice vinegar until it stops smoking, and then stir-frying it again. When done, the mixture is broken up with a mallet made from willow wood and finely crushed with a roller. It is stir-fried again until it takes on the color of "bluish bricks" (令青磚色為度), which should take about six hours, and then finely crushed again with a roller. The product is now called qīngjīntóumò. Given the fact that it is unlikely for a contemporary reader to replicate the compounding of cinnabar from sulfur and mercury because of the known toxicity of any fumes released when heating mercury, I will spare you the finer details.

薑合丸

療中脘停寒，胸膈結痞，嘔吐惡心，不思飲食。

木香	各一兩
肉桂	
附子	
硇砂(紙上飛)	
陳皮	各一兩
丁香	
沉香	
蓽澄茄	
青皮(去白)	
茴香(炒)	一分

上為細末，次入硇砂研，酒煮麵糊為丸。每一兩作二十丸，每服一丸。

以生薑一塊，剜如盒子，安藥在內，濕紙裹煨，令香，去紙放溫，細嚼鹽湯送下。

Jiāng Hé Wán
(Ginger-Encased Pill)

A cure for cold collecting in the middle stomach duct, binding *pǐ* Glomus in the chest and diaphragm, and retching and vomiting with nausea and lack of interest in eating and drinking.

mùxiāng	
ròuguì	1 *liǎng* each
fùzǐ	
náoshā (sublimate on paper)	
chénpí	
dīngxiāng	
chénxiāng	1 *liǎng* each
bìchéngqié	
qīngpí (remove white parts)	
huíxiāng (stir-fry)	1 *fēn*

Process the above ingredients into a fine powder and then add the náoshā and grind it. Boil with rice wine, make a paste with flour, and form pills. Each 1 *liǎng* should make 20 pills. Take 1 pill per dose.

Hollow out a chunk of fresh ginger to form a box-like container and place the medicine inside. Wrap this in moistened paper and roast it over embers until it starts to smell. Remove the paper and let it rest until warm. Chew it well and drink it down in hot salty water.

Formula Note

For readers not well trained in the technical terminology of traditional Chinese medicine, a brief explanation may be helpful on the term 痞 *pǐ*, which I translate throughout this book as "*pǐ* Glomus." Being a combination of the character 否 *pǐ*, which can mean "standstill" or "blockage," and the disease radical 疒 nì, Wiseman explains it as follows in the entry on this term in his *Practical Dictionary of Chinese Medicine*:

> A localized subjective feeling of fullness and blockage. In the chest (glomus in the chest), it can be associated with a feeling of oppression in severe cases; hence the terms fullness in the chest, distention in the chest, glomus in the chest, and oppression in the chest are largely synonymous. In the abdomen, glomus is the sensation of a lump that cannot be detected by palapation. Hard glomus below the heart, which can be subjectively felt and objectively palpated, is a sign of evil heat with water collecting in the stomach. Any palpable abdominal mass is referred to as a glomus lump, although in texts predating *On Cold Damage*, these were referred to as glomus. Glomus lump in traditional literature are labeled differently, according to shape, behavior, and pathomechanism; see Concretions, Conglomerations, Accumulations, and Gatherings; Deep-Lying Beam; Strings and Aggregations; Inquiry; Palpation.

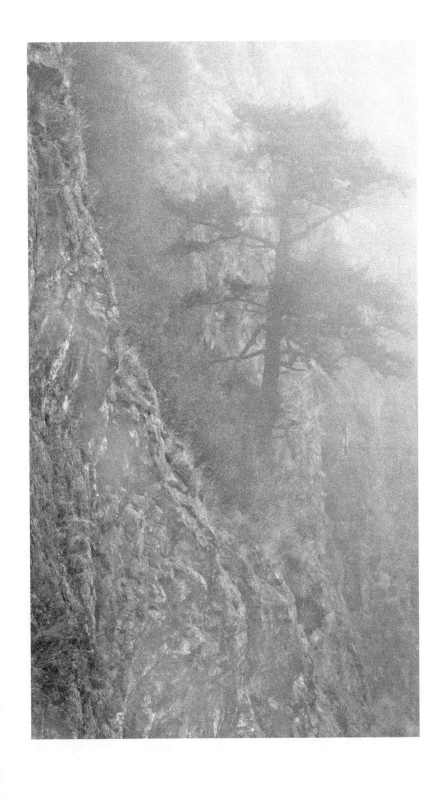

第二十問

婦人之病多因氣生者，何也？

答曰：氣以形載，形以氣充。惟氣與形，兩者相待，氣和則生，氣戾則病。

結為積聚，氣不舒也。逆為狂厥，氣不降也。宜通而塞則為痛，氣不達也。宜消而息則為痞。嬰之為癭，留之為瘤，亦氣之凝耳。

內經曰：「怒則氣上，喜則氣緩，悲則氣消，恐則氣下，寒則氣收，熱則氣泄，勞則氣耗，思則氣結，驚則氣亂。」九氣不同，故婦人之病，多因氣之所生也。

QUESTION TWENTY

What is the Reason for Women's Diseases Being Predominantly Engendered Due to Qì?

ANSWER: Qì is carried about by the physical body, and the physical body is made plentiful by Qì. As we ponder Qì in relationship to the physical body, these two depend on each other. When Qì is harmonious, life results; when Qì is in rebellion, disease results.

Binding and forming masses, this means that Qì is not relaxed. Moving counter-current and forming *kuáng* mania and Reversal, this means that Qì fails to descend. When it should flow through but is congested instead, the result is pain and failure of Qì to break through. When it should dissipate but instead halts in one place, the result is Dissipation Disease. When it encircles like a necklace, this constitutes goiters. When it lodges, this constitutes tumors, which likewise means congealing of Qì.

The *Nèijīng* states: "Anger results in ascent of Qì, elation in laxness of Qì, grief in the dissipation of Qì, fear in descent of Qì, cold in constriction of Qì, heat in leakage of Qì, taxation in exhaustion of Qì, pondering in binding of Qì, and panic in Qì chaos." These nine [forms of] Qì are different from each other, and as such women's diseases are predominantly engendered due to Qì.

Discussion

The term 形 *xíng*, which I have translated above as "physical body," literally means shape or form, in the sense of the outside contour that throws a shadow 彡. It is essential that we do not read the contrast between Qì and *xíng* in the sense of our Cartesian dualism as between the immaterial mind and the material body or between "energy" and "matter," as beginning students and popular accounts of Chinese medicine often do. There is a very good reason why well-trained professionals of Chinese medicine tend to carefully avoid the term "energy" and use the Chinese term Qì instead. Yes, energy is one aspect of Qì, but the Chinese concept includes so much more, as suggested by its etymology of steam rising up from cooked rice. Depending on context, Qì might more narrowly refer also to the breath that we inhale and exhale, or the basic "stuff" that makes up the universe, which is condensed into an infinite number of constantly changing gaseous, fluid, or solid forms. Qì is what animates the *xíng*, which has led some translators to use the phrase "vital stuff" to render it in English. While more accurate than "energy," that translation is too general and so devoid of the powerful associations of Qì, especially in a medical context, as to be almost meaningless.

The third paragraph of the answer contains four plays on words that are impossible to reflect in a literal translation: First, the two terms 通 "flow through" and 痛 "pain" are closely related etymologically, only differing by the semantic aspect or "radical" of the character. The intimate relationship between pain and lack of flow is one of the most basic concepts in the Chinese understanding of how the body works and how pain is generated and treated. It is eloquently expressed in the famous saying:

通則不痛；痛則不通。

Tōng zé bú tòng; tòng zé bù tōng.

Flow-through means absence of pain; pain means absence of flow-through.

The second instance of a play on words is much more challenging to translate and involves the character that I have translated as "dissipate" in the present context: 消 *xiāo*. It is the etymological source for the character 痟 *xiāo*, which I have translated a bit awkwardly as "Dissipation Disease." Most readers who are familiar with Nigel Wiseman's terminology in his *Practical Dictionary of Chinese Medicine* should recognize the term in the context of pathology from the compound "dissipation (or in his terminology "dispersion") thirst" (消渴 *xiāokě*), usually rendered in English TCM literature as "diabetes." In traditional Chinese dictionaries, the character is explained with two groups of meanings as "soreness and headache" or as "diabetes." The *Zhōngyī dàcídiǎn* 《中醫大辭典》 (Great Dictionary of Chinese Medicine), for example, offers two different meanings: First, as a symptom that is related to the notion of dissolution or dissipation, of melting away, in the sense of Dissipation Emaciation (痟瘦), as in the compounds Dissipation Thirst 消渴 and Dissipation of the Center 痟中. Second, this dictionary defines 痟 *xiāo* as a disease name characterized by headache.

The third and fourth instances of a play on words work in a similar fashion: Both are disease names that are etymologically related to the state of the Qì described by the source character. First there is the relationship between the character 嬰 *yīng*, which means "necklace" or "to wear around the neck," and 癭 *yǐng*, literally "encircling-the-neck disease," or in other words, goiters. And then we find the character 留 *liú* "to lodge" that is used inside the character for "tumor," which is a combination of "to lodge" with the disease radical: 瘤, also pronounced *liú*. In all of these cases, it is obvious how knowledge of the character's etymology provides important insights into the etiology of the disease.

The quotation from the *Nèijīng* at the end of this Question is from *Sùwèn* Chapter Thirty-Nine, which is the famous treatise on pain. In that chapter, no reference is made to women being more prone to these diseases than men, and even after the explanation in the present answer above, it is not clear to me how these nine types of Qì explain why women are more prone to disease engendered by Qì. A much more convincing answer to that question is offered by Sūn Sīmiǎo in his famous introductory essay on his gynecological formulas:

然而女人嗜欲多於丈夫，感病倍於男子，加以慈戀，愛憎，嫉妒，憂恚，染著堅牢，情不自抑，所以為病根深，療之難瘥。

This being so, women's predilections and desires exceed those of men, and they contract diseases at twice the rate of men. In addition, when they are affected by compassion and attachment, love and hatred, envy and jealousy, and worry and rancor, these become firmly lodged and deep-seated. Since they are unable to control their emotions by themselves, the roots of their diseases are deep, and it is difficult to obtain a cure in their treatment.

It is up to the individual reader to decide how to interpret this statement: My feminist students tend to view it as an offensive and patronizing attempt by an elite man to explain women's frustrations that were due to their difficult lives in a time, society, and culture that did not allow them to express themselves fully. I tend to be reluctant to pass judgment on the supposed misogyny of early Táng society because it is simply too difficult, in my opinion, to get a true sense of the lived experiences of women, varied as they were by class, region, individual circumstances, and even the meaning of male-female hierarchical relationships in such a distant time. In the context of that essay, I read it as part of Sūn Sīmiǎo's effort to convince his contemporaries of the importance of taking care of women as the true foundation of "nurturing life" by creating and maintaining healthy families, in all meanings of that word.

To return to the question here and to Qí Zhòngfǔ's answer, his explanation on the basis of the *Sùwèn* quote makes sense when we assume that the connection between women and emotionality was something so self-evident to medical authors of the Sòng period that it did not need to be spelled out. Since, in their minds, women were obviously much more strongly affected by emotional upheaval than men, the answer here merely explains the specific effects of these emotions, subdivided into nine different kinds to emphasize the comprehensiveness of this emotional profile and all the various ways in which the flow of Qì could be disrupted. With its reference to the "Seven Qì," which can be interpreted here as identical to the "Seven Emotions," the first formula following the present answer also supports this emphasis on the emotions as the link between women and Qì disorders.

大七氣湯

治驚恐恚怒相搏而痛。

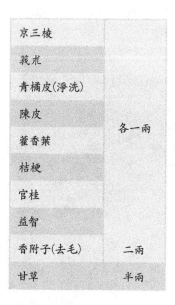

京三棱	
莪朮	
青橘皮(淨洗)	
陳皮	
藿香葉	各一兩
桔梗	
官桂	
益智	
香附子(去毛)	二兩
甘草	半兩

上為粗末散，每服五錢，水二盞，薑三片，棗一枚，煎至一盞，去滓溫服。

Dà Qī Qì Tāng
(Major Seven Qì Decoction)

A treatment for panic, fear, rage, and anger assaulting each other and causing pain.

jīngsānléng	
ézhú	
qīngjúpí (wash clean)	
chénpí	1 *liǎng* each
huòxiāngyè	
jiégěng	
guānguì	
yìzhì	
xiāngfùzǐ (remove hairs)	2 *liǎng*
gāncǎo	0.5 *liǎng*

Process the ingredients above into a coarse powder and take 5 *qián* per dose. Simmer in 2 cups of water with three slices of ginger and 1 jujube until reduced to 1 cup. Remove the dregs and take warm.

Formula Note

The "seven Qì" in the name of this formula refer to emotional upheaval that disorders the Qì flow in general, or specifically to cold, heat, anger, rage, sorrow, elation, and worry. The earliest known reference to this list is found in the entry on the "Seven Qì" in Cháo Yúanfāng's *Zhūbìng yuánhòu lùn*. There Cháo explains that when these seven Qì gather into masses and harden, the key signs for this pathology are excruciating pain below the heart and in the abdomen and inability to eat and drink which occur in intermittent episodes that bring the patient to the brink of death. A Míng period text defines the Seven Qì strictly as emotional causes, and it is possible that by Sòng times this psychological definition of the Seven Qì was already prevalent, as the introductory line to this formula suggests. Similarly, it could be a reference to the famous "Seven Emotions" (七情 qī qíng), for which the *locus classicus* is the seven emotional causes of Qì disruption included among the Nine Qì cited in Qí Zhòngfǔ's answer to Question Twenty in his quotation from *Sùwèn* Chapter Thirty-Nine.

As is often the case with Chinese formula names, several formulas with this name exist, including one in the *Bèijí qiānjīn yàofāng*, that are not directly related to the present one. I have, however, been able to find an almost identical version of this formula with the same name in a text called *Quánshēng zhǐmí fāng* 《全生指迷方》 (Confusion-Evincing Formulas for All of One's Life) by Wáng Kuàngzhuàn 王貺撰, which appears to be roughly contemporaneous with the *Hundred Questions on Gynecology*. At this point, it is impossible to determine which of these two sources is the earlier one. In that text, it is also called "Major Confusion-Evincing Seven Qì Decoction" and is indicated for "mutual assault of the seven emotions, for Yīn and Yáng rising and falling, for congestion and stagnation in the pathways of Qì, and for aggressive surging causing pain."

木香順氣散

理衛氣，順三焦。

烏藥
木香
香附子
薑黃
砂仁
甘草

上為吹咀，每服半兩。水二鐘，薑五片，棗二枚，煎至八分，去滓溫服，不拘時。

Mùxiāng Shùn Qì Sǎn
(Costusroot Powder that Restores the Proper Direction of the Qì Flow)

[A formula that] restores the correct pattern of the *wèi* Qì and the proper direction of flow in the Sānjiāo.

wūyào
mùxiāng
xiāngfùzǐ
jiānghuáng
shārén
gāncǎo

Pound the ingredients above and take 0.5 *liǎng* per dose. Simmer in 2 goblets of water with 2 slices of ginger and 2 jujubes until reduced to 80 percent. Discard the dregs and ingest warm. Do not restrict the timing.

紫金丹

治氣癖，氣瘕，蠱脹病。

針砂	十兩
餘糧	各二兩
石硫黃	

上先用藥三件，同好醋入鐵鍋內煮乾，碾為末。

平胃散	十兩	白茯苓	
莪朮	二兩	大黃	
縮砂仁		黃連	
丁香		黑牽牛	
木香	各一兩	甘草	各三兩
獨活		茱萸	
黃耆		檳榔	
枳殼		破故紙	
干漆(須好者生漆二兩亦得)	一兩		

上件為細末，同前藥末用酒糊為丸，桐子大。每日三五服，不拘數，如病重則多服。忌鹽醬油麵生冷等物。

Zǐ Jīn Dān
(Precious Gold Elixir)

A treatment for Qì Aggregations, Qì Conglomerations, and the disease of *gǔ* toxin distention.

zhēnshā	10 *liǎng*
yúliáng	
shíliúhuáng	2 *liǎng* each

First take the three ingredients above and boil them together with good vinegar in an iron wok until the medicinals are dry. Crush them with a roller into a powder.

Píngwèisǎn	10 *liǎng*	báifúlíng	
ézhú	2 *liǎng*	dàhuáng	
suōshārén		huánglián	
dīngxiāng		hēiqiānniú	3 *liǎng* each
mùxiāng	1 *liǎng* each	gāncǎo	
dúhuó		zhūyú	
huángqí		bīnláng	
zhǐké		pògùzhǐ	
gānqī (must be high quality. Otherwise, 2 *liǎng* of shēngqī is also acceptable)	1 *liǎng*		

Process the ingredients above into a fine powder. Combine with the previous medicinals, use rice wine to make a paste, and form into pills the size of *wútóng* seeds. Every day take 3-5 doses and do not restrict the number [of pills]. If the condition is serious, take more. Avoid salt, soy sauce, noodles, and raw and cold foods.

Formula Note

It is interesting to ponder why a formula for Qì Aggregations and *gǔ* distention is listed under this question on women's propensity to suffer from Qì disorders based on their emotional volatility. It may serve as a useful reminder of the inseparability in traditional Chinese medicine of what in biomedicine is neatly divided into physiological and psychological disorders, or disorders of the body and disorders of the mind. The present discussion of Qì disorders is a perfect illustration of the different conception of the Chinese medicine body as a seamless unit of its material and immaterial, tangible and intangible, or formed and formless aspects, of flesh and blood and Essence and Qì and Shén, which are impossible to diagnose and treat in isolation. In this body, Qì is central as the basic substance that the body is constructed of and animated by, but also disordered by due to the influence of internal or external imbalances and disharmonies of Qì. It is no wonder that the Chinese character for "to treat" (治 *zhi*) has the water radical as its semantic component, originally meaning to manage the flow of water to irrigate, moisten, drain, and fertilize the land and make agriculture possible. Like a sagely ruler and skilled farmer who manage water and resources, the physician directs, regulates, and facilitates the proper distribution of Qì, preventing blockages and stagnation but also excessive and counter-current surging, flooding, and leaking. Regardless of the tangible physiological signs and symptoms that a patient might present with, we must never forget that especially in women the emotions are the key internal factor, next to taxation, that causes any disordered flow of Qì. Reflecting the view of emotion already common in the early classical period, the *Lǚ shì chūnqiú* 《呂氏春秋》 (Spring and Autumn Annals of Master Lü) from 239 BCE emphasizes the significance of the emotions as the foundation of life and death:

天生人而使有貪有欲。欲有情，情有節。聖人修節以止欲，故不過行其情也。故耳之欲五聲，目之欲五色，口之欲五味，情也。此三者，貴賤、愚智、賢不肖欲之若一，雖神農、黃帝，其與桀、紂同。聖人之所以異者，得其情也。由貴生動，則得其情矣；不由貴生動，則失其情矣。此二者，死生存亡之本也。

Heaven gives birth to us humans and causes us to have cravings and desires. Desires mean the existence of emotions, and emotions mean the existence of moderation. The sages cultivate moderation and thereby stop desire. This is the reason that they do not mishandle their emotions. As such, the ears' desire for the five sounds, the eyes' desire for the five colors, and the mouth's desire for the five flavors, these are the emotions. These three are desired by all alike, whether noble or vulgar, foolish or wise, worthy or unworthy. Even the Divine Farmer and the Yellow Emperor did not differ in this from the evil Jié and Zhòu (the corrupt last rulers of the Xià and Shāng dynasties). What makes the sages different in this regard is that they were able to obtain their desires. When we act on the basis of valuing life, we obtain our desires. When we act not on the basis of valuing life, we lose our desires. These two conditions are the foundation of life and death, of survival and perishing!

第二十一問

猝然而死，少間復蘇者，何也？

答曰：世言氣中者，雖不見於方書，然暴喜傷陽，暴怒傷陰，亦氣中之源也。況憂愁不意，氣多厥逆，往往多得此疾。便覺涎潮昏塞，牙關緊急，若概作中風候用藥，非止不相當，多致殺人。

經云：「無故而瘖，脈不至，不治，自已。」謂氣暴逆也。氣復則已。故猝然而死，少間復蘇者，正謂此也。

QUESTION TWENTY-ONE

What is the Reason for Dying Abruptly and Shortly Thereafter Coming Back to Life?

ANSWER: Even though what people call Qì strike is not something that you see in the formula texts, still, fulminant elation damages the Yáng, and fulminant anger damages the Yīn, and both are also sources of Qì strike. Furthermore, unanticipated grief and worrying and the [resulting] tendency of Qì to reverse its flow and move counter-current frequently cause a propensity to contract this condition. In that case, if the perception of surging saliva, clouded consciousness, and clenched jaw are interpreted as symptoms of wind strike and addressed accordingly with medicinals, this is not just inappropriate but will most likely kill the patient!

According to the Classic, "Muteness without a cause with a pulse that fails to arrive will end on its own without treatment." This is referred to as "fulminant counter-current flow of Qì." When the Qì returns [to its proper direction of flow], the disease will end. As such, dying abruptly and shortly thereafter coming back to life refers to exactly this condition.

DISCUSSION

The first difficult issue in translating the answer above concerns the term 氣中 qìzhōng/zhòng. Depending on the translation and context, the character 中 can mean either "center" (in which case it is pronounced with the first tone as zhōng), or it can mean "to hit the mark" or "to strike" (in which case it is pronounced with the fourth tone as zhòng). In the compound 中氣, "center Qì" can refer to the Qì in the center of the body, or to Qì in the Middle Jiāo, the Center Burner, in the sense of spleen and stomach Qì, tasked with the function of upbearing the clear and downbearing the turbid. This is the most commonly seen meaning of the compound term in clinical literature, especially in the context of physiology or the pathology of "insufficiency of center Qì" 中氣不足. Alternatively, it can refer to the Qì that is situated between the trunk 本 and the branches 標. What the trunk and the branches, and hence the middle in between them, refer to differs yet again depending on context, but can even be interpreted in etiology as the trunk of the six climatic Qì (wind, heat, dampness, dryness, cold and fire) and the branches of the six conformations (Shàoyáng, Tàiyáng, Yángmíng, Shàoyīn, Tàiyīn, Juéyīn), with the center Qì being situated in the middle, between these two concepts.

That being said, in the present case, I have chosen to read 中 in the fourth tone, as zhòng in the meaning of "to strike," both because of the order of the characters and because of the context. To start with, the present question concerns abrupt death followed by recovery, and then mentions increased salivation, clouded consciousness, and clenched jaw, which are classic signs of wind strike. The attached formula below also includes many symptoms that are best explained by the etiology of pathogenic factors (whether wind or ghosts etc.) "striking" the patient. In addition, as I explain below, the original source of the explanation from the "classic" mentioned in the answer above may have been lost, but is quoted in what appears to be a potentially more literal version in a chapter on Wind Strike (中風 zhòngfēng) in another text, albeit several centuries later.

Most of the answer given here appears to be a slightly altered quotation from the Pǔjì běnshì fāng 《普濟本事方》 (Original Formulas for Popular

Relief), published in 1132 by Xǔ Shūwēi 許叔微 (1079-1154), a famous Sòng dynasty medical author who specialized in the *Shānghán lùn*. There, Xǔ adds a case study of a lady who tragically died from such a condition after being wrongly treated for Wind Strike by a village doctor and given Dà Tōng Wán, which caused numerous bouts of severe diarrhea and death on that same evening. My attribution of this passage to Xǔ Shūwēi is supported by the fact that an almost identical passage with a bit of additional information is found in a Míng dynasty text called *Gǔjīn yītǒng dàquán* 《古今醫統大全》 (Compendium of Ancient and Modern Medicine) by Xú Chūnfǔ 徐春甫, where it is identified as a quotation from a "Scholar Xǔ" 許學士, presumably referring to Xǔ Shūwēi. In that text, this passage is included in Volume Nine on Wind Strike under the heading "Pathomechanism." I am sharing the full entry here since the text goes on to discuss Sūhéxiāng Wán (Storax Pill), which is also the formula that is attached to Question Twenty-One of the *Hundred Questions*.

許學士云：世言氣中者，雖不見方書，然暴怒傷陰，暴喜傷陽，憂愁不已，氣多厥逆，往往得此疾。便覺涎潮昏塞，牙關緊急。若便作中風用藥，多致殺人。惟宜蘇合香丸灌之便醒。然後隨寒熱虛實而調之，無不愈者。

經曰：無故而喑，肺不至，不治自已，謂氣暴逆也，氣複則已。審如是，雖不服藥亦可。

《玉機微義》云：中氣即七情內火之動，氣厥逆，由其本虛故也。用蘇合香丸，通行經絡，其決烈之性，如摧枯拉朽，恐氣血虛者，非所宜也。後云不治自複之意，蓋警用藥之失，實勝誤於庸醫之所為也。

According to Scholar Xǔ, even though what people call Qì strike is not something that you see in the formula texts, still, fulminant anger damaging the Yīn, fulminant elation damaging the Yáng, endless grief and worries, and the [resultant] propensity of Qì to reverse its flow and move counter-current frequently lead to the contraction of this disease. In that case, if the perception of surging saliva, clouded consciousness, and clenched jaw is interpreted as wind strike and addressed with medicinals accordingly, this will most likely kill the patient! It is only appropriate to force Sūhéxiāng Wán down their throat to revive them. Then afterwards, if you attune their condition on the basis of vacuity or repletion of cold or heat, not a single patient will fail to recover!

According to the Classic, "Muteness without a cause, with a pulse that fails to arrive will end on its own without treatment." This is referred to as "fulminant counter-current flow of Qì." When the Qì returns [to its proper flow], the disease will end. Having examined the condition like this, even if you do not give the patient medicine, [the condition] can be resolved.

According to the text *Yùjī wéiyì*, Qì Strike means that the inner fire of the seven emotions is stirring and that Qì has reversed flow to move counter-current. This is caused by the patient's root vacuity. Use Sūhéxiāng Wán to free the flow in the channels and network vessels. Its abrupt and violent nature is like snapping a piece of rotten wood, but fearing the vacuity of Qì and blood is not called for! When people later say that this condition should not be treated and that the patient will recover on their own, this must be seen as a warning against the [often fatal] misapplication of medicinals. In reality, we must overcome the mistakes caused by the actions of charlatan physicians.

The key issue discussed in this question is thus the vital need to distinguish between a diagnosis of Wind Strike and one of Qì Strike, with the key difference being that in the case of Qì Strike the pulse fails to arrive at all. The Sòng dynasty text *Chábìng zhǐnán* 《察病指南》 (Guide to Scrutinizing Disease, published in 1241) by Shī Guìtáng 施桂堂, for example, in the volume on "Method for Examining the Life- and Death-Pulse of the Various Diseases) identifies "muteness without a cause, with a pulse that fails to arrive" as a sign of "fulminant Reversal of Qì" (氣暴厥 qì bào jué) and contrasts it with the pulses for Wind Strike:

中風口噤。脈遲浮者生。急實大數者死。

In Wind Strike with clenched jaw, a slow superficial pulse means life, and a tight, replete, large, and rapid pulse means death.

To shed light on Qí Zhòngfǔ's answer above and the quotation from the unidentified "classic" there, allow me to quote *Sùwèn* Chapter Forty-Eight:

肝脈鶩暴，有所驚駭，脈不至若喑，不治，自已。

When the liver pulse is galloping fulminantly, the patient has been [exposed to] fright and panic. When the pulse fails to arrive, if the patient is mute, [this condition] will end on its own without treatment.

According to Zhāng Jièbīn, fright or panic cause a fulminantly galloping pulse, which is associated with the liver. In severe cases, this condition may lead to the pulse failing to arrive and to muteness. This sudden counter-current movement of Qì is temporary, however, and should not be treated medically since the patient will recover as soon as the flow of Qì returns to its proper direction. The muteness is due to the fact that the liver channel runs through the throat.

The main message to take away from this answer is that it is essential for the skilled physician to not treat all cases of sudden loss of consciousness or apparent death (manifesting in an absence of movement in the vessels) aggressively as wind strike but to carefully consider the possibility of Qì strike, which needs to be treated differently and with great caution. This is due to the severity of the underlying vacuity of Qì and blood, which makes any erroneous aggressive treatment aimed at eliminating the wind through drastic purgation far too risky and potentially fatal. The reason for finding this discussion here in a textbook on gynecology is presumably that women are seen by Sòng dynasty medical authors as having a propensity to panic (see Question Fifteen) and to suffering from Qì disorders related to emotional upheavals (Question Twenty) but are also likely to be treated for wind strike, especially in the extremely dangerous state of postpartum recovery when they are exhausted and open and therefore highly susceptible to wind invasion.

蘇合香丸

療傳屍骨蒸，肺痿疰忤，鬼猝心痛，霍亂吐利時氣，鬼魅瘴瘧，赤白暴利，瘀血月閉。痃癖下腫，驚癇鬼忤中人。小兒吐利乳，大人狐狸等病。

蘇合香油(入安息香膏內)	
薰陸香(另研)	一兩
龍腦(研)	
白朮	
丁香	
朱砂(水飛研)	
安息香(另為末，用無灰好酒一升熬膏)	
木香	
白檀香	
沉香	二兩
烏犀屑	
蓽茇	
香附子(炒)	
訶梨勒(煨，去核，取皮)	
麝香(另研)	

上為細末研藥和，用安息膏並煉白蜜和劑，每服旋丸如梧桐子大，早朝取井華水，溫冷任意，化服四丸。

Sūhéxiāng Wán
(Storax Pill)

A cure for Corpse Transmission and Bone Steaming, Lung Wilting and Infixation Upset, demonic abrupt heart pain, Sudden Turmoil with vomiting and diarrhea and seasonal Qì, Miasmic Malaria from demons and goblins, red and white fulminant diarrhea, static blood and blocked menses, Strings and Aggregations with swelling in the lower body, panic seizures and demonic upset striking the person, vomiting and diarrhea of breastmilk in small children, and Fox and similar diseases in adults.

sūhéxiāngyóu (add to the ānxīxiāng paste)	
xūnlùxiāng (grind separately)	1 *liǎng*
lóngnǎo (grind)	
báizhú	
dīngxiāng	
zhūshā (water grind)	
ānxīxiāng (process separately into a powder and boil with high-quality lime-free rice wine into a paste)	
mùxiāng	
báitánxiāng	2 *liǎng*
chénxiāng	
wūxīxiè	
bìbá	
xiāngfùzǐ (stir-fry)	
hēlílè (roast over embers, remove the stone and skin)	
shèxiāng (grind separately)	

Process the above into a fine powder and grind the medicinals until well-mixed. Use the Ānxīxiāng paste and refined honey to compound the preparation. For each dose, roll pills about the size of *wútóng* seeds and take 4 pills with wellflower water freshly drawn in the early morning, warm or cool as you wish.

FORMULA NOTE

The conditions of Corpse Transmission, Bone Steaming, Lung Wilting, and Infixation Upset are all related to and often subsumed under what is now usually called 癆瘵 *láozhài* in more contemporary literature and usually translated as "consumption" in English. As we can see from the name, each term emphasizes a different aspect of "consumption" in accordance with the definition from the *Merriam-Webster Online Dictionary* as "a progressive wasting away of the body especially from pulmonary tuberculosis."[1] To begin with, Corpse Transmission is clearly a dreadful disease of a highly contagious nature. In the *Wàitái mìyào* 《外台秘要》 (Essential Secrets from the Outer Terrace/Palace Library, completed by Wáng Tāo 王燾 in 752), it is described as a debilitating condition that affects men and women, old and young equally and is marked by fullness and oppression in the heart and chest, pain in the back and shoulders, lack of strength especially in the lower extremities, tension in the spine, pain in the knees, wanting to sleep but being unable to fall asleep, progressive exhaustion from morning until night, night sweats, dreams of intercourse with ghosts, intermittent coughing, etc.

The same text explains that Bone Steaming is a condition where the marrow in the bones is struck by heat. The *Zhūbìng yuánhòu lùn* states:

夫蒸病有五：一曰骨蒸，其根在腎。旦起體涼，日晚即熱，煩躁，寢不能安，食無味，小便赤黃，忽忽煩亂，細喘無力，腰疼，兩足逆冷，手心常熱，蒸盛過，傷內則變為疳，食人五臟。

---

1 Merriam-Webster.com, 2019, https://www.merriam-webster.com.

There are five types of Steaming disease. The first is called Bone Steaming, and its roots are in the kidney. It is marked by a cool body upon rising in the morning but heat in the evening, with vexation and agitation, inability to sleep quietly, lack of appetite, reddish yellow urine, sudden vexing confusion, faint forceless panting, lumbar pain, counter-current cold in the feet, constant heat in the palms of the hands, and eventual internal damage when the steaming becomes intense, transforming into *gān* malnutrition and consuming the person's five *zàng* organs.

According to the *Zhōngyī dàcídiǎn*, Bone Steaming is caused by Yīn vacuity and internal heat and should be treated by nurturing Yīn and clearing heat with formulas like Qínjiāo Biējiǎ Sǎn (Large Gentian and Turtle Shell Powder). This modern reference also states that it is identical to 癆瘵 *láozhài* "consumption."

Lung Wilting is first mentioned in the *Jīnguì yàolüè* chapter on the "Pulses, Patterns, and Treatments of Lung Wilting, Lung Welling-Abscess, and Coughing with Ascent of Qì":

問曰：熱在上焦者，因咳為肺痿。肺痿之病，從何得之？

師曰：或從汗出，或從嘔吐，或從消渴，小便利數，或從便難，又被快藥下利，重亡津液，故得之。

曰：寸口脈數，其人咳，口中反有濁唾涎沫者何？

師曰：為肺痿之病。 若口中辟辟燥，咳即胸中隱隱痛，脈反滑數，此為肺癰，咳唾膿血。 脈數虛者為肺痿，數實者為肺癰。

Question: "Heat in the Upper Jiāo leads to coughing and constitutes Lung Wilting. Where is this disease of Lung Wilting contracted from?"

The teacher's answer: "It is contracted from sweating, or from retching and vomiting, or from dispersion thirst with frequent disinhibited urination, or from severe loss of fluids due to [inappropriate] treatment of constipation by purgation with quick medicinals."

[Question:] "What [does it mean when you find] a rapid *cùnkǒu* pulse in a patient who, when coughing, has turbid spittle and foamy drool in the mouth?"

The teacher's answer: "This is the disease of Lung Wilting. If the mouth is sapless and dry and the coughing causes dull pain in the chest, but the pulse is slippery and rapid, this means Lung Welling-Abscess, which manifests with coughing and spitting of pus and blood. A pulse that is rapid and vacuous means Lung Wilting. A pulse that is rapid and replete means Lung Welling-Abscess.

Infixation is another dreaded condition that is aptly described by its name. The first character 疰 zhù consists of the disease radical with the character 主 underneath, which, in the sense that is most commonly written as 住, indicates the dreaded abiding, persisting character of this condition. I therefore translate this character in the medical context as "Infixation Disease." The alternate version of this character that is also used to refer to the disease, 注, means "to pour" or "to stream," thus emphasizing the contagious nature of the condition, characterized by the sudden invasion of some evil Qì that upsets (the meaning of 忤 wǔ) the normal and proper physiology of the body. In other words, the compound 疰忤 denotes a situation of upset, of the normal order being turned upside down as the result of an influx of evil Qì that stubbornly takes up residence in the body. The Qīng Dynasty text *Jīnguì yì* 《金匱翼》 (Appendix to the *Jīnguì*), published in 1768 by Yóu Yí 尤怡, defines it in this way:

疰者，住也，邪氣停住而為病也。皆因精氣不足，邪氣乘之，伏於筋脈，流傳臟腑，深入骨髓，經久不已，時發時止，令心昏悶，無不痛處。

其因風邪所觸者，則為風疰。臨喪哭泣，死氣所感者，則為屍疰。鬼邪所擊者為鬼疰。其風疰之去來擊痛，游走無常者，又謂之走疰。其他又有氣血溫涼勞泄等疰之名，病各不同，其為停住不去則一也。

"Infixation" means to lodge and refers to evil Qì lodging and causing this disease. It is always due to an insufficiency of Essence Qì, allowing evil Qì to exploit it, hiding in the sinews and vessels, streaming into the *zàngfǔ* organs, and deeply entering into the bones and marrow. This situation persists for a long time without stopping, sometimes erupting and then stopping, causing clouding oppression in the heart and nowhere in the body to escape the pain.

If it was caused by an assault by wind evil, it is Wind Infixation. If contracted through the Qì of death from vicinity to a funeral and crying and weeping, it is Corpse Infixation. If it is the result of an attack by demonic evil, it is Demonic Infixation. Because of the coming and going nature of Wind Infixation and its violent pain that roams all over without a constant location, this [variety of Infixation] is also called Roaming Infixation. In addition, there are also [varieties of Infixation] named after Blood, Qì, Warm, Cool, Taxation, Draining, etc. While they differ by name, they are all identical in the persistent, chronic nature of the condition.

After a host of other conditions, many with connotations of an intrusion of demonic Qì, the last indication for the present formula is literally translated, "fox and other diseases in adults." Unfortunately, the author fails to explain what specifically he means by this mentioning of Fox Disease. Other historical sources that list this formula merely repeat the same expression. Given the demonic nature of most of the other indications for the formula, "fox disease" is likely to be literally a reference to possession or affliction by a fox spirit. This would then mean that the treatment is indicated as an exorcistic formula to expel this presence of malign Qì. Any reader familiar with popular Chinese culture should know that fox spirits, as presented in late imperial and contemporary ghost stories, movies, and other popular sources, are associated with erotic temptation and tend to transform themselves into beautiful maidens who bewitch and ensnare unsuspecting young men. Nevertheless, historical sources suggest that this identification of fox spirits with beguiling feminine beauty may be a later development and was originally not gender-specific. Thus we find the following citation of the now lost *Xuánzhōng jì* 《玄中記》 (Records from Amidst the Obscure), purportedly authored by Guō Pú 郭璞 in the Jìn dynasty (265-420 CE), in the *Tàipíng guāngjì* 《太平廣記》 (Comprehensive Records from the Tàipíng Era), which was completed in 978 under the direction of Lǐ Fǎng 李昉:

狐五十歲，能變代為婦人。百歲為美女，為神巫，或為丈夫與女人交接。能知千里外事，善蠱惑，使人迷惑失智。千歲則與天通，為天狐。

When foxes are fifty years old, they are able to transform themselves into women. At a hundred years of age, they can become beautiful women or divine spirit-mediums and sometimes have sexual intercourse with either men or women. They are able to know of things happening more than a thousand miles away, they excel at deception by *gǔ* toxin, and they can cause humans to become confused and lose their wits. At a thousand years of age, they communicate with heaven and become heavenly foxes.

Dreams of intercourse with ghosts (see Question Forty-Seven below) was an established gynecological condition already in early medieval China, as evidenced by the entry in the *Zhūbìng yuánhòu lùn*.

It is, however, also possible that Fox Disease is here used in a more technical medical sense to refer to what is usually called 狐疝 *húshàn* ("Fox Mounding"), a particular variety of Mounding. Already mentioned in the *Jīnguì yàolüè* as "Yīn Fox Mounding Qì" (陰狐疝氣), this condition is described eloquently in the *Rúmén shìqīn* 《儒門事親》 (Confucians Serving Their Parents) from 1228:

狐疝，其狀如瓦，臥則入小腹，行立則出小腹入囊中。狐則晝出穴而溺，夜則入穴而不溺。此疝出入，上下往來，正與狐相類也。

Fox Mounding has an appearance like a roof tile. When lying down it enters the smaller abdomen and when standing or walking it exits the smaller abdomen and enters the scrotum. The fox leaves its den during the day to urinate and enters its den at night and does not urinate. The behavior of this form of Mounding, alternatingly exiting and entering and moving up and down, is just like that of the fox.

Lastly, a brief note is necessary on the term "well-flower water" for readers unfamiliar with early Chinese medical or religious literature. This expression refers to the first water drawn from a well in the morning, which the *Běncǎo gāngmù* 《本草綱目》 (Classified Materia Medica, published in 1596) classifies as "sweet, balanced, and non-toxic" and recommends for the following conditions:

主治酒後熱痢，洗目中膚翳，治人大驚九竅四肢指歧皆出血，以水喫面。和朱砂服，令人好顏色，鎮心安神。治口臭，堪煉諸藥石。投酒醋，令不腐（《嘉》）。宜煎補陰之藥（虞摶）。宜煎一切痰火氣血藥。

It is indicated for heat dysentery after alcohol, for washing the skin screens in eyes, for treating a person bleeding after great panic from all the nine orifices, four limbs, digits and other divergences, by squirting water into the face. Take it together with cinnabar for a beautiful facial complexion, and for settling the heart and putting the Shén at ease. It treats bad breath and makes alchemical preparations of all the various medicinal stones tolerable. Added to liquor or vinegar, it prevents it from going bad. It is suitable for brewing Yīn-supplementing medicinals and for all phlegm and fire Qì and blood medicinals.

As the following explanation in this text details, freshly drawn well water is purer and more potent than regular water, because it contains the genuine heavenly Qì that floats on the surface, similar to snow melt. In addition, wells and springs are the channels of the earth, and the water from these sources thus resonates with the blood in the channels of the human body and therefore has special potency. For all these reasons, it is often specified for alchemical preparations and for Yīn-supplementing medicines.

第二十二問

病非瘧之邪，四時多病寒熱者，何也？

答曰：風者，陽之氣也。寒者，陰之邪也。陰氣上升入陽中則發寒。陽氣下陷入陰中則發熱。陰陽偏勝，寒熱互作。經曰：「夏傷於暑，秋必病瘧者，是也。」

婦人之病，證見寒熱邪非暑氣者，皆由營衛之兆作也。且衛者氣也，氣為陽，陽微則惡寒。營者血也，血為陰，陰弱則發熱。故婦人寒熱，多因氣血之所使也。或勞傷而體弱，或經閉而寒熱，若此之類，久而不已，則成虛損之疾也。

QUESTION TWENTY-TWO

What is the Reason for the Propensity to Fall Ill with [Alternating Aversion to] Cold and Heat [Effusion] in the Four Seasons When the Disease is not Malaria Evil?

ANSWER: Wind is a Yáng Qì, and cold is a Yīn evil. When Yīn Qì rises to enter into Yáng, [aversion to] cold erupts. When Yáng Qì descends to sink into Yīn, heat [effusion] erupts. As Yīn or Yáng prevail unilaterally, alternating cold and heat arise. This is what is meant by the quotation from the Classic that "Damage from summer-heat in summer inevitably leads to malaria disease in the fall."

In women's disease, when you see the sign of [alternating] cold and heat but the evil is not summer-heat Qì, it is always due to the portentous activity of *yíng* Provisioning and *wèi* Defense. In addition, *wèi* Defense is Qì, and since Qì is Yáng, a faintness of Yáng results in aversion to cold. *Yíng* Provisioning is blood, and since blood is Yīn, a weakness of Yīn results in heat effusion. For this reason, alternating cold and heat in women is in most cases a condition caused by Qì and blood. Whether it is a case of general weakness from taxation damage or of blocked menstruation resulting in [alternating] heat and cold, if it is of this type and persists for a long time without stopping, it will form the critical condition of vacuity detriment.

Discussion

The present question concerns the symptom of alternating aversion to cold and heat effusion in cases that are not related to malaria. Given its inclusion in the present book on gynecology, Sòng dynasty medical authors must have thus considered this symptom to have a gendered component. Perhaps surprisingly given that the question in the title specifically asks for an explanation in cases that are not related to malaria, the first phrase about wind being Yáng and cold being Yīn is an almost literal quotation from Sùwèn Chapter Thirty-Five, the "Discourse on Malaria." Similarly, the quotation from the classic at the end of the first paragraph refers loosely to the explanation in the same chapter, that malaria in the fall can be caused by severe heat damage in the summer causing great sweating and open interstices, which allow wind, the main pathogenic factor in malaria, to enter in the following season.

When the text discusses Yīn ascending into Yáng, and Yáng descending into Yīn, this could refer to a vertical movement of the pathogen, with the evil rising into the upper and sinking into the lower part of the body, respectively, since above is associated with Yáng and below with Yīn. Alternatively, it could refer to an inward-outward movement, since Yáng is associated with the more exterior parts of the body and Yīn with the interior. At first sight, the choice of directional terms suggests that we are looking at a standing body and that "above" and "below" do refer to the upper and lower parts thereof, respectively, as is often the case in medical literature. After reading the second half of Qí Zhòngfǔ's answer, however, we may want to rethink our reading of this first sentence. It is interesting that the first half of the answer does not contain any direct reference to women's physiology or pathology but instead appears to repeat well-known general ideas about the etiology and manifestations of malaria. This being said, Sòng dynasty readers would have most likely shared the common sentiment that women are particularly susceptible to invasions of wind and cold.

One brief side-note concerns the character 發 fā, which I translate, depending on context, as "erupt" or "effuse." In a medical context, it most commonly refers to the upward and outward movement of a pathological factor, as exemplified by the compound 發熱 *fārè*, "heat effusion." As such, it should not automatically be considered a negative term, like the English word "fever," which this compound is often rendered as in modern translations, since the Chinese term implies an ultimately positive development in a condition when the pathogenic factor of heat leaves the body through the surface. The character 發 *fā* is also often used to describe a treatment goal, namely to cause internal pathogens to be released through the surface to the outside and, conversely, denotes a serious pathology in its negated version as 不發 *bù fā* ("fails to effuse"), when a pathogenic factor fails to be discharged in this way. The relevancy for the present question is that the manifestation of alternating cold and heat at the surface of the body should be to be understood not as indicating the presence of cold and heat as pathological factors in the body but in a neutral sense as an indication of an underlying imbalance of Yīn and Yáng, *yíng* Provisioning and *wèi* Defense, and blood and Qì. The ramifications of this insight for treatment should be obvious.

必應散

治久寒熱，如瘧狀。

熟地	
檳榔	
陳皮	
草果(去皮)	以上各等分
當歸	
砂仁	
甘草(炙)	
柴胡	

上為粗末，每服三錢。水二盞，薑五片，煎八分，去滓，無時溫服。

合藥時，忌雞犬婦人見。

Bì Yīng Sǎn
(Inevitable Response Powder)

A treatment for long-term [alternating] heat and cold that appears like malaria.

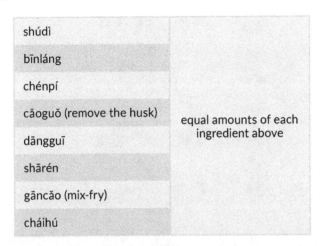

shúdì	
bīnláng	
chénpí	
cǎoguǒ (remove the husk)	equal amounts of each ingredient above
dāngguī	
shārén	
gāncǎo (mix-fry)	
cháihú	

Process the ingredients above into a coarse powder and take 3 *qián* per dose. Simmer in 2 cups of water with 5 slices of ginger until reduced to 80 percent, and remove the dregs. Ingest warm and do not restrict the timing.

When compounding the medicine, beware of letting chickens, dogs, and women see [it].

神健飲子

治婦人寒熱。

赤芍		柴胡	
白术	各二兩	黃芪	
赤茯		秦艽	
當歸		桔梗	
肉桂		橘紅	
鱉甲		甘草	各一兩
川芎		木香	
枳殼			

上為㕮咀，每服三錢。水二盞，薑五片，棗一枚，煎至八分，去滓溫服。不拘時。

Shén Jiàn Yǐnzi
(Divine Health Drink)

A treatment for [alternating] cold and heat in women.

chìsháo		cháihú	
báizhú	2 *liǎng* each	huángqí	
chìfú		qínjiāo	
dānguī		jiégěng	
ròuguì		júhóng	
biējiǎ		gāncǎo	1 *liǎng* each
chuānxiōng		mùxiāng	
zhǐké			

Pound the ingredients above and take 3 *qián* per dose. Simmer in 2 cups of water with 5 slices of ginger and 1 jujube until reduced to 80 percent. Remove the dregs and ingest warm. Do not restrict the timing.

FORMULA NOTE

All the editions of the *Hundred Questions* that are available to me replicate what must be a typographical error in the list of ingredients. Mùxiāng is missing information on the required amount for this formula, which could mean two things: It could be placed below gāncǎo because its dosage differs from 1 *liǎng* indicated for the preceding ingredients, or the phrase "1 *liǎng* each" is placed incorrectly and should also include mùxiāng.

第二十三問

因咳嗽，經候不行者，何也？

答曰：咳嗽之說，古書有咳而無嗽，後人兼言之。大抵皆從肺出。其聲響亮，不因痰涎而發者，謂之咳，言其聲音聞於人。痰涎上下隨聲而發者，謂之嗽，如水之嗽蕩，能蕩其真氣也。況肺主乎氣？

經云：「營氣之行，常與衛氣相隨。」久嗽損氣，則血亦不足，遂致經閉不行，時發寒熱。久久成勞者，氣血俱損之故也。

QUESTION TWENTY-THREE

What is the Reason for Stopped Menstrual Flow Because of Coughing?

ANSWER: Regarding the term *késòu* ("productive cough"), the ancient texts only speak of *ké* ("dry cough") but not of *sòu* ("gurgling"). People have subsequently started talking about these two concepts together. In general, [this condition] always comes out of the lung. When its sound is clear and bright and its emission is not due to phlegm, it is referred to as "dry cough," which speaks to the fact that its sound is heard by others. When it erupts as phlegm-rheum rising and falling along with the sound, it is referred to as "gurgling," like the gurgling sweeping of water. This refers to its ability to sweep away the person's genuine Qì! How much more so since the lung is in charge of the Qì!

The Classic states: "The movement of *yíng* Provisioning Qì consistently follows along with the *wèi* Defense Qì." When long-term gurgling injures the Qì, the blood also become insufficient. This in turn causes blocked menstruation and lack of flow, with intermittently erupting cold and heat. The reason why it turns into taxation when occurring over a very long period of time is that both Qì and blood are injured.

DISCUSSION

Apparently there was already broad agreement in the Sòng dynasty that the early medical texts tended to not differentiate between the two characters 咳 *ké* and 嗽 *sòu*, which to this day are used in combination to mean "cough." Chapter Twenty-One on Cough in the *Sùwèn bìngjī qìyí bǎomìng jí* 素問病機氣宜保命集 ("Collected [Comments on] Pathomechanisms, Appropriateness of Qì, and Safeguarding Life from the *Sùwèn*," completed in 1186) by Liú Wánsù 劉完素 explains the difference between the two terms:

> 咳謂無痰而有聲，肺氣傷而不清也。嗽是無聲而有痰，脾濕動而為痰也。咳嗽謂有痰而有聲，蓋因傷於肺氣，動於脾濕，咳而為嗽也。脾濕者，秋傷於濕，積於脾也。故內經曰：「秋傷於濕，冬必咳嗽。」

> *Ké* refers to sound with no phlegm, which indicates the lung Qì is damaged and not clear. *Sòu* means the presence of phlegm with no sound, which indicates that spleen dampness is stirred, producing phlegm. *Késòu* refers to the presence of phlegm together with sound, which presumably means that *ké* then forms *sòu* because of damage to lung Qì and stirring of phlegm dampness. Spleen dampness means damage from dampness in the autumn that has gathered in the spleen. For this reason, the *Nèijīng* says that "damage by dampness in the autumn must result in cough in the winter."

How does this information on cough address the issue about which Qí Zhòngfǔ is asking, namely the reason for the connection between cough and stopped menstrual flow and therefore for a woman-specific approach to the treatment of cough? To make sense of the second paragraph, we must remember that this question follows up on the previous one that discussed the identification of *yíng* Provisioning with blood, and of *wèi* Defense with Qì, in the context of alternating cold and heat. The first paragraph explains cough as an indication of lung Qì being damaged, complicated by the presence of phlegm due to spleen dampness perhaps, but most importantly as a sign of the state of Qì in general since the lung rules the Qì. Over time, this damage to Qì affects the blood, and thereby the menstrual cycle in women, because of the direct linkage between *yíng* Provisioning and *wèi* Defense, and between blood and Qì.

In addition, the gendered component of coughing and its linkage to menstruation may be influenced by women's tendency towards dampness, or rather "moistness," as a constitutional factor. This association is stated by Qí Zhòngfǔ in his answer to Question Three on the reasons why "women contract illness at double the rate of men":

夫婦人者，眾陰之所集，常與濕居。

Women are the site of multitudes of Yīn accumulating, and they are constantly inhabited by moistness.

As I explain in that discussion,[2] this statement, which is an almost literal quotation from Sūn Sīmiǎo's introductory essay to his gynecological writings, is quite likely to be of foreign origin and have been imported in the early medieval period into Chinese medical theory from early Indian or Greek notions. Given the association of both women and moistness with Yīn though, it does make sense also from a classical Chinese perspective and had most likely become an integrated part of the way in which gynecologists in the Sòng period viewed the female body.

The so-called statement from the Classic quoted in the answer above about the relationship between *yíng* Provisioning and *wèi* Defense is once again unfortunately not a literal statement that can be traced to a passage from the *Huángdì nèijīng*. In this case, the closest precursor I have found is the title of Question Thirty in the *Nànjīng* 《難經》 (Classic of Difficulties), which simply asks whether the movement of *yíng* Provisioning Qì consistently follows after that of *wèi* Defense Qì or not and then proceeds to explain why and how it does:

---

2 *Channeling the Moon, Part One*, pp. 90-99

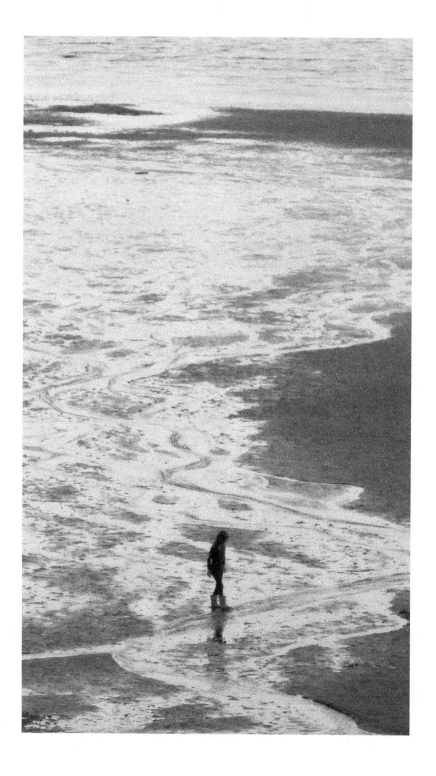

三十難曰：榮氣之行，常與衛氣相隨不？

然。經言：人受氣於穀。穀入於胃，乃傳與五臟六腑，五臟六腑皆受於氣。其清者為榮，濁者為衛。榮行脈中，衛行脈外。榮周不息，五十而復大會，陰陽相貫，如環之無端，故知榮衛相隨也。

Thirtieth Difficulty: Does the movement of *yíng* Provisioning Qì consistently follow along after the *wèi* Defense Qì or not?

Answer: According to the Classic, humans receive Qì from grain. Grain enters the stomach and is then transmitted to the five *zàng* and six *fǔ* organs, so all of them receive Qì. Its clear [aspect] constitutes *yíng* Provisioning, and the turbid constitutes *wèi* Defense. *Yíng* Provisioning moves inside the vessels and *wèi* Defense moves outside the vessels. *Yíng* Provisioning circulates without stopping, fifty times before it returns for a great meeting. Yīn and Yáng are linked together, like a ring that has no end. Thus we know that *yíng* Provisioning and *wèi* Defense follow each other.

By the Sòng dynasty, this relationship between *yíng* Provisioning and *wèi* Defense was no longer a question since the *Nànjīng* had presented the affirmative answer with sufficient clarity. And because cough rattles the genuine Qì, it eventually is bound to affect the state of blood as well.

六神散

治婦人熱勞咳嗽，月水不通。

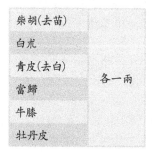

柴胡(去苗)	
白朮	
青皮(去白)	各一兩
當歸	
牛膝	
牡丹皮	

上為粗末，每用六兩，入蜜四兩，炒令焦。入酒並童便各一碗，煎八九沸，去滓。分作六服，空心食前。

Liù Shén Wán
(Six Spirits Powder)

A treatment for women's heat taxation, productive cough, and a failure of the menstrual fluids to flow through.

cháihú (remove sprouts)	
báizhú	
qīngpí (remove any white parts)	1 *liǎng* each
dāngguī	
niúxī	
mǔdānpí	

Process the ingredients above into a coarse powder. For each use, prepare six *liǎng*, add 4 *liǎng* of honey and stir-fry until it is dry. Add 1 bowl each of rice wine and boys' urine, and simmer, bringing it to a boil 8 or 9 times. Remove the dregs. Divide it to make six doses and take before meals on an empty stomach.

Formula Note

The *Shèngjì zǒnglù* 聖濟總錄 ("Encyclopedia of Sagely Benefaction," compiled under the direction of Sòng emperor Huīzōng 徽宗 in 1117) describes the condition of heat taxation in this way:

> 熱勞之證，心神煩躁，面赤頭疼，眼澀唇焦，身體壯熱，煩渴不止，
> 口舌生瘡，食飲無味，肢節酸疼，多臥少起，或時盜汗，日漸羸瘦者
> 是也。

The pattern of heat taxation is this: vexation and agitation of the heart Shén, red face, headache, dry eyes, scorched lips, severe heat all over the body, vexing thirst that will not stop, sores forming in the mouth and on the tongue, lack of appetite for food and drink, soreness in the limbs and joints, sleeping more and being less active, occasional night sweats, and gradually progressing emaciation.

It is interesting that the first formula presented here prominently features heat in the term "heat taxation," when Qí Zhòngfǔ's answer above merely mentions alternating heat and cold as an eventual side-symptom of a basic condition of Qì injury leading to an insufficiency of blood. In addition, both women's general physiology and the symptoms of coughing and stopped menstrual flow are normally associated with cold pathologies rather than with conditions due to heat. The constellation of ingredients in this formula, with the exception of mǔdānpí, which clears heat, also makes it clear that we are not dealing with a condition of internal heat causing taxation but with a condition where vacuity taxation (a common condition in gynecological writings) has caused heat effusion as an external symptom.

紫菀丸

治肺氣咳嗽。

紫菀	
防風	
桑白皮(炙)	
木香	
貝母	
人參	各一兩
款冬花	
葶藶(隔紙炒)	
檳榔	
杏仁(炒)	
天門冬(去心)	
甘草	

上為細末，蜜丸桐子大，每服三十九。清米飲送
下，食後服。

Zǐwǎn Wán
(Aster Pill)

A treatment for lung Qì cough.

zǐwǎn	
fángfēng	
sāngbáipí (mix-fry)	
mùxiāng	
bèimǔ	
rénshēn	1 *liǎng* each
kuǎndōnghuā	
tínglì (stir-fry on top of paper)	
bīnláng	
xìngrén (stir-fry)	
tiānméndōng (remove the core)	
gāncǎo	

Process the ingredients above into a fine powder and make honey pills the size of *wútóng* seeds. Take 30 pills per dose and ingest them after meals by chasing them down with clear thin rice gruel.

FORMULA NOTE

In the list of ingredients presented in the text, there is obviously a typographical error since the instructions on measurements do not make sense. Unfortunately, I have been unable to find another version of this exact formula and we therefore have to guess the amounts or, better yet, adjust them to each patient's particular condition at the moment.

第二十四問

咳嗽有紅痰者，何也？

答曰：經稱「五臟六腑皆令人咳」，原其至理，雖因寒邪之為患，當分內外所傷。《難經》云：「形寒飲冷則傷肺。」肺主皮毛，自皮毛而入中者，謂之形寒；胃脈絡肺，食寒而為嗽者，謂之飲冷。水飲停積於胸膈，所以為痰。

痰中有血者，乃心肺之相剋也。肺屬金而主氣，心屬火而行血。以五臟而言之，心肺皆居膈上；以五行論之，金火應乎相制。故痰中有血者，此火克乎金，心勝乎肺。久而不已，亦變成勞。《難經》所謂「七傳者死」，亦此之類也。

《褚氏遺書》云：「喉有竅，則咳血殺人。腸有竅，則便血羸人。便血猶可止，咳血不易醫。」所以咳嗽有紅痰者，多成虛勞之疾也。

Question Twenty-Four

What is the Reason for the Presence of Red Phlegm in the Cough?

Answer: The Classic states that the five *zàng* and six *fǔ* organs can all cause a person to suffer from cough. The original principle behind this statement is that even though it is cold evil that causes this trouble, we must differentiate between internal damage and external damage. As the *Nànjīng* states, "A cold body and cool drinks damage the lung." Since the lung is in charge of the skin and body hair, [the process of cold] entering the center of the body through the skin and body hair is here referred to as "a cold body." Since the stomach vessel connects to the lung, [the process of] a productive cough resulting from eating something cold is here referred to as "cool drinks." Phlegm is formed because pathological fluids collect in the chest and diaphragm.

When there is blood in the phlegm, this means that the heart and lung are restraining each other. The lung belongs to Metal and is in charge of Qì. The heart belongs to Fire and moves the blood. Speaking about this situation in terms of the five *zàng* organs, the heart and lung both reside above the diaphragm. Discussing this in terms of the five Dynamic Agents, Metal and Fire should restrain each other. As such, when there is blood in the phlegm, this means that Fire is restraining Metal and that the heart is prevailing over the lung. If this situation persists for a long period of time without stopping, this will transform into taxation. The *Nànjīng* discussion on "the seven transmissions that mean death" also falls into this category.

The *Chǔ shì yíshū* states: "A hole in the throat results in coughing with blood, which kills the person. A hole in the intestines results in blood in the urine, which emaciates the person. Blood in the urine is something that can still be stopped, but coughing with blood is not easy to cure." For this reason, the presence of red phlegm when coughing is a sign that in most cases turns into the critical condition of vacuity taxation.

This Question includes a number of quotations from the Hàn dynasty classics that all need to be unpacked here so that we can understand them in their original context. The first mention of the classic refers to the well-known "Treatise on Cough," which is *Sùwèn* Chapter Thirty-Eight. The introductory paragraph is worth citing in full:

黃帝問曰：肺之令人咳何也？ 岐伯對曰：五臟六腑皆令人咳，非獨肺也。帝曰：願聞其狀。

岐伯曰：皮毛者肺之合也，皮毛先受邪氣，邪氣以從其合也。其寒飲食入胃，從肺脈上至於肺則肺寒，肺寒則外內合邪因而客之，則為肺咳。五臟各以其時受病，非其時各傳以與之。

The Yellow Emperor asked: "How is it that the lung causes people to cough?" Qí Bó answered: "The five *zàng* and six *fǔ* organs all cause people to cough. It is not only the lung that does so." The Emperor said: "I would like to hear what this looks like."

Qí Bó said: "The skin and body hairs are the match of the lung. The skin and body hair first receive the evil Qì, and the evil Qì thereby follows its match. Cold drinks and foods [consumed by] the patient enter the stomach and follow the lung vessels up until they reach the lung, making the lung cold. Coldness of the lung then results in a situation where evil causes from the outside and the inside match up and take up residence there. Hence, they cause lung cough. The five *zàng* organs each receive illness during their associated season. When it is not the season associated with the lung, any [of the other *zàng* organs] transmit it and thereby give it to the lung.

In other words, while coughing is generally associated with cold as the external pathogenic factor, another dimension needs to be taken into account in diagnosis and treatment, namely the association of coughing with one or more of the *zàng* and *fǔ* organs as an internal cause of the condition.

The second quotation, identified as coming from the *Nànjīng*, is found in Chapter Forty-Nine of that text. This Difficulty discusses how to differentiate between direct illness in the channels themselves and damage from the "five evils," which are in the text defined as wind, summer-heat, winter-cold, dampness, and diet and exhaustion. A cold body and cool drinks damaging the lung is the second example in the text of a pathogen directly damaging a channel.

The third reference to a classic, namely to the *Nànjīng* discussion of death from the seven transmissions, directs us to Difficulty Fifty-Three of this classic. This chapter explains the difference between disease transmission along the cycle of conquest or "restraint" (剋 *kè*), which results in death, and disease transmission along the cycle of creation (生 *shēng*), which results in survival. Heart disease that is being transmitted to the lung is the first example in that text of the seven transmissions that result in death. Thus this quotation here serves to emphasize the critical nature of this condition, alerting the careful reader to the fact that finding blood in a female patient's coughed up sputum is a sign of impending death.

Lastly, the answer to this question cites a passage from the *Chǔ shì yíshū* 褚氏遺書 (Posthumous Writings of Master Chǔ), a now lost text from the Southern Qí dynasty (479-502 CE). Based on the context of the cited passage in that text, I have decided to translate the term 便 *biàn*, which can refer to either defecation (大便 *dàbiàn*) or urination (小便 *xiǎobiàn*) in medical literature but is usually translated as "blood in the feces" in the compound 便血 *biànxuè*, here as "urination." It is found in the middle of a paragraph on "moistening" and is worth citing in full, so that you, dear reader, can make up your own mind on whether the term here refers only to urine or to both urine and stool. Valid arguments can be made for both answers, but the presence of the character 溺 *niào* ("urine") in the following sentence strongly suggests a focus on urination. Ultimately, this distinction is not essential for our topic here, namely for understanding Qí Zhòngfǔ's answer to the question of the meaning of blood in the sputum.

天地定位，而水位乎中，天地通氣，而水氣蒸達。土潤膏滋，雲興雨降，而百物生化。人肖天地，亦有水焉，在上為痰，伏皮為血，在下為精。從毛竅出為汗，從腹腸出為瀉，從瘡口出為水。痰盡死，精竟死，汗枯死，瀉極死，水從瘡口出不止，干即死。

至于血，充目則見明，充耳則聽聰，充四肢則舉動強，充肌膚則身色白，漬則黑，去則黃。外熱則赤，內熱則上蒸喉，或下蒸大腸，為小竅。喉有竅，則咳血，殺人；腸有竅則便血，殺人。便血猶可止，咳血不易醫。

喉不停物，毫髮必咳，血滲入喉，愈滲愈咳，愈咳愈滲。飲溲溺則百不一死，服寒涼則百不一生。血雖陰類，運之者，其和陽乎。

Heaven and earth are fixed in their position, and water is positioned in the middle. Heaven and earth are connected through Qì, and water Qì reaches its destination by steaming. When the soil is moist, rich, and fertile, and clouds and rain descend, the hundred things are born through transformation. We humans resemble heaven and earth and also have water within us. Above, it is phlegm; lying hidden in the skin, it is blood; and located below, it is Essence. Leaving from orifices in the body hair, it is sweat; leaving from the abdomen and intestines, it is diarrhea; and leaving from open wounds, it is water. Phlegm being exhausted means death; Essence being finished means death; sweat drying up means death; diarrhea reaching its extreme means death; water leaving from open wounds without stopping means death when it dries out.

As for blood, when it fills the eyes, the vision is bright; when it fills the ears, the hearing is acute; when it fills the four limbs, lifting and actions are strong; when it fills the skin, the complexion on the body is white. Soaked, it becomes black, and when gone it becomes yellow. External heat results in redness, internal heat in steaming upward into the throat or downward into the large intestine and the formation of small holes. Holes in the throat result in coughing up blood, which kills the person; holes in the intestine results in blood in the urine/feces, which kills the person. Blood in the urine/feces is something that can still be stopped, but coughing with blood is not easily cured.

The throat does not have anything retained in it and even a tiny hair must cause cough. When blood seeps into the throat, the more it seeps in, the more the person coughs, and the more the person coughs, the more seeping occurs. When fluids are excreted through the urine, of a hundred patients, not a single one dies, but when you give cold and cooling [medicinals in this condition], of a hundred patients, not a single one lives. Even though blood belongs to the category of Yīn, for its movement, it must harmonize with Yáng.

The crux of Qí Zhòngfǔ's answer here, and the reason for the inclusion of this question on the presence of red phlegm when coughing, is that bloody sputum is an extremely serious and important diagnostic sign. On the one hand, it indicates the involvement of the heart, as the organ of Fire, which is prevailing over lung Metal. On the other, it is a key sign that the condition has evolved into one of a life-threatening state of vacuity that will be difficult, if not impossible, to treat, which is vitally important information for the physician treating such a patient. A third dimension that Qí Zhòngfǔ does not mention explicitly but presumably just expects all of his readers to know and that we must remember is the color associations of white with cold and red with heat. In other words, cough is generally a sign of a cold pathology and therefore manifests with white sputum (or with yellow, which also may indicate the involvement of the spleen and stomach), but if it manifests with redness, this can indicate the presence of pathogenic heat, which must be addressed in treatment. The following formulas point to such a problematic as well.

平肺湯

定喘治嗽。

五味子	杏仁(泡去皮尖)
紫菀(洗去土)	半夏(湯浸七次)
陳皮(去白)	紫蘇子
甘草(炙)	桑白皮

上為末，每服二錢，水一盞薑四片，煎至七分。去
滓，溫服食後。

Píng Fèi Tāng
(Calming-the-Lung Decoction)

To settle panting and treat cough.

wǔwèizǐ	xìngrén (steep and remove skin and tips)
zǐwǎn (rinse and remove dirt)	bànxià (steep in hot water seven times)
chénpí (remove white parts)	zǐsūzǐ
gāncǎo (mix-fry)	sāngbáipí

Process the ingredients above into a powder and take 2 *qián* per dose. Simmer in 1 cup of water with 4 slices of ginger until reduced to 70 percent. Remove the dregs and ingest warm after meals.

立驗丸

治肺熱而咳，上氣喘急，不得坐臥，身面浮腫，不下飲食，消腫下氣，止嗽。

葶藶(研，炒，為末)	十分
貝母	三分
杏仁(炒，去皮尖)	一兩半
赤茯苓	
紫菀	各三分
五味子	
人參	一兩
桑白皮(炙)	一兩

上為細末，蜜丸梧桐子大。每服十丸，日二服。甚者夜一服，加至三十丸，棗湯下。腫盛者食後服。

Lì Yàn Wán
(Instant Efficacy Pill)

A treatment for lung heat and cough with Qì ascent and urgent panting, inability to sit or lie down, puffy swelling of the body and face, and inability to get down food and drink, by dissolving swelling and moving down Qì, and stopping productive coughing.

tínglì (grind, stir-fry, and pulverize)	10 *fēn*
bèimǔ	3 *fēn*
xìngrén (stir-fry and remove the skin and tips)	1.5 *liǎng*
chìfúlíng	
zǐwǎn	3 *fēn* each
wǔwèizǐ	
rénshēn	1 *liǎng*
sāngbáipí	1 *liǎng*

Process the ingredients above into a fine powder and turn into the honey pills the size of *wútóng* seeds. Take 10 pills per dose, 2 doses per day. In severe cases, take an[other] dose at night, and increase the dosage [as needed] to up to 30 pills. Down them in jujube decoction. In cases with exuberant swelling, take them after meals.

止紅散

治心肺客熱，咳嗽吐血。

柴胡(去苗)	一兩
胡黃連	各半兩
宣連	

上為末，入朱砂少許，研和。每服二錢，水一盞，
煎半盞，通口服。

Zhǐ Hóng Sǎn
(Stopping-the-Red Powder)

A treatment for intrusive heat in the heart and lung, [causing] cough with expectoration of blood.

cháihú (remove sprouts)	1 *liǎng*
húhuánglián	
xuānlián	0.5 *liǎng* each

Process the ingredients above into a powder. Add a small amount of zhūshā and grind it together until well mixed. Take 2 *qián* per dose and simmer in 1 cup of water until reduced to 0.5 cup. Ingest orally.

第二十五問

吐血，衄血，齒衄，舌上出血，汗血者，何也？

答曰：氣屬乎陽，血屬乎陰，陰盛則陽虧，陽盛則
陰虧。經所謂「陽勝則陰病，陰勝則陽病。」

諸吐血衄血，由陽氣勝，陰之氣被傷，血失常道，
或從口出，或從鼻出，皆謂之妄行。其脈洪數者
逆，微細者順。

陽明之經，行絡於頤頷，陽明受邪，熱血從齒出
也。脾氣通於口，心氣通於舌，心脾二經被傷，血
故從舌出也。營血內通於臟腑，外縈於經絡，藏則
舍於肝經，行則出於心臟，又心之液為汗，令肝心
二臟俱虛，血隨汗液出也。

QUESTION TWENTY-FIVE

What is the Reason for Expectorating Blood, Nosebleed, Bleeding Gums, Bleeding from the Top of the Tongue, and Sweating Blood?

ANSWER: Qì belongs to Yáng; blood belongs to Yīn. When Yīn exuberates, Yáng wanes; and when Yáng exuberates, Yīn wanes. This is what the Classic refers to as "Yáng prevailing results in Yīn falling ill; Yīn prevailing results in Yáng falling ill."

The various forms of expectorating blood and nosebleeds are caused by Yáng Qì prevailing, so that Yīn Qì sustains damage and blood loses its normal pathways, exiting either through the mouth or through the nose. Both of these situations are referred to as frenetic movement. When the patient's pulse is surging and rapid, it means counter-current movement; when it is faint and fine, it means movement in the direction of the current.

A branch of the Yángmíng channel connects to the jaw. Thus, when Yángmíng contracts an evil, hot blood exits from the gums. Spleen Qì connects to the mouth, and heart Qì connects to the tongue. Thus, when the two channels of the heart and spleen sustain damage, the blood consequently exits from the tongue. *Yíng* Provisioning blood connects internally to the *zàng* and *fǔ* organs and externally is encompassed by the channels and network vessels. When stored, it resides in the liver channel; when moving, it exits from the heart *zàng* organ. Moreover, the fluid of the heart is the sweat. This causes blood to exit along with sweat when both the liver and heart *zàng* organs are vacuous.

DISCUSSION

This line once again reminds us that all of Chinese medicine can ultimately be reduced to the simple guideline of restoring the equilibrium of Yīn and Yáng, here expressed in terms of the dynamic between blood and Qì. This interaction between Yīn and Yáng at the foundation of all change in the universe is the topic of one of the most important classical texts: the "Great Treatise on the Resonant Manifestations of Yīn and Yáng" (*Yīnyáng yìngxiàng dàlùn* 《陰陽應象大論》), *Sùwèn* Chapter Five.[3] Thus, it is no coincidence that Qí Zhòngfǔ cites this treatise. Here is the original line, following a discussion of Qì and flavor:

氣味，辛甘發散為陽，酸苦湧泄為陰。

陰勝則陽病，陽勝則陰病。陽勝則熱，陰勝則寒。重寒則熱，重熱則寒。

In terms of Qì and Flavor, acridity and sweetness effuse and scatter, and are Yáng; sourness and bitterness gush up and drain down, and are Yīn.

When Yīn prevails, Yáng falls ill; when Yáng prevails, Yīn falls ill. When Yáng prevails, Heat results; when Yīn prevails, Cold results. Extreme/double Cold results in Heat; extreme/double Heat results in Cold.

In the context of women's bodies, which are associated with Yīn and "ruled by blood," as we are reminded of again and again throughout this text, it makes perfect sense that we see a tendency to disorders of the blood. The association of the female body with Yīn in Chinese medicine theory is expressed in such notions as Sūn Sīmiǎo's statement that "women are constantly inhabited by moistness" or their susceptibility to Yīn conditions like demonic possession and cold. What is important to note in the present question is the fact that this physiological predominance of Yīn in women's bodies does not lead to a tendency to pathologies of Yīn prevalence and

---

3 Translated by Sabine Wilms and published by Happy Goat Productions as *Humming with Elephants* in 2018.

thus damage to the Yáng aspect here, as one would expect on the basis of Chinese medicine theory, but rather to its opposite, namely damage to Yīn Qì with the result that "blood loses its normal pathways," as the result of Yáng prevailing over Yīn.

The most likely explanation for this conundrum, from my perspective, is that the present question is concerned specifically with pathologies of bleeding, or in other words with abnormal manifestations of excessive blood flow, which is only one kind of blood-related disorder. Nevertheless, more commonly seen in clinic than the disordered blood flow discussed here are disorders associated with a lack of healthy flow, or in other words with the absence or inhibition of physiological bleeding, most notably in the form of menstrual pathologies, even if only subtly expressed as slight premenstrual discomfort or delayed timing. Unfortunately for women's health, such conditions do not greatly concern biomedical doctors or popular culture in the West, unless and until the woman desires to become pregnant and finds herself unable to do so. As Chinese medicine practitioners, it is our responsibility to raise awareness around this issue of women's bleeding, both in physiological and pathological terms, in excess and in deficiency, as the result of either Yáng exuberance or, more commonly, Yīn exuberance, on the basis of our understanding of Chinese medicine theory in terms of the dynamic equilibrium of Yīn and Yáng.

Differentiating further between specific manifestations of abnormal bleeding, Qí Zhòngfǔ notes that bleeding can result from a flow that is either in the direction of the current or moving counter-current, which can be diagnosed by means of the pulse. In addition, the location of the bleeding indicates which aspects of the body are damaged: The Yángmíng channel in the case of bleeding from the jaw, the spleen and heart in the case of bleeding from the mouth and tongue. Lastly, bleeding through the sweat indicates that the liver is affected, due to its impaired function of storing the blood, as well as the heart because "sweat is the fluid of the heart" and because the heart is in charge of the movement in the vessels.

內補芎歸湯

治婦人血氣羸弱，或崩傷過多，少氣傷絕，腹中拘急，四肢煩熱，面目無色，及唾血吐血。

芎藭	各四兩
熟地	
白芍	五兩
桂心	二兩
甘草	各三兩
乾薑	
大棗	四十枚
當歸	二兩

上為粗末，每服五錢，水一盞半，煎至八分。去滓，溫服，不拘時。

Nèi Bǔ Xiōng Guī Tāng
(Internally-Supplementing Chuānxiōng and Chinese Angelica Decoction)

A treatment for women who suffer from marked weakness of blood and Qì, possibly due to excessive damage from Landslide Collapse, scanty breath with Reversal damage, gripping tension in the abdomen, vexing heat in the four limbs, lack of color in the face and eyes, as well as blood in the spittle and expectoration of blood.

xiōngqióng	4 *liǎng* each
shúdì	
báisháo	5 *liǎng*
guìxīn	2 *liǎng*
gāncǎo	3 *liǎng* each
gānjiāng	
dàzǎo	40 pieces
dāngguī	2 *liǎng*

Process the ingredients above into a coarse powder. Take 5 *qián* per dose and simmer it in 1.5 cups of water until reduced to 80 percent. Remove the dregs and ingest warm, with no restrictions on timing.

FORMULA NOTE

For a thorough discussion on the serious condition of Landslide Collapse (崩 *bēng*), see p. 132 in *Channeling the Moon: A Translation and Discussion of Qí Zhòngfǔ's Hundred Questions on Gynecology, Part One.*

柔脾湯

治吐血下血衄血。

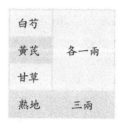

白芍	
黃芪	各一兩
甘草	
熟地	三兩

上為㕮咀，每服三錢。水酒各一盞，煎八分，去
滓，通口服。不拘時。

Róu Pí Tāng
(Spleen-Softening Decoction)

A treatment for expectorating blood, bleeding from the lower
orifices, and nosebleed.

báisháo	
huángqí	1 *liǎng* each
gāncǎo	
shúdì	3 *liǎng*

Pound the ingredients above and take 3 *qián* per dose.
Simmer with 1 cup each of water and rice wine until reduced
to 80 percent, remove the dregs, and ingest it orally. Do not
restrict the timing.

FORMULA NOTE

It is interesting that the formula here is intended to "soften the spleen," to treat not just the condition addressed in the present question but also the symptom of bleeding from the orifices of the lower body, which we would ordinarily think of as quite a different condition. Literally translated, the Chinese expression (下血 xiàxuè) means "descent of blood" in the sense of downward movement. The term can also mean "to cause the blood to descend" in different contexts, such as in the formula name Xià Yū Xuè Tāng 下瘀血湯 (Blood-Stasis-Precipitating Decoction) from the *Jīnguì yàolüè*. The downward movement of blood is generally seen as a sign of health and of balanced Qì and blood in women in the form of a regular abundant menstrual flow, with the key problem, especially in the context of fertility, being its retention.

In the present case, though, the discharge of blood from the openings in the lower body (another way of translating the expression 下血) indicates a pathology that is explained in the first part of this question as Yáng Qì prevailing over Yīn Qì and thereby causing the blood to move frenetically. For this presentation, the association with the spleen in the present formula makes sense when we recall that "the spleen stores *yíng* Provisioning" (*Língshū* 《靈樞》, Chapter Eight) and that *yíng* is associated with Yīn blood. The term "soften" (柔 *róu*) strikes me as a little unusual since it is usually associated with the liver rather than the spleen. The spleen is not an organ that tends to be in need of softening, of being mollified and made pliable. My best guess is that the character 柔, in its function as a verb, carries the implication of moistening and irrigating, like what you do to make a tender bean sprout thrive.

The condition of bleeding below is already discussed in the *Zhūbìng yuánhòu lùn* under the heading "The Symptom of Red Discharge Below the Belt" (帶下赤候 *dàixià chì hòu*):

> 勞傷血氣，損動衝脈、任脈。衝任之脈，皆起受於胞內，為經脈之海；手太陽小腸之經也，手少陰心之經也，此二經主下為月水。若經脈傷損，衝任氣虛，不能約製經血，則與穢液相兼而成帶下。然

五臟皆稟血氣，其色則隨臟不同。心臟之色赤，帶下赤者，是心臟虛損，故帶下而挾赤色。

Taxation damage to the blood and Qì injures and stirs the Chōngmài and Rènmài. Both of these vessels start inside the womb and constitute the sea of the channels. The Hand Tàiyáng Small Intestine Channel and the Hand Shàoyīn Heart Channel are in charge of the descent of the menstrual fluids. If these channels and vessels are injured and the Qì in the Chōng and Rèn is vacuous and unable to restrain the blood in the channels, it combines with filthy fluids and forms discharge below the belt. This being so, the five *zàng* organs all contribute Qì and blood, and its color differs depending on the *zàng* organ involved. The color of the heart is red, and when the discharge below the belt is red, this means vacuity injury in the heart. This is the reason why the discharge harbors the color red.

The standard translation for the term 帶下 *dàixià* is "vaginal discharge," which is also a translation I choose in certain passages where this narrower meaning is clear. Whether Cháo Yuánfāng and his contemporaries were sophisticated enough in their understanding of the medical body to differentiate between vaginal bleeding and bleeding from the urethra and anus or to differentiate between red vaginal discharge as part of the menstrual cycle and as blood being mixed into vaginal discharge for other reasons is not clear. As such, I prefer to err on the side of caution and make sure that I do not read more specificity into the term than was intended by the authors of our sources and thereby inadvertently narrow the focus of the text too much. In our mind, there may be a great difference between blood in the urine and feces and blood that exits from the vagina. Given that an unequivocal expression exists in classical Chinese that Qí Zhòngfǔ could have used to refer specifically to blood in the urine and feces (便血 *biànxuè*), I have chosen to retain the ambiguity of the original Chinese and translated the symptom literally as "bleeding from the lower orifices."

琥珀散

治小便出血。

琥珀	
豬苓（去皮）	
茯苓	各一兩
澤瀉	
滑石	
阿膠（炒）	三兩
車前子	一兩

上為粗末，每服五錢，水二盞，煎一盞。去渣，溫
服。

Hǔpò Sǎn
(Amber Powder)

A treatment for blood in the urine.

hǔpò	
zhūlíng (remove the skin)	
fúlíng	1 *liǎng* each
zéxiè	
huáshí	
ējiāo	3 *liǎng*
chēqiánzǐ	1 *liǎng*

Process the ingredients above into a coarse powder and take
5 *qián* per dose. Simmer in 2 cups of water until reduced to
1 cup. Discard the dregs and ingest warm.

第二十六問

婦人偏喜酸物，或嗜冷者，何也？

答曰：天食人以五氣，地食人以五味者，酸苦甘辛鹹是也。五味各有所入，酸入肝、辛入肺、苦入心、甘入脾、鹹入腎，是謂五入也。

肝藏血，婦人以血為主。所以偏喜酸物食者，酸入肝而養血，血得其酸物，所以含藏也。

血虛多熱，邪熱蓄於上焦，煩躁內生，婦人虛煩，往往多嗜冷物也。

QUESTION TWENTY-SIX

What is the Reason for Women Having a Particular Fondness for Sour Substances and Sometimes Craving Cold?

ANSWER: Heaven feeds humanity with the Five Qì, and earth feeds humanity with the Five Flavors. These are sour, bitter, sweet, acrid, and salty. The Five Flavors each have an organ that they enter: Sour enters the liver, acrid enters the lung, bitter enters the heart, sweet enters the spleen, and salty enters the kidney. This is what we call the Five Entries.

The liver stores the blood, and women are ruled by blood. This is the reason why they have a particular fondness for eating sour substances. Sour enters the liver and nourishes the blood. Because the blood obtains these sour substances, it remains in storage there.

Blood vacuity means increased heat. This evil heat amasses in the Upper Jiāo, and vexation and agitation form internally. When women suffer from vacuity vexation, they commonly have an increased craving for cold substances.

DISCUSSION

Continuing the theme from the previous question, we have a simi-lar correlation between specific *zàng* organs and resonating signs and symptoms that can provide guidance in treatment. Question Twenty-Five discusses pathological bleeding in such forms as from the mouth and tongue as indicators of pathology in the spleen and heart, or in the sweat as a weakness of the heart (which rules the movement of blood and is associated with sweat) and of the liver (in charge of blood storage). The present question again emphasizes the special role that the liver plays in women due to its function of storing blood.

Because "women are ruled by blood," women have a craving for sour substances, which "nourish the blood" and allow it to "remain in storage" in the liver.

Not directly related to this resonance between women, the liver, blood storage, and a liking of sour foods, Qí Zhòngfǔ next explains why women have a craving for cool substances, presumably referring to food and drink. The connection between these two pathologies must be that both condi-tions are ultimately rooted in a vacuity of blood, which can express with either or both of these symptoms and can be addressed, like the majority of gendered conditions, by supplementing the blood as the foundation of their health.

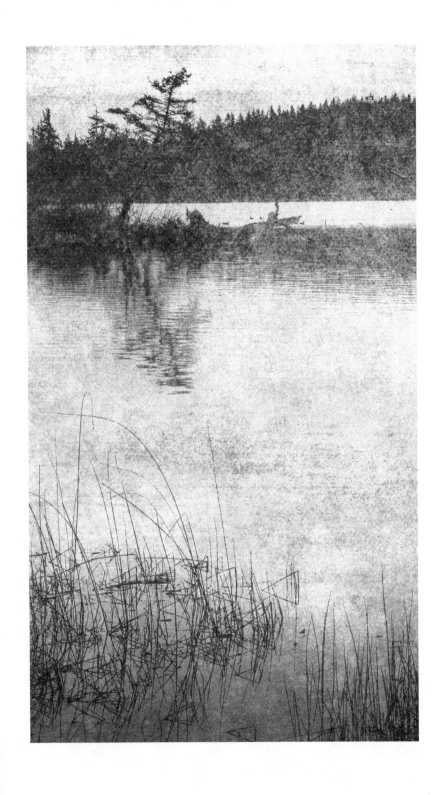

茯苓半夏湯

治妊娠惡阻，心中憒悶，嘔吐惡心，好啖鹹酸物。

旋復花	
陳皮	
桔梗	
白芍	各半兩
人參	
甘草(炙)	
芎藭	
赤茯苓	三分
干熟地	一兩一分
半夏(湯洗十遍)	

上為粗末，每服二錢，水盞半，薑四片，煎八分，去滓，食前稍熱服。

Fúlíng Bànxià Tāng
(Poria and Pinellia Decoction)

A treatment for nausea in pregnancy; irritation and oppression in the heart; retching, vomiting, and nausea; and a taste for salty and sour substances.

xuánfùhuā	
chénpí	
jiégěng	
báisháo	0.5 *liǎng* each
rénshēn	
gāncǎo (mix-fry)	
xiōngqióng	
chìfúlíng	3 *fēn*
shúdìhuáng (dry)	1 *liǎng* 1 *fēn*
bànxià (rinse ten times in hot water)	

Process the ingredients above into a coarse powder and take 2 *qián* per dose. Simmer it in 0.5 cup of water with 4 slices of ginger until reduced to 80 percent, remove the dregs, and take before meals, slightly heated.

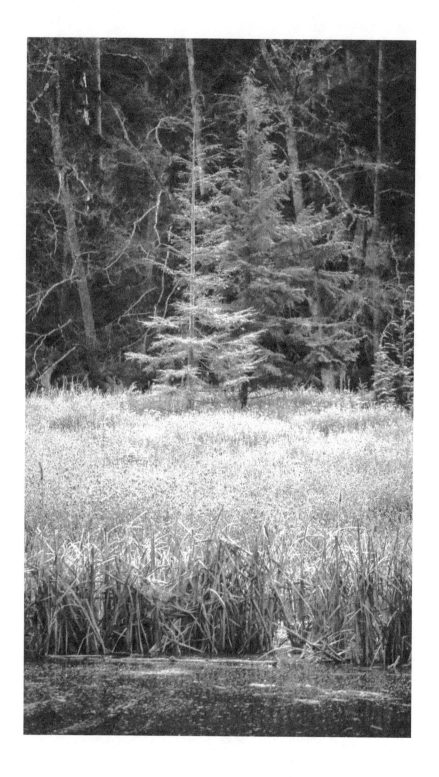

Formula Note

The measurements in the formula above are clearly in need of correction or clarification. There are many other versions of Fúlíng Bànxià Tāng that are somewhat related but not identical with the one above and therefore not helpful here. In the interest of historical accuracy, I have translated the text literally and not introduced changes. Nevertheless and fortunately for us, the same formula, complete with almost literally identical indications and instructions for preparation and the exact same ingredients, listed in the same order, is found in Volume Nine (on gynecology) of the *Tàipíng Huìmín Héjìjú fāng* from 1078, one of Qí Zhòngfǔ's treasured sources. That text instructs us to use 0.5 *liǎng* each of the first seven ingredients, as in the formula above, and then 3 *fēn* each of the fúlíng and dìhuáng, and 1 *liǎng* and 2 *fēn* of bànxià.

In a final note to the formula instructions of interest to readers, that text adds the advice to follow up with Fúlíng Wán 茯苓丸 (Poria Pill), which will result in the dispersal and elimination of phlegm and water enabling the patient to eat again. That formula consists of 2 *liǎng* each of gégēn, zhǐshí, báizhú, gāncǎo, and 1 *liǎng* each of chìfúlíng, rénshēn, gānjiāng, ròuguì, chénpí, and bànxià. These ingredients are processed into a fine powder, mixed with honey to form pills the size of *wútóng* seeds, and ingested by drinking down 30 pills per dose in warm rice gruel on an empty stomach.

As a side note, it is interesting that Qí Zhòngfǔ chose to place this formula in the section for miscellaneous gynecological conditions in his text, rather than in the section on pregnancy as the first indication of this formula (nausea in pregnancy) and also the indications for Fúlíng Wán in the *Tàipíng Huìmín Héjìjú fāng* would suggest. The lack of punctuation in classical Chinese formulas often makes it quite difficult to decide how formula indications in a list relate to each other. In the present case, I have resisted the temptation to add explanatory English language in my translation to give my readers the space to make up their own minds, but suggest that we should interpret the list of indications as "treatment for nausea in pregnancy WITH irritation and oppression in the heart, retching, vomiting, and nausea, and a taste for salty and sour substances."

清平湯

治血虛口燥，咽乾，喜飲。

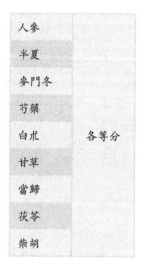

人參	
半夏	
麥門冬	
芍藥	
白朮	各等分
甘草	
當歸	
茯苓	
柴胡	

上咬咀，每服二錢。水盞半，燒生薑一塊切破，薄荷少許，同煎七分，去滓，熱服。不拘時。

Qīng Píng Tāng
(Peace and Balance Decoction)

A treatment for blood vacuity with dry mouth, dry throat, and a fondness for drinking fluids.

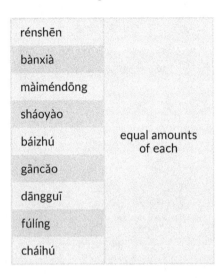

rénshēn	
bànxià	
màiméndōng	
sháoyào	
báizhú	equal amounts of each
gāncǎo	
dāngguī	
fúlíng	
cháihú	

Pound the ingredients above and take 2 *qián* per dose. Simmer in 0.5 cup of water with one piece of roasted fresh ginger, sliced and broken up, and a small amount of bòhé until reduced to 70 percent. Remove the dregs and take hot, with no restricton on the timing.

第二十七問

婦人喜少怒多，悲泣不止者，何也？

答曰：婦人無故悲泣不止，象如神靈或以祟，祈禱終不應，《金匱》謂之燥臟是也。

為所欲不稱其意，大棗湯主之。

QUESTION TWENTY-SEVEN

What is the Reason for Women Experiencing Less Joy and More Anger, and Weeping Incessantly?

ANSWER: When women weep incessantly for no reason and appear as if [possessed by] spirits or suffering from an evil spell for which no prayer ever brings any response, this is precisely what the *Jīnguì yàolüè* calls "visceral agitation."

Failing to weigh their intentions because of their desires, Dàzǎo Tāng rules this condition.

DISCUSSION

As suggested by the named quotation from the *Jīnguì yàolüè*, the answer here refers directly to the well-known passage in Volume Twenty-Two of that text:

婦人臟躁，喜悲傷欲哭，象如神靈所作，數欠伸，甘麥大棗湯主之。

Women's visceral agitation [manifests in] a tendency to sorrow and desire to weep, as if possessed by spirits, and frequent yawning and stretching. Gān Mài Dàzǎo Tāng (Licorice, Wheat, and Jujube Decoction) rules this condition.

With some hesitation, I have chosen to identify the compound 燥臟 *zàozàng* as an alternate version of the technical term 臟躁 *zàngzào*, and have translated it, following Wiseman's terminology, as "visceral agitation" because this wording elegantly and accurately reflects the intended clinical as well as literal meaning of the characters. It is my hope that well-educated readers will immediately recognize the close parallels between the two passages. It should be noted that in this answer Qí Zhòngfǔ reverses the order of the characters and uses a different but closely related character with the same pronunciation of *zào*: The original passage contains the character 躁, which means "rashness" or "restlessness," or in Wiseman's rendition "agitation," and is marked by the radical 足 meaning "foot." By contrast, Qí Zhòngfǔ uses the character 燥, pronounced identically but with the literal meaning of dryness. As such, a literal translation of 燥臟 would be "parched *zàng* organ." My choice is due to the clear textual parallel and reference to Zhāng Zhòngjǐng's text, and hence to the clinical meaning of the term, which is associated with symptoms of irritability and agitation, but is also ultimately associated with dryness, as Genevieve LeGoff's commentary shows. Both versions of the character, 燥 and 躁, were used interchangeably in early medical literature to refer to this condition, so it is not the case that Qí Zhòngfǔ intentionally and consciously changed a character to express a different shade of meaning. It is interesting that the following formula repeats the compound with the characters placed in the more common order as 臟燥 *zàngzào*.

Lastly, I find the final sentence of Qí Zhòngfǔ's statement, that this condition is related to "failing to weigh their intentions because of their desires," a fascinating addition to Zhāng Zhòngjǐng's explanation. It does contrast Zhāng Zhòngjǐng's description of weeping "for no reason" and makes me wonder about the social dimension of this disease. Pushed by popular historical accounts and even many feminist and Women's Studies publications, most modern readers in the West are all too familiar with China's supposed misogynistic history and the oppression and powerlessness that women in China are said to have suffered throughout its long (and varied) history. From that perspective, it makes immediate sense that this disease would be viewed and treated as gendered by the dominant male medical practitioners and authors. In that context, the phrase "for no reason" can be interpreted as a man's perspective on women's unhappiness to the point of exhibiting serious physical symptoms.

Two questions remain in my mind: First, is that all there is to the story? And second, how are we to translate this diagnosis and subsequent treatment into contemporary clinical practice? Regarding the first question, I would like to remind the reader once again of Sūn Sīmiǎo's famous statement, from his introduction to his writings on women's formulas (see *Channeling the Moon, Part One*, Question Three):

然而女人嗜欲多於丈夫，感病倍於男子，加以慈戀，愛憎，嫉妒，憂恚，染著堅牢，情不自抑，所以為病根深，療之難瘥。

Women's predilections and desires exceed those of men, and they contract illness at double the rate of men. In addition, when they are affected by compassion and attachment, love and hatred, envy and jealousy, and worry and rancor, these anchor themselves firmly. Since they are unable to control their emotions by themselves, the roots of their diseases are deep, and it is difficult to obtain a cure in their treatment.

As Sūn Sīmiǎo points out here, women's diseases are "ten times more difficult to treat" than men's because of their emotionality, which is broken down into three factors: because they have greater "predilections and desires" than men, because their emotions are "firmly anchored," and because they are "unable to control their emotions by themselves."

How are we to read this statement, and where did it come from? Is it an expression of a common attitude in early Táng China, akin to women's association with cold and wind? Or is it rooted in Master Sūn's personal experience and was perhaps influenced by his deep immersion in Buddhism? This non-indigenous religion had arrived from India several centuries earlier and had by Sūn's times exerted so much influence on Chinese culture that it is difficult, if not impossible, to tease out indigenous from Indo-European concepts from medieval times on. In addition to religious teachings and practices, the vibrant trade along the Silk Road had also brought in medical theories and treatments, along with philosophy, cosmology, food, music, medicinal and dietary substances, and many other aspects of Indo-European culture. Buddhism viewed women's bodies as more "material" than mens', related to their reproductive functions and the agonies of childbirth and pollution of female bleeding, and therefore an impediment to the pursuit of the spiritual path and eventual enlightenment. At this point, it is most likely impossible to reconstruct at this point to what extent Sūn Sīmiǎo's famous statement, and the frequent repetition of this attitude by subsequent medical authors, was rooted in Indo-European views of the female body, in traditional Chinese views, or even in Sūn's personal experience.

It is probably equally impossible to state conclusively whether his statement should be read as a patronizing, condescending, and ultimately misogynistic attitude by a man towards women as emotionally unstable, and therefore indirectly as a medical justification for the patriarchal structures that grew more and more restrictive throughout Chinese history. To remind Western readers of our own history, women were kept from voting because of their "hysterical" (derived from the Greek word for "uterus") nature, explained by the medical "fact" that they possessed a uterus that was in need of being kept occupied through pregnancies to prevent it from wreaking havoc with their bodies and minds. Is it fair and accurate to accuse Sūn Sīmiǎo and his later colleagues of a similar attitude? Or is there another way to read his statement, related perhaps to his previous statement, which Qí Zhòngfǔ also cited in his response to Question Three:

十四以上，陰氣浮溢，百想經心，內傷腑臟，外損姿容。月水去留，前來交互，瘀血停凝，中道絕斷，其中傷墮，不可具論。冷熱臟腑，虛實交錯，惡血內滿，氣脈耗竭。

From their fourteenth year on, Yīn Qì floats up and spills over, and a hundred thoughts pass through their hearts. Internally, this damages their *fǔ* and *zàng* organs; externally it injures their outward appearance. The menstrual fluids are now discharged and now retained, their arrival all mixed up; static blood collects and congeals; and the central pathways are cut off. The damage and destruction in all these areas is impossible to discuss in their entirety. Cold and heat and vacuity and repletion in the *zàng* and *fǔ* organs alternate with each other, malign blood fills the inside, and the Qì flow in the vessels is exhausted.

In other words, is there another way to look at statements about women's emotionality by Chinese medical authors, one that is related not to a supposedly misogynistic social environment but to male medical authors' sensitivity to women's reproductive processes, especially in regard to menstruation? Given how much the status and lives of women varied from one dynasty to the next, we should always be very careful about passing judgment on statements from such a different time and place. Here, it is also important to recall the continuity and equal weight placed by Chinese medicine on material and immaterial processes, on signs of the body and the heart and the Shén, and on Qì as a factor that expresses itself in a range of symptoms from tangible masses to emotional outbursts or hot flashes.

In this context, the monthly process of bleeding, which causes Yīn Qì to "float up and spill over," is a complicating factor to be taken into account in the diagnosis and treatment of women's illness, making them "ten times more difficult to treat" and therefore justifying the development of a professional specialization with separate institutionalized training, separate textbooks, and separate professors and practitioners. From this perspective, women's propensity toward greater emotionality and the resulting illnesses can just be seen, and treated, as the logical result of physiological processes that affect women in a way that men do not experience. Not better or worse, but different. And therefore in potential need of special treatment. I am quite certain that countless teenage girls in contemporary Western society who are suffering from menstrual conditions and emotional outbreaks would benefit from a doctor's compassionate care on the basis of this perspective.

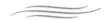

CLINICAL COMMENTARY BY GENEVIEVE LEGOFF

I interpret Zhāng Zhòngjǐng's comment about crying "without a reason" as a clinical clue. There may very well be societal reasons, but I think he is trying to nail down that the crying is disproportionate to the circumstances. Of course no one can really judge anyone's circumstances, but as a doctor one has to judge situations and make decisions based on that judgment all the time. When I see a Gān Mài Dàzǎo Tāng patient, there is definitely an element of excessive weepiness or easy crying, --in other words, a very thin skin.

To a certain extent, the circumstances don't matter to me for writing the prescription — what matters is that certain stimuli are having an effect because there is organ dryness. By moistening the organs, I cannot change the stimuli, but I can help the person withstand them better.

Of course, in my opinion, being a good doctor involves more than prescribing formulas with precision, and I would also try to understand any societal aspects and offer guidance if I can. Not to say that Zhāng Zhòngjǐng did not do that in his practice, which we will never know. I think his text is worded this way because the *Shānghán zábìng lùn* is a practical and succinct handbook and he simply wants to convey the key symptom.

大棗湯

治婦人臟燥。

甘草	一兩
小麥	三合

上㕮咀，每服三錢，水盞半，棗五枚，煎八分，去
渣，溫服。

Dàzǎo Tāng
(Jujube Decoction)

A treatment for women's visceral agitation.

gāncǎo	1 *liǎng*
xiǎomài	3 *gě*

Pound the ingredients above and take 3 *qián* per dose. Simmer in 0.5 cup of water with 5 jujubes until reduced to 80 percent, remove the dregs, and ingest warm.

Formula Note

The gentle, soothing quality of this formula with its mild sweet ingredients and absence of harsh medicinals can tell us a lot about the way in which this condition was interpreted.

第二十八問

咽中狀如梅核，或如炙肉者，何也？

答曰：有喉嚨，有咽門，二者各有所司。

喉嚨者，空虛也，肺之系，氣之道路也。肺應天，故屬天氣所生，有九節以通九竅之氣。

咽者，咽也。言可咽物，為胃之系。胃屬土，地氣所生，謂之嗌也。

或陰陽之氣痞結，咽膈噎塞，狀若梅核，妨礙飲食。久而不愈，即成翻胃。或胸膈痰結，與氣相搏上逆，咽喉之間結聚，狀如炙肉之臠也。

QUESTION TWENTY-EIGHT

What is the Reason for a Feeling as If a Plum Pit or Roasted Meat [Were Stuck] in the Throat?

ANSWER: There is the larynx, and then there is the pharynx. These two each are in charge of their own area.

The larynx is empty. It is the link to the lung and the pathway of air. The lung resonates with heaven and therefore is associated with what is generated by the Qì of heaven. It has nine joints, thereby facilitating the through-flow of the Qì of the nine orifices.

The [term for the] pharynx means "to swallow." As such it means that this is the part that is able to swallow things. It is the link to the stomach. The stomach is associated with Earth [as one of the Five Dynamic Agents] and with what is generated by the Qì of earth [in the pairing of heaven and earth]. This is referred to as the upper opening of the esophagus.

Perhaps the Qì of Yīn and Yáng has formed *pǐ* Glomus binds and caused choking and obstruction in the throat and diaphragm that [feels] like a plum pit and impedes eating and drinking. If this is left untreated for a long time, it turns into stomach reflux. Or there is phlegm binding in the chest and diaphragm that is battling the Qì, causing counter-current upward movement and binding and gathering in the space of the larynx and pharynx. This feels like bits of roasted meat.

DISCUSSION

While I am usually careful not to translate classical Chinese terms with highly specific modern Western anatomical terms, in the present context it actually works to translate the term 喉嚨 *hóulóng* not in the broader sense of "lower part of the throat," as some translators do, but specifically as "larynx." In anatomical terms, the larynx is the upper part of the trachea and, in contrast to the pharynx above it, only has air flowing through it, while food and drink pass from the pharynx into the esophagus. And this is exactly what the text above describes. We can even go so far as to identify the "nine joints" mentioned above with the nine laryngeal cartilages: the epiglottic, thyroid, and cricoid, and the paired arytenoid, corniculate, and cuneiform cartilages.

The "nine orifices" mentioned next are usually a reference to the seven Yáng orifices in the upper body (two eyes, two ears, two nostrils, and mouth) and two Yīn orifices (urethra and anus), but here are perhaps more likely to refer to the nine orifices outlined in the thirty-seventh difficult issue of the *Nànjīng*:

五臟者，當上關於九竅也。故肺氣通於鼻，鼻和則知香臭矣；肝氣通於目，目和則知黑白矣；脾氣通於口，口和則知穀味矣；心氣通於舌，舌和則知五味矣；腎氣通於耳，耳和則知五音矣。五臟不和，則九竅不通.

The five *zàng* organs are gated above by the nine orifices. Thus, the lung's Qì is connected to the nose, and when the nose is harmonious, we know good and bad smells. The liver's Qì is connected to the eyes, and when the eyes are harmonious, we know black and white. The spleen's Qì is connected to the mouth, and when the mouth is harmonious, we know the flavor of grains. The heart's Qì is connected to the tongue, and when the tongue is harmonious, we know the five flavors. The kidney's Qì is connected to the ears, and when the ears are harmonious, we know the five sounds. When the five *zàng* organs are not harmonious, the nine orifices are not passable.

In this text, the lung is connected to the nostrils, the liver to the eyes, the spleen to the mouth, the heart to the tongue, and the kidney to the ears. To make this list add up to a total of nine, commentators have had to engage in some mental gymnastics. To complicate matters further, it is obvious that the tongue is not, strictly speaking, an orifice and is usually counted as part of the mouth, but supplemented by the throat, to arrive at a total of seven orifices. We can count the mouth as two, in the sense of the upper and lower lips, which still only brings us to a total of eight, or we can interpret the phrase here as including the two hidden Yīn orifices, which is also how some commentators explain the list in the *Nànjīng* passage. Most likely, the text here is using the expression "nine orifices" to emphasize the fact that the larynx is the place where the Qì of heaven, as air, enters the body and from where it is conveyed to the internal organs. As such, it is an essential passageway that can give diagnostic clues to internal processes in the hidden *zàng* organs.

Qí Zhòngfǔ's explanation for the term that I have translated as pharynx, namely 咽門 *yànmén*, hinges on the fact that the character 咽 literally means "to swallow" and his term for pharynx therefore is literally the "swallowing entrance." He even provides an alternate term at the end of this line: 嗌 *yì*, which the *Shuōwén jiězì* dictionary simply explains as identical with 咽 and which has another meaning of "to choke" or "obstruction in the throat." In the present context, however, the two terms are simply meant as equivalent terms to refer to the part of the throat that connects the mouth to the esophagus, or in other words, the pharynx.

Please note that in the explanation of the functions of the pharynx, the Chinese text uses two distinct but etymologically related terms that unfortunately both translate into English as "earth": 地 *dì*, the earth that is the Yīn counterpart to Yáng heaven, and 土 *tǔ*, which is one of the Five Dynamic Agents (五行 *wǔxíng*) and refers to earth in the sense of soil, dirt, humus, the stuff that plants grow in and we can stick our hands in. To distinguish these two terms and to mark the Five Dynamic Agents as the important key terms they are, I capitalize Earth as a translation of the Dynamic Agent 土, associated with the center, yellow, and the spleen/stomach, while leaving the Yīn earth that is paired with Yáng heaven, expressed in Chinese as 地, in lower case.

This brings us to the last paragraph and the question of the meaning of the term "Qì of Yīn and Yáng." Contemporary explanations of "plum-pit Qì" generally equate it with the feeling of pieces of roasted meat being stuck in the throat and present these two sensations as symptoms for the same condition: a subjective sensation of something stuck in the throat that the patient is neither able to cough up nor swallow down but that does not impede the ingestion of food and drink. They also emphasize its etiology in emotional oppression or excessive stimulation that have negatively affected the Qì dynamic. The locus classicus for this condition is invariably cited as Volume Twenty-Two of the *Jīngguì yàolüè*:

婦人咽中如有炙臠，半夏厚朴湯主之。

When a woman has a [feeling] in the throat like a lump of roasted meat, Bànxià Hòupò Tāng (Pinellia and Officinal Magnolia Bark Decoction) rules this condition.

It is noteworthy that, while some modern editions of that text even include the headline "Plum-Pit Qì" for this entry, that term is nowhere to be found in the original text. As a matter of fact, modern explanations of Plum-Pit Qì invariably cite classical sources, yet those sources describe the sensation as "roasted meat." I am unaware of any sources pre-dating the Sòng period that use the term Plum-Pit Qì.

Regardless of the history of the term, the last paragraph of Qí Zhòngfǔ's answer above finally addresses the topic of this question, namely the reasons for a feeling as if a plum pit or bits of roasted meat were stuck in the throat. It is not clear in my mind whether the differentiation in the middle paragraph between the larynx, associated with channeling the Qì from heaven (i.e., air) to the lung, and the pharynx, associated with channeling the Qì from earth (i.e., food and drink) to the stomach, is relevant to a parallel differentiation between the feeling of plum-pit versus bits of roasted meat in the following section. The second half of Qí Zhòngfǔ's explanation in this last paragraph, which discusses the etiology of the sensation of roasted meat in the throat as due to phlegm binding and causing counter-current ascent into the throat, is taken almost literally from the seventh-century text *Zhūbìng yuánhòu lùn* by Cháo Yuánfāng. So what we have, then, is a classical explanation for a feeling of roasted meat in the throat that is associated with phlegm binding in the diaphragm and counter-current ascent of Qì. As the following formula suggests and contemporary descriptions of Plum-Pit Qì emphasize, the phlegm in turn is associated with the Seven Emotions, which is the likely reason for the placement of this condition in gynecological texts, even though later texts make clear that it is not limited strictly to women.

Given the other characteristic of this condition that is emphasized in later accounts, namely the fact that it does not impede the ingestion of food and drink, we should most likely associate the sensation of roasted meat with an obstruction in the larynx and the passage of the Qì of heaven in the second paragraph of Qí Zhòngfǔ's answer above.

It is possible that the root of the categorical confusion between plum pit and roasted meat lies in the fact that texts from the Sòng period and later associated the condition that had earlier been identified with the sensation of roasted meat with what had by then become the technical term Plum-Pit Qì while ignoring the difference that Qí Zhòngfǔ was trying to make here between the two sensations. The condition that he associated with plum pit is something quite different, namely a *pǐ* Glomus bind that is actually causing a physical obstruction in the throat with choking and obstructed intake of food and drink, to the point of causing the serious disease of "stomach reflux," with regurgitation and vomiting of food, which is associated not with the lung but with the stomach. In light of these insights, can we now form a better understanding of the term "Qì of Yīn and Yáng"? I have translated the expression as literally as possible to allow my readers to make up their own minds and shall leave it at that.

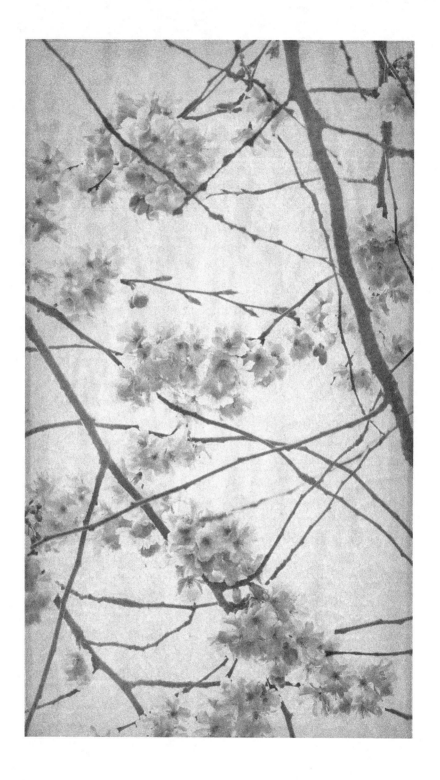

One final note is necessary on the accuracy of "plum pit" as a translation for the Chinese 梅核 *méihé*. Following Wiseman's terminology and the widely accepted habit of generations of English-speaking Chinese medicine teachers, practitioners, and students, I reluctantly translate the Chinese 梅 *méi* in the context of this famous indication as "plum," even though this most definitely does not refer to our European varieties of plum but should properly be referred to as a "sour apricot." In the context of formulas where *méi*, or more commonly, 烏梅 *wūméi* is mentioned as an ingredient, I identify it as Prunus mume and render it by its common English name as "mume plum," even though that plant is in the subgenus of "Armeniaca" or "apricot" rather than plum. Western readers who like Japanese food may actually be more familiar with this species through its use as umeboshi ("pickled plum") or umeshū ("plum wine") in Japan. I have two reasons for maintaining the potentially misleading name of "plum-pit Qì" here: First, the English word "plum" also has the more general sense of referring to the large genus Prunus, of which Prunus mume is a subspecies. In addition, for the purpose of describing this sensation, it is irrelevant whether somebody feels like they have swallowed the pit of a Greengage plum, a Mirabelle, a regular apricot, or a "mume plum." Obviously, this does not hold true when the same substance is used not to describe a sensation but as a medicinal or dietary ingredient. In that case, we must clearly identify the subspecies used, and distinguish it from the Chinese 李 *lǐ*, which refers to Prunus salicina and is in the same family as our Western varieties of plum. I am indebted to Dr. Eugene Anderson for insisting that "*méi* is a sour apricot, but early translators misidentified it as a plum, and thus it has the established translation as 'plum' in Western languages, though actual plums are *lǐ* in Chinese."

四七湯

治喜怒悲思憂恐驚之氣，結成痰涎，狀如破絮或如梅核在咽喉，咯不出，咽不下，此七氣所為。或中脘痞滿，氣不舒快；或痰涎壅盛，上氣喘急；或因痰飲節注，嘔吐惡心。

半夏	五兩
茯苓	四兩
厚朴	三兩
紫蘇葉	二兩

上為㕮咀，每服四錢，水盞半，薑七片，棗一枚，煎六分，去滓熱服。不拘時。

Sì Qī Tāng
(Four Seven Decoction)

A treatment for the Qì of elation, anger, grief, pondering, worry, fear, and panic, binding to form phlegm-drool that appears like broken silk floss or plum pit in the throat, impossible to cough out or swallow down. This is caused by the Seven Qì. Possibly [this is accompanied by] *pǐ* Glomus fullness in the middle stomach duct and constrained Qì flow; or phlegm-drool congestion with ascent of Qì and urgent panting; or a rhythmic outpouring of phlegm-rheum with retching, vomiting, and nausea.

bànxià	5 *liǎng*
fúlíng	4 *liǎng*
hòupò	3 *liǎng*
zǐsūyè	2 *liǎng*

Pound the ingredients above and take 4 *qián* per dose. Simmer in 0.5 cup of water with 7 ginger slices and 1 jujube until reduced to 60 percent. Remove the dregs and ingest hot. Do not restrict the timing.

FORMULA NOTE

This is an almost literal quotation from the imperially sponsored *Tàipíng Huìmín Héjìjú fāng*, where the formula is found under the same name at the very end of Volume Four on "Treating Phlegm-Rheum." As in the formula indications above, the feeling is described there not as roasted meat but as plum pit. As an alternate formula name, that text gives the name Dà Qī Qì Tāng 大七氣湯 (Major Seven-Qi Decoction), which suggests that we should interpret the "Seven" in the formula name above as a reference to the Seven Emotions that it addresses. We could thus translate the name above as "Four-Ingredient Decoction for the Seven Emotions."

Comparing the formula indications above with the indications listed in that text, from which many of Qí Zhòngfǔ's formulas originated, a discrepancy stands out that sheds some light on a curious phrase in our text above: The last indication listed is 因痰飲節注，嘔吐惡心, which I have translated to the best of my ability and in an effort to stay faithful to the text as "rhythmic outpouring of phlegm-rheum with retching, vomiting, and nausea." The expression 節注 *jié zhù* in particular caused me a bit of a headache, until I found the parallel passage in the *Tàipíng Huìmín Héjìjú fāng*:

因痰飲中結，嘔逆噁心。

Due to phlegm-rheum binding in the center, retching counter-current flow and nausea.

That source thus uses 中結 *zhōng jié* ("binding in the center") in the place of 節注 *jié zhù* ("rhythmic outpouring"). Based on this discrepancy between two texts that are otherwise almost literally identical, it seems most likely that the character 節 ("rhythmic," or literally "bamboo node") in Qí Zhòngfǔ's text is a typographical error and should be replaced with the character 結 ("to knot" or "bind"), which has the exact same pronunciation. It is a good reminder for later readers, editors, and translators, to always keep in mind the possibility of mistakes in classical Chinese written sources. Following this line of reasoning, you may want to read the expression above simply as "phlegm-rheum binding and pouring out" instead of as "rhythmic outpouring of phlegm-rheum."

Lastly, a brief note is in order on the various kinds of pathological fluids mentioned in this question: 痰 *tán* is familiar to most readers as the most general term for pathological fluids in the human body and is translated consistently in Western medical literature on Chinese medicine as "phlegm." In a more specific meaning, it is a thick, sticky, turbid substance that manifests visibly when expectorated from the lung. In Chinese medicine, however, it can also form and lodge elsewhere in the body. In addition to the involvement of the lung, it is most commonly caused by an impairment of the spleen, which is in charge of moving and transforming water-dampness. It tends to be associated with pathological heat that is concentrating the fluids to the point where they are no longer able to flow freely. In contrast to phlegm, "drool" (涎 *xián*) is a thin clear liquid and is associated with the spleen. *Sùwèn* Chapter Twenty-Three lists "drool" as one of the Five Humors, which are the five kinds of fluids formed from the Five Flavors and exiting the body in association with the five *zàng* organs:

五臟化液。心為汗。肺為涕。肝為淚。脾為涎。腎為唾。是謂五液。

The five *zàng* organs form the humors: The heart makes sweat, the lung snivel, the liver tears, the spleen drool, and the kidney spittle. These are what we call the Five Humors.

Additionally, the indications above also include the term 飲 *yǐn*, which I follow Wiseman in translating as "rheum." Like "drool," it is often used in opposition to or in combination with "phlegm," to connote the thin aspect of all pathological fluids in the body. Moreover, in contrast to phlegm, it tends to be associated with cold pathologies and therefore suggests the need for a warming treatment.

二氣散

治陰陽痞結，咽膈噎塞，狀若梅核，妨礙飲食。久
而不愈，即成翻胃。

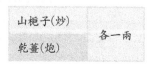

山梔子(炒)	各一兩
乾薑(炮)	

上為粗末，每服二錢，水一盞，煎五分，去滓熱服。食遠。

Èr Qì Săn
(Two Qì Powder)

A treatment for Yīn Yáng Glomus bind, with choking and
congestion in the neck and diaphragm that feels like a plum
pit and obstructs drinking and eating. Left untreated for a
long time, [this condition will] turn into stomach reflux.

shānzhīzi (stir-fry)	1 *liǎng* each
gānjiāng (blast-fry)	

Process the ingredients above into a coarse powder and take
2 *qián* per dose. Simmer in 1 cup of water until reduced
to 50 percent, remove the dregs, and ingest hot. Take it in
between meals.

Formula Note

The sixteenth-century text *Chìshuǐ xuánzhū* 《赤水玄珠》 (Dark Pearl of Red Water), although composed several centuries later, offers insight into the pathology of *pǐ* Glomus but unfortunately does not directly mention "Yīn and Yáng Glomus." It states that it is located below the heart, in the center, and is always a disease of Earth. Often caused by a physician's erroneous precipitation treatment, it can also be associated with vacuity of center Qì and failure to move and transform the Subtle Essences. Lastly, diet-related phlegm accumulation causes *pǐ* Glomus from damp heat, when Earth assails the heart. Dampness and Glomus should be treated identically, with a need to distinguish the location in both cases, so as to disperse it either above or below. The *Zhōngyī dà cídiǎn* 《中醫大辭典》 (Dictionary of Chinese Medicine) adds that we must distinguish in diagnosis and treatment between Qì and phlegm Glomus, vacuity and repletion Glomus, and upper, center, and lower Glomus.

I have been unable to find literary precedents or explanations for the expression "Yīn Yáng Glomus bind." The term can be read as "Yīn-Yáng Glomus bind," as "Yīn AND Yáng Glomus bind," or even as "Yīn OR Yáng Glomus bind," in the sense of this formula being indicated for either Yīn Glomus bind or Yáng Glomus bind. The compound Yīn-Yáng can also suggest a condition with alternating Yīn and Yáng characteristics or can have the connotation of sexual intercourse. The disease 陰陽易 *yīnyáng yì* ("Yīn-Yáng Change"), for example, can refer to a condition that is transferred or "exchanged" (a possible meaning of 易) between Yīn and Yáng in the sense of female and male partners, as in line 392 of the *Shānghánlùn*. Or it can refer to a condition where a Yáng pulse manifests in a Yīn location or a Yīn pulse in a Yáng location, as in *Sùwèn* Chapter Twenty-Two. Without additional evidence, I read "Yīn Yáng Glomus bind" here to mean that the formula is indicated as a treatment for both Yīn and Yáng conditions.

第二十九問

婦人足十指痛如油煎，覆之則熱痛，
風吹則冷痛者，何也？

答曰：孫真人云有腳氣之人，先從腳起，或先緩弱，起行忽倒，或兩脛腫滿，或膝枯細，或心中忪悸，或小腹不仁，或舉動轉筋，或見食嘔逆，惡聞食氣，或胸滿氣急，或遍體酸痛，皆腳氣候也。

黃帝所謂緩氣濕痺是也。頑弱名緩風，疼痛為濕痺，寒中三陽，所患必冷，暑中三陰，所患必熱。

婦人足十指如熱油煎者，此由營衛氣虛，濕毒之氣留滯經絡，上攻心則心痛，下攻腳則腳疼。其腳指如熱油所煎，亦氣之類。經云熱厥是也。

QUESTION TWENTY-NINE

What is the Reason for Women Suffering from Pain in the Ten Toes as If They Were Being Fried in Oil, and Experiencing Heat Pain When Covered up and Cold Pain When Exposed to Blowing Wind?

ANSWER: According to the words of the Realized Master Sūn, people who have Lower-Leg Qì [have the following characteristics: The condition] first rises from the lower legs, possibly with slackening and weakness first, suddenly falling over when getting up or walking, or swelling and fullness in the shins, or withered and delicate knees, or palpitations in the heart, or numbness in the lower abdomen, or cramping sinews when moving, or retching counter-current flow when seeing food and aversion to the smell of food, or fullness in the chest and urgent breathing, or soreness and pain all over the body. All of these are the signs of Lower-Leg Qì.

What the Yellow Emperor refers to as "slackened Qì damp *bì* Impediment" is precisely this. Unresponsive softness is called "slackening wind"; the pain constitutes damp *bì* Impediment. In the winter, it strikes the three Yáng [channels], and the ailment must be cold, while in the summer it strikes the three Yīn [channels] and the ailment must be heat.

When women [suffer from pain] in the ten toes as if they were being fried in hot oil, this is caused by Qì vacuity in *yíng* Provisioning and *wèi* Defense and by the retention of the toxic Qì of dampness in the channels and network vessels. When this [damp Qì] attacks the heart above, heart pain results; when it attacks the lower legs below, pain in the lower legs results. The feeling as if the ten toes were being fried in hot oil also falls into the category of Qì [disorder]. What the Classic refers to as "heat Reversal" is precisely this.

DISCUSSION

As the first line in the answer makes clear, Question Twenty-Nine is concerned with a condition called Lower-Leg Qì (脚氣 jiǎoqì). Despite Qí Zhòngfǔ's claim that the first part of his answer is a quotation from Sūn Sīmiǎo, I have been unable to confirm that. It should be noted that Sūn's *Bèijí qiānjīn yàofāng* devotes an entire volume to the topic of "Wind Toxin Lower-Leg Qì," so it must have been a medical category of great diagnostic and therapeutic significance in the early Táng period. Supporting this, the slightly earlier *Zhūbìng yuánhòu lùn* by Cháo Yuánfāng 巢元方 also contains abundant information in Volume Thirteen on "The Various Signs of Lower-Leg Qì Disease." Reviewing the historical information on this condition and explaining the quite tenuous relationship to the biomedical condition beriberi, as it is quite inaccurately translated in most contemporary TCM literature, is beyond the scope of this book. For more information, the reader is referred to Hilary Smith's outstanding book on the topic, *Forgotten Disease: Illnesses Transformed in Chinese Medicine.*

The key points to take away from earlier medical literature on the disease of Lower-Leg Qì are as follows: It is a condition that can express itself in numerous ways and does not have a single cause or even key symptoms. Nevertheless, it was originally, associated with pathological wind that invades the body through the feet. As such, texts warned against prolonged standing, sitting, or lying on damp, wet, and cold or hot ground. From the feet, this evil Qì is seen as rising up in the body, often without the patient's notice. Expressing itself primarily in weakness and slackening, pain and soreness, swelling, or numbness as it traveled upward, it eventually affects the heart, at which point it has reached a critical point and become difficult to treat. In addition to the patient's carelessness in protecting themselves from an invasion of pathological Qì through the feet, and the dangers of wet or damp locations, diet and emotion are also mentioned as contributing factors.

Concerning the affected channels, Sūn Sīmiǎo mentions that while wind toxin can strike a person anywhere in the body, the fact that the three channels of the liver, kidney, and spleen start in the feet means that these are the most likely vectors for wind toxin Qì rising up from the ground. In contrast to this etiology, the middle section of the answer above offers an alternative explanation related to the seasons, namely that the three Yīn and Yáng channels are the place where damp *bì* Impediment strikes in summer and winter, respectively. This is a much simpler concept than the explanation on seasonal variations of *bì* Impediment found in *Sùwèn* Chapter Forty-Three, the "Treatise on *Bì* Impediment:"

黃帝問曰：痺之安生？

岐伯對曰：風寒濕三氣雜至，合而為痺也。其風氣勝者為行痺，寒氣勝者為痛痺，濕氣勝者為著痺也。

帝曰：其有五者何也？

岐伯曰：以冬遇此者為骨痺，以春遇此者為筋痺，以夏遇此者為脈痺，以至陰遇此者為肌痺，以秋遇此者為皮痺。

The Yellow Emperor asked: "How is it that *bì* Impediment is created?"

Qí Bó replied: "When a medley of the three Qì of wind, cold, and dampness reaches the body and blends together, it forms *bì* Impediment. In this condition, if the wind Qì prevails, the patient develops moving *bì*; if the cold Qì prevails, the patient develops painful *bì*; if the dampness Qì prevails, the patient develops adhesive *bì*."

The Emperor said: "How is it that there are five types of this *bì*?"

Qí Bó said: "Encountering this condition in the winter causes bone *bì*. Encountering this condition in the spring causes sinew *bì*. Encountering this condition in the summer causes vessel *bì*. Encountering this condition at the time of "reaching/apex yīn" causes muscle *bì*. Encountering this condition in autumn causes skin *bì*.

In the following paragraph, these physiological features are related to the associated *zàng* organs in accordance with standard Chinese medicine theory, "when the condition becomes chronic and fails to leave": As such, chronic bone *bì* is related to the kidney, sinew *bì* to the liver, vessel *bì* to the heart, muscle *bì* to the spleen, and skin *bì* to the lung. The section concludes, "what we refer to as *bì* is this multi-layered contraction of the Qì of wind, cold, and/or dampness, each in its respective season."

To complicate matters further, the last paragraph mentions a third etiology, namely "heat Reversal." This condition is explained in the "Treatise on Reversal," which is *Sùwèn* Chapter Forty-Five:

黃帝問曰：厥之寒熱者何也？

岐伯對曰：陽氣衰於下，則為寒厥；陰氣衰於下，則為熱厥。

帝曰：熱厥之為熱也，必起於足下者何也？

岐伯曰：陽氣起於足五指之表，陰脈者集於足下而聚於足心，故陽氣勝則足下熱也。

The Yellow Emperor asked: 'What is the reason for the cold and heat forms of Reversal?'

Qí Bó replied: 'Debilitation of Yáng Qì below results in cold Reversal. Debilitation of Yīn Qì below results in heat Reversal.'

The Yellow Emperor said: 'Why is it that when heat Reversal causes heat, it must rise up from the underside of the feet?'

Qí Bó said: 'Yáng Qì arises from the exterior of the five toes, while the Yīn vessels come together on the underside of the foot and gather in the center of the foot. Thus, the soaring of Yáng Qì results in heat on the underside of the feet.'

To conclude this discussion and bring it back to the topic of Lower-Leg Qì, let me mention an interesting side note on this condition from a much later text from Japan, *Zábìng guǎngyào* 《雜病廣要》 (Comprehensive Essentials about the Various Diseases) by Tanba no Genken 丹波元堅 from 1853. The volume on "External Causes" includes the following paragraph on women's particular association with this disease. Because this text is obviously much later and originated in Japan, it was thus most likely influenced by localized understandings of the disease and must be treated with caution in its proper historical context. I have included it here solely because it may be of clinical interest. This text identifies the statement below as a quotation from a text called *Jìshēng* 《濟生》 (Rescuing Life), which presumably refers to the Sòng dynasty text *Yán shì jìshēng fāng* 《嚴氏濟生方》 (Life-Saving Formulas by Master Yán), completed in 1253. That text in turn contains a whole section on formulas for Lower-Leg Qì and mentions briefly that this disease also affects women and must be due to blood, but the following is by no means a literal quotation and thus must be seen as an expression of a nineteenth-century Japanese understanding of the disease.

婦人腳氣因血虛。觀乎腳氣，皆由腎虛而生；然婦人亦有病腳氣者，必因血海既虛，宿懷嗔恚，複感悲傷，遂成斯疾。今婦人病此者甚眾，則知婦人以血海虛而得之，與男子腎虛類矣。治婦人之法，與男子用藥固無異，但兼以治憂恚藥，無不效也。

Women's Lower-Leg Qì is caused by blood vacuity. Looking at Lower-Leg Qì, it is always engendered as the result of kidney vacuity. This being so, there are also women who fall ill with Lower-Leg Qì, and this is invariably caused by vacuity in the Sea of Blood and a habit of harboring anger and worry, which is further complicated by contracting sorrow and subsequently forms this disease. Because there are currently great multitudes of women suffering from this condition, we know that women contract it from a vacuity of the Sea of Blood, which falls into the same category as kidney vacuity in men. The treatment method for women is certainly no different from the medicinals used for men. Nevertheless, you will most definitely see results if you concurrently use medicinals that treat [the female patients'] worry and rage.

換腿丸

治一切腳氣，即石楠丸。

石楠葉	
天南星(炮)	
金釵石斛	
草薢	
牛膝(酒浸一宿)	
薏苡仁	
羌活(不蛀者)	
川續斷	
天麻(銼)	
防風(去蘆)	
當歸	
黃芪	
甘草	各一兩
檳榔	二兩半
乾木瓜	四兩

上為細末，酒糊為丸，桐子大。每服五十丸，漸加
至一百丸，溫酒或木瓜湯下。空心食前。

Huàn Tuǐ Wán
(Leg-Changing Pill)

A treatment for all cases of Lower-Leg Qì. This is identical with Shínán Wán (Photinia Pill).

shínányè	
tiānnánxīng (blast-fry)	
jīnchāshíhú	
bìxiè	
niúxī (steep in rice wine for one night)	
yìyǐrén	
qiānghuó (no wormy pieces)	
chuānxùduàn	
tiānmá (chop coarsely)	
fángfēng (remove shoots)	
dāngguī	
huángqí	
gāncǎo	1 *liǎng*
bīnláng	2.5 *liǎng*
gānmùguā	4 *liǎng*

Process the ingredients above into a fine powder, make a thick paste with rice wine, and form into pills the size of *wútóng* seeds. Take 50 pills per dose, gradually increasing the dosage to a maximum of 100 pills, and down in warm rice wine or Mùguā Tāng (Chaenomeles Decoction). Take on an empty stomach before meals.

萬靈散

治婦人腳氣。

當歸	
赤芍	
烏藥	各一兩
青皮	
白朮	
肉桂	各半兩
黑牽牛	二兩

上為粗末，每服三錢，水盞半，酒少許，煎八分，
去滓溫服，食前。

Wàn Líng Sǎn
(Ten-Thousandfold Magic Powder)

A treatment of Lower-Leg Qì in women.

dāngguī	
chìsháo	1 *liǎng* each
wūyào	
qīngpí	
báizhú	0.5 *liǎng* each
ròuguì	
hēiqiānniú	2 *liǎng*

Process the ingredients above into a coarse powder. Take 3 *qián* per dose, simmer in 0.5 cup of water and a little rice wine until reduced to 80 percent. Remove the dregs and ingest warm before meals.

活血丹

治婦人脾血久冷。諸般風邪濕毒之氣，留滯經絡，流注腳手，筋脈拳攣，或發赤腫，行步艱辛，腰腿沉重，腳心吊痛，及上沖脅腹膨脹，胸膈痞悶，不思飲食，沖心悶亂，及一切痛風走注，渾身疼痛。

川烏	
草烏	
地龍	
天南星	一兩
牛膝	
木瓜	
乳香(另研)	一錢半
沒藥(另研)	三錢半

上為細末，入研藥，酒糊丸，梧子大。每服二十丸，空心日午冷酒下，或荊芥湯清茶亦得。

Huó Xuè Dān
(Blood-Enlivening Elixir)

A treatment for women suffering from long-term cold of
spleen blood and all sorts of wind evil damp toxin Qì, stagnating in the channels and network vessels and streaming
into the lower legs and hands, with sinew spasms, possible
outbreaks of red swelling, difficulty walking, heaviness in
the lumbar area and legs, dropping pain in the center of the
feet, and upward surging causing inflation in the rib-sides
and abdomen, pǐ Glomus and oppression in the chest and
diaphragm, no interest in food and drink, and surging into
the heart to cause oppression and chaos, as well as all roaming influxes of painful wind with pain all over the body.

chuānwū	
cǎowū	
dìlóng	
tiānnánxīng	1 liǎng
niúxī	
mùguā	
rǔxiāng (grind separately)	1.5 qián
mòyào (grind separately)	3.5 qián

Process the ingredients above into a fine powder, add the
[separately] ground medicinals, and mix with rice wine into
a thick paste to form pills the size of wútóng seeds. Take 20
pills per dose, downing them on an empty stomach at noon
with cold rice wine. Alternatively, you can also ingest them
with Jīngjiè Tāng (Schizonepeta Decoction) or green tea.

第三十問

婦人少年髮少者，何也？

答曰：足少陽膽之經，其榮在髮；足少陰腎之經，其華在髮。

衝任之脈為十二經之海，謂之血海，其脈絡上唇口。

若血盛，則榮於頭，鬢髮美。若血海弱，則經脈虛竭，不能榮潤，故髮少而禿，或有純赤黃者。

QUESTION THIRTY

What is the Reason for Women's Lack of Head Hair in their Youth?

ANSWER: The Foot Shàoyáng Gallbladder Channel has its fruition in the head hair. The Foot Shàoyīn Kidney Channel has its flowering in the head hair.

The Chōngmài and the Rènmài are the sea of the twelve channels, what we call the "Sea of Blood," and their vessels form a network around the lips and mouth above.

If blood is exuberant, it comes to fruition in the head, and the hair of the temples and on the head is beautiful. If the Sea of Blood is frail, the channels are exhausted and thus unable to bear fruit and moisten. For this reason, we see scant head hair and baldness, or possibly pure red or yellow [hair].

DISCUSSION

The entire answer to this question is an almost literal quotation from Cháo Yuánfāng's *Zhū Bìng Yuán Hòu Lùn*. Like the rest of this entire section, the first phrase of the answer above, stating that the fruition of the Foot Shàoyáng Gallbladder Channel is seen in the hair of the head, is a nearly exact citation from the introductory essay to the section on "The Various Signs of Disease of the Hair on the Body and Head" in that text, but with some subtle yet interesting changes. Let me first cite the original in full:

足少陽膽之經也，其榮在鬚。 足少陰腎之經也，其華在髮。
衝任之脈為十二經之海，謂之血海，其別絡上唇口。
若血盛，則榮於鬚髮，故鬚髮美。若血氣衰弱，經脈虛竭，不能榮
潤，故鬚髮禿落。

The Foot Shàoyáng Gallbladder Channel has its fruition in the beard. The Foot Shàoyīn Kidney Channel has its flowering in the head hair.

The Chōngmài and the Rènmài are the sea of the twelve channels, what we call the "Sea of Blood," and their diverging vessels form a network around the lips and mouth above.

If blood is exuberant, it comes to fruition in the beard and head hair, and hence the beard and head hair are beautiful. If the Sea of Blood is frail, the channels are exhausted and thus unable unable to bear fruit and moisten. For this reason, the beard and head hair turn bald.

The key difference between Qí Zhòngfǔ's version and Cháo's original, which is clearly the precedent for Qí Zhòngfǔ's statement, is that the manifestation of the Foot Shàoyáng Gallbladder Channel is described as being in the "head hair" 髮 in our text but as "beard" 鬚 in Cháo's text. Similarly, in the last phrase, the character 鬚 xū (beard) is replaced with a very similar-looking character, 鬢 bìn, which means temple hair. The reason for this substitution is obvious when we recall that our present text is aimed at treating specifically female disorders. Is it therefore reasonable to explain this discrepancy as an intentional alteration by our author, to emphasize the close relationship between women and blood that became more and more central to the gynecological theory developing in the Sòng period? Given how awkward the first line turns out in Qí's version and how Cháo's text also discusses the role of the beard as an indication of health in the Foot Shàoyáng Channel in two other entries in this section, I suspect that Qí took creative license here to adapt the statement from the well-known *Zhūbìng yuánhòu lùn* for his gynecology text.

Now that we have established the origin of this quotation, allow me to unpack the theoretical foundations of this answer more carefully: The second half of the first sentence establishes the connection between the Foot Shàoyīn Kidney Channel and the head hair. Seasoned practitioners of Chinese medicine should recall the following line from *Sùwèn* Chapter Ten on the "Engendering and Completing of the Five *Zàng* Organs":

腎之合，骨也；其榮，髮也。

The match of the kidney is in the bones, and its fruition is in the head hair.

Similarly, we are all aware of the central role of the kidney in the developmental processes of the human body, and of the fact that its general state of health is reflected in the formation, growth, decline, and loss of the head hair. This is expressed most famously in the description of human development and aging, for women and men in multiples of seven and eight respectively, in the "Treatise on Heavenly Perfection in the Ancient Past," which is the first chapter of the *Sùwèn*.

Regarding the connection between the gallbladder and the head hair, Chinese medicine theory clearly associates the liver with the storage of blood, and the liver and gallbladder are linked in an interior-exterior *zàng-fǔ* relationship. Additionally, the condition of the blood is reflected in the health of the head hair since, as the common saying goes, "the head hair is the remainder of the blood" (髮為血之餘也). The unquestioned acceptance of this close relationship between the liver-gallbladder and the head hair is also reflected in ubiquitous popular contemporary advice for improving the health of the hair, such as the practice of tapping the gallbladder channel daily for a certain number of times. Furthermore, the Five-Agent association of the gallbladder with the Yáng aspect of Wood can also explain its importance in the earlier stages of human life and thus its importance in the current question, which addresses the lack of head hair in a person's youth.

Lastly, we can cite *Língshū* Chapter Two to support the link between the gallbladder and the head hair, since the head hair is the visible manifestation of Essence in Chinese medical theory:

肝合膽；膽者，中精之府。

> The liver matches up with the gallbladder. The gallbladder is the palace of central Essence.

Regarding the last phrase of Qí's answer above, "For this reason, we see scant head hair and baldness, or possibly pure red or yellow [hair]," I have intentionally translated it literally to avoid reading my own interpretation into it. It is striking at first glance, since we are more accustomed to seeing a liver blood or kidney Essence deficiency, or any other sort of age-related decline, described as manifesting in hair becoming sparse and desiccated and white, not "pure red or yellow." We can, however, interpret the description here as a browning of originally black hair, a decrease in the natural shine and luster and loss of the deep dark black color typical of healthy Chinese hair, which slowly turns into white hair with age but passes through "red" and "yellow" as intermediary stages. Of course, this statement has to be adapted in the context of Caucasian hair colors and does not mean that blond hair turns red or brown but that the hair loses sheen and appears lighter in color than it would in a physiological state.

The character 純, pronounced *chún*, usually means pure or unmixed, which certainly works well here grammatically as a modifier for the colors red and yellow. As a noun, however, it can also mean "strand of silk," so perhaps it could refer here to something like streaks of red and yellow, which would make more clinical sense but would be a grammatical stretch.

生髮藥

蔓荊子	
青葙子	各一兩
蓮子草	
附子	二字
頭髮灰	一匙

上為末。以酒漬，納瓷器中，封閉經二七日，藥
成。以烏雞脂和，塗之。先以米泔洗髮，然後敷
之，數月生長一尺也。

Shēng Fà Yào
(Hair-Sprouting Medicine)

mànjīngzǐ	
qīngxiāngzǐ	1 *liǎng* each
liánzǐcǎo	
fùzǐ	2 *zì*
tóufǎ (ash)	1 spoonfull

Process the ingredients above into a powder. Drench in rice wine,
place in a ceramic vessel, seal tightly, and wait for 14 days until the
medicine is finished. Mix it with the fat from a black-boned chicken
and spread it on [the hair]. First wash the hair with rice-rinsing water
and then apply this [paste]. After several months, the hair will have
grown 1 *chǐ* in length.

生眉毛

七月七日烏麻，陰乾為末，烏麻油和塗，眉即生妙。

Shēng Méimāo
(Making the Eyebrows Sprout)

On the seventh day of the seventh month, take raven-black sesame. Dry it in the shade and process into a powder. Mix it with black sesame oil and spread it on. The eyebrows will sprout miraculously!

滋陰養血丸

治勞虛血弱，肌肉枯燥，手足多煩，肢節酸疼，鬢
髮脫落，面少顏色，腹拘急痛引腰背，去血過多，
崩傷內竭，胸中短氣，晝夜不能眠，情思不樂，怔
忡多汗。

熟地	各一兩
當歸	
鹿茸(酥炙)	二兩

上為細末，蜜丸桐子大。每服五十丸，米飲湯任
下，不拘時。

Zī Yīn Yǎng Xùe Wán
(Yin-Saturating Blood-Nourishing Pill)

A treatment for taxation vacuity and blood frailty, with desiccated flesh and bones, much vexation in the hands and feet,
soreness in the limb joints, loss of temple and head hair,
a lack of color in the face, hypertonicity and pain in the
abdomen stretching into the lower back, excessive bleeding, damage from Landslide Collapse and critical internal
exhaustion, shortness of breath in the chest, inability to sleep
day or night, lack of joy, and fearful throbbing with much
sweating.

shúdì	1 *liǎng* each
dāngguī	
lùróng (mix-fry in ghee)	2 *liǎng*

Process the ingredients above into a fine powder and form
with honey into pills the size of *wútóng* seeds. Take 50 pills
per dose and down them in thin rice gruel at will, with no
restriction on the timing.

第三十一問

四肢如故，但腹脹者，何也？

答曰：身腫及四肢者，本起於水。手足瘦削腹大者，本起於脾。或脹滿或散者，氣也。

然腹脹之狀，上下膨亨，或鼓之有聲，喘息不便，由上者不降，下者不升，氣痞於中，無所歸息，三焦渾亂。

若猝然脹滿，餘無所苦，此由脾胃不調，冷氣暴折，客乘於中。寒之，則氣收聚，壅遏不通，是以脹滿。

《內經》云：「臟寒生滿病」是也。

若臍凸者難治，大便利者為逆。

QUESTION THIRTY-ONE

What is the Reason for Abdominal Distention as a Single [Symptom] but Without Any Symptoms in the Four Limbs?

ANSWER: Any generalized swelling that reaches the four limbs originally arises from water. Gauntness in the hands and feet with an enlarged abdomen originally arises from the spleen. Distention that now arises and now scatters is related to Qì.

This being so, if the appearance of the abdominal distention is such that the upper and lower part are inflated through-out, possibly making a sound when you drum on it, with discomfort from panting, this is due to the fact that what is above is unable to descend and what is below is unable to ascend, that the Qì is obstructed in the middle, that there is no place to return the breath to, and that the Sānjiāo is in a state of chaos.

If there is abruptly occurring distention that is not accom-panied by any other problems in the rest [of the body], this is caused by a lack of attunement in the spleen and stom-ach and fulminant snapping of cool Qì, which has intruded upon and overwhelmed the center. If [you add] cold to this, Qì gathers together and becomes congested to the point of failing to flow through. For this reason, there is distention.

The quotation from the *Nèijīng* that "Cold in the *zàng* organs engenders fullness," refers exactly to this.

If the navel protrudes outward, it is difficult to treat. If defe-cation is disinhibited, it means counter-current movement.

DISCUSSION

Qí Zhòngfǔ's answer first offers a diagnostic guideline to differentiate three different causes of swelling: Generalized swelling indicates a problem with water; abdominal swelling with emaciated limbs points to a spleen issue; and intermittently occurring distention is a condition related to the Qì. Each of these signs can be helpful in diagnosing swelling, and of course conditions are usually a combination of several factors, as the third paragraph suggests. The rest of Qí's answer explains that suddenly appearing distention without other symptoms, which is what the question is asking about, is due to lack of attunement in the spleen and stomach that is complicated by the presence of pathogenic cold in the center, which prevents the Qì from moving freely.

The term 歸息 guī xī can be read in different ways, based on the meaning of both characters individually and as a compound. Literally translated, 歸 means "to return," in the sense of a movement to the proper place where a person or substance belongs. As such, it is used to describe a hermit withdrawing into the mountains for retreat or a newly married maiden entering her new husband's home, which in the traditional Chinese perspective is the place where she belongs, instead of her natal family. It can also be used in the transitive sense of "to return," in the sense of giving something back. The second character, 息, means "to breathe" in its narrowest meaning, but can also mean "to rest" or "to stop," "to give up something." As a compound, 歸息 has the established meaning of "to rest" or "to stop," in both the sense of stopping in a location and of ceasing an activity. Rather than reading it in this compound meaning as "the condition has no way to abate," I interpret the phrase here as "to return the breath." I am indebted to Leo Lok for assistance on this line.

Another difficult phrase in this section is the expression 客乘於中寒之則氣收聚. As most readers are aware, classical texts originally do not possess punctuation, and modern editions of early texts can differ substantially in this regard. All contemporary editions I am aware of punctuate this phrase as 「客乘於中寒之，則氣收聚。」 I have chosen a different punctuation for grammatical reasons. In the reading advocated by modern editions, it is impossible to make grammatical sense of the character 之, which can be a verb "to go to" but most commonly functions as a direct object. If we read 中寒 as a compound meaning "cold strike," it is impossible to fit 之, either as a second direct object or as a verb, into the sentence, and ignoring the character is not an option I am comfortable with. Instead, I suggest reading 寒 ("cold") here as a verb in the causative sense of "to cause to be cold," whether by accidentally exposing the patient to additional cold through diet or the outside environment or by erroneous medical treatment with cold medicinals.

Lastly, the phrase that is attributed to the *Néijīng* is in fact a literal citation from *Sùwèn* Chapter Twelve. This treatise discusses the different treatment methods appropriate for the five regions of China: lancing stones for the east, because of the prevalence of abscesses related to the salty and fishy diet of the people who live in the coastal region, which causes heat and blood problems; toxic medicinals for the west because the land is windy and hard and its people are robust and less receptive to external invasion but prone to internally generated illnesses; moxibustion for the north, which is cold and icy and where the people love the wilderness and eat dairy, to treat the fullness disorders associated with cold in the *zàng* organs; fine needles for the south, the land of abundant Yáng, of frail geography and low elevations full of fog and dew, where people love sour things and suffer from convulsions and *bì* Impediment; and lastly massage and stretching for the center, a land of plains and moisture, full of abundant and varied foods where people do not have to exert themselves and are prone to Wilting Reversal and cold and heat.

沉香導氣丸

順氣消腫。

黑白牽牛(各一兩，炒，共取末)	一兩
青皮(去白同巴豆)	
陳皮(去白同巴豆)	
檳榔(銼碎，用巴豆五十粒，去皮膜，將三味炒黃色，去巴豆不用)	半兩
沉香	
全蠍(炒)	
蓽澄茄	
丁香	
胡椒	各半兩
續隨子(研)	一錢
蘿卜子(炒)	三兩
甘遂(銼，炒黃色)	半兩

上為細末，用蔥白研如膏，和丸，桐子大。每服二十丸。炒酒醱煎湯下。醋湯亦得。

Chénxiāng Dǎo Qì Wán
(Agarwood Resin Qì-Conducting Pill)

Restores the flow of Qì in the proper direction and dissipates swelling.

qiānniú (1 *liǎng* each of black and white seeds and stir-fry, altogether take a total of 1 *liǎng* and pulverize)	1 *liǎng*
qīngpí (remove the white parts and combine with bādòu)	
chénpí (remove the white parts and combine with bādòu)	
bīnláng (crush into pieces. Use 50 seeds of bādòu and remove the skin, stir-fry with the three formula ingredients until yellow, and then remove the bādòu and do not use it!)	0.5 *liǎng*
chénxiāng	
quánxiē (stir-fry)	
bìchéngqié	
dīngxiāng	
hújiāo	1 *liǎng* each
xùsuízǐ (grind)	1 *qián*
luóbózǐ (stir-fry)	3 *liǎng*
gānsuì (crush and stir-fry until yellow)	0.5 *liǎng*

Process the ingredients above into a fine powder. Grind the white part of scallions into a paste-like consistency and mix [with the powdered herbs] to form pills the size of *wútóng* seeds. Take 20 pills per dose. Make a decoction with stir-fried rice wine leaven and down the pills in this. Taking it in a hot vinegar decoction is also possible.

神助丸

治四肢瘦，肚大。

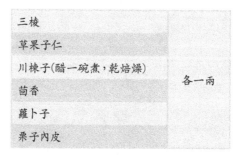

三棱	
草果子仁	
川楝子(醋一碗煮，乾焙燥)	各一兩
茴香	
蘿卜子	
栗子內皮	

上為末，醋糊丸，桐子大。蘿卜湯送下五十丸。虛者三十丸。

Shén Zhù Wán
(Divine Assistance Pill)

A treatment for emaciation of the four limbs with an enlarged belly.

sānléng	
cǎoguǒzǐrén	
chuānliànzǐ (boil [the three ingredients above] with 1 bowlful of vinegar until evaporated, dry and roast gently on a slab)	1 *liǎng* each
huíxiāng	
luóbózǐ	
lìzǐnèipí	

Process the ingredients above into a powder and mix with vinegar into a paste to form pills the size of *wútóng* seeds. Down 50 pills [per dose] in radish decoction. In cases with vacuity, take 30 pills.

Formula Note

The instructions in this formula are a little ambiguous in the original Chinese text. To make sense of the repeated measurement in the table above, I interpret the "each" (各 gè) in the first measurement as referring not just to the measurement, but also to the instructions to boil each of the substances above in vinegar and dry-roast them. The reason for this confusion is likely that in some editions, as in my own layout above, the measurement is listed after the instructions on how to prepare each substance. It therefore appears as if the "each" refers only to the measurement. In other editions, however, and presumably in the original source for our current text, the measurement precedes the preparation details, and in that case it makes sense that the instructions for preparation apply to all the previous ingredients. I have expressed this by adding "the three ingredients above" in square brackets. If we were to read the preparation instructions as referring only to the chuānliànzǐ, but not to the previous substances, it would make no sense to give the measurement here and then again in the last line of the table unless there was a scribal error for one of the measurements. None of the modern editions suggest such an interpretation and it thus seems unlikely, while the explanation of the confusion as resulting from the editorial variations is entirely plausible.

As a side note, it is interesting that this formula includes "emaciation of the four limbs" when the actual question inquires about abdominal distention with no other symptoms. This formula thus addresses the condition that he has mentioned in his answer above as "gauntness in the hands and feet with an enlarged abdomen," explained as arising from the spleen.

第三十二問

病有血分，有水分，何以別之？

答曰：婦人月經通流，流則水血消化。

若風寒搏於經脈，血結不通，血積為水，故曰血分。

若先病，於後經水或斷，名曰水分。其病易治，去其水，經自下也。

若病人覺腹內脹，外視如常，大便黑，小便赤，是其証也。

QUESTION THIRTY-TWO

Disease Can Be in the Blood Aspect or in the Water Aspect. How Do We Distinguish Between Them?

ANSWER: Regarding the flow of women's menstrual period, as a result of the flow, water and blood dissipate through transformation.

If wind and/or cold have assaulted the channels, the blood binds and fails to flow through. Blood amasses to become Water. Thus, we call this the blood aspect.

If there was a pre-existing illness and then afterwards the menstrual fluids were perhaps interrupted, we call this the water aspect. These conditions are easy to treat. Get rid of her Water, and the menstrual period will descend again on its own accord.

If the patient feels distention inside the abdomen but appears healthy from the outside, with black feces and red urine, these are the signs for this condition.

Discussion

To make sense of Qí Zhòngfǔ's explanation, we first need to unwrap the multiple meanings and definitions of the word "water" in Chinese medicine, especially in its juxtaposition with blood. I have consistently translated the Chinese term 水 shuǐ literally as "water," even though I was at first tempted to render it more elegantly as "fluids" or "liquid," in some contexts, and in others as "Water [Qì disease]". To avoid overinterpreting the original source and introducing my own interpretation, I suggest these different meanings only by capitalizing the term when I am certain that it must refer to the disease of "Water Qì."

It is obvious that the meaning of the term here far exceeds the narrowest meaning of the English "water." As we contemplate the answer above, it also becomes obvious that the Chinese term 水 here cannot possibly refer to "fluids" in the general sense of liquid substances, as it frequently does in other contexts in Chinese literature. In Qí Zhòngfǔ's answer here, and in many other occurrences in Chinese medical literature, it must mean something other than the physiological fluids in the human body, such as blood, saliva, tears, sweat, and so on, that we usually see referred to as 津液 jīnyè, a compound that includes (in Wiseman's terminology) the thinner "fluids" and the thicker "humors" respectively.

Instead, we have to read this passage with a more specific technical meaning of "water" in mind, namely one that is often expressed in medical texts in the compound 水氣 shuǐqì ("Water Qì"). This is similar to the way in which the Chinese term for the English "blood," namely 血 xuè, does not refer only or precisely to the narrow biomedical definition of blood either, but includes a much more specific and at the same time broader range of meanings related to the menstrual cycle, the role of blood in nurturing the fetus, and its transformation into various entities or substances that are only tangentially related to its biomedical meaning, like breastmilk or palpable or impalpable abdominal masses. This is the reason why some English writers of books on Chinese medicine, especially ones with a more academic historical or anthropological background, prefer to capitalize the English Blood for 血 when they discuss it in this specialized meaning. For the same reason, one could argue for capitalizing "Water" in the present question, to alert the reader that we are not just talking about water in the common English sense but as a technical term in Chinese medicine. As I assume that any serious student or practitioner of Chinese medicine learns about the different meanings of blood in the context of Chinese medicine in general and in gynecology in particular, I decided a long time ago to leave that word in lower case. In regard to the innocuous-looking term "water," though, how many Western students and practitioners are similarly aware of its technical meanings in the classical Chinese medicine literature? To differentiate between at least two of the meanings relevant in the answer above, I leave "water" in lower case when it refers to fluids but capitalize it when it refers to the disease of Water Qì. Lastly, I should warn the careful reader that I also capitalize water in the third sense of being one of the Five Dynamic Agents, seen below as the Agent associated with the kidney and in charge of managing lower-case water.

In the classics, our earliest theoretical reference to Water Qì and to disease in the "water aspect" is, as so often, the *Jīnguì yàolüè*. Interestingly, this also happens to be the source for Qí Zhòngfǔ's answer above and clearly addresses a gynecological condition there as well, even though we find this explanation not in the gynecological volumes but in the volume on "Pulses, Signs, and Treatments of Water Qì Disease." Here is the literal quotation from that text:

問曰：病有血分、水分，何也？

師曰：經水前斷，後病水，名曰血分，此病難治；先病水，後經水斷，名曰水分，此病易治。何以故？去水，其經自下。

Question: "Disease can be in the blood aspect or in the water aspect. What does that mean?"

The teacher answered: "When menstruation is interrupted first and then Water disease occurs afterwards, this is called blood aspect. This disease is difficult to treat. When the patient first suffers from Water [disease] and then afterwards from interrupted menstruation, this is called water aspect. This disease is easy to treat. What is the reason for this? As soon you get rid of the water, the patient's menstrual period will descend on its own accord."

In other words, the key to proper diagnosis in conditions that combine an interrupted menstrual period with signs of Water Qì disease is to detect which one came first. If you can find an answer to that question, this will give you important therapeutic and prognostic information.

To gain a better understanding of the meaning of Water Qì, two excerpts from Volume Twenty-One of the *Zhūbìng yuánhòu lùn*, in the section that covers the "Various Signs of Water Swelling," provide important insights. The introduction explains the general etiology of Water Disease:

腎者主水，脾胃俱主土，土性克水。脾與胃合，相為表裡。胃為水穀之海。

今胃虛不能傳化水氣，使水氣滲溢經絡，浸漬腑臟。脾得水濕之氣加之則病，脾病則不能制水，故水氣獨歸於腎。三焦不瀉，經脈閉塞，故水氣溢受於皮膚而令腫也。其狀：目裡上微腫，如新臥起之狀，頸脈動，時咳，股間冷，以手按腫處，隨手而起，如物裡水之狀，口苦舌乾，不得正偃，偃則咳清水；不得臥，臥則驚，驚則咳甚；小便黃澀是也。

The kidney is in charge of Water, and the spleen and stomach are together in charge of Earth. It is the nature of Earth to overcome Water. The spleen and stomach are a matching unit and stand in an exterior-interior relationship to each other. The stomach is the Sea of Water and Grain.

In the present case, the stomach is vacuous and unable to transform Water Qì, which causes Water Qì to spill over into the channels and network vessels and soak into the *zàng* and *fǔ* organs. The spleen receives the Qì of water damp, and when this is added to, it falls ill. Because the spleen is unable to control water as the result of illness, Water Qì only returns back to its home in the kidney. Because the *Sānjiāo* is not drained and the channels are blocked, Water Qì spills out into the skin and causes swelling. It looks like this: Slight swelling above inside the eyes as in a person who has just risen from sleep; stirring in the vessels of the neck; occasional coughing; coolness in the area of the thighs; a rising response when you push on the swollen area with the hand, like water inside something; bitterness in the mouth and a dry tongue; inability to lie flat on the back and coughing up of clear water when you do lie down; inability to sleep, sleep resulting in panic, and panic in aggravated coughing; and yellow and rough urination.

Later on in the same section, Cháo Yuánfāng explains:

水病者，由腎脾俱虛故也。腎虛不能宣通水氣，脾虛又不能製水，故水氣盈溢，滲液皮膚，流遍四肢，所以通身腫也。

Water disease is caused by dual vacuity in the kidney and spleen. Because the kidney is vacuous and therefore unable to promote the free movement of water Qì, and because the spleen is vacuous and unable to control water, water Qì spills over and seeps into the skin, streams into the four limbs, and thus causes swelling all over the body.

As we can see, Water Qì is the name of a disease that is caused by impaired spleen and kidney function and manifests with the primary sign of generalized swelling due to the accumulation of fluids in the skin. There are two reasons why this condition is discussed here in a textbook on women's diseases:

First, Cháo mentions in the introduction that blocked channels are one of the effects of Water Qì when the spleen and stomach are unable to manage the free flow and elimination of fluids from the body, as Earth fails to overcome Water in the cycle of the Five Dynamic Agents. Whether as a direct result of the presence of water, or as a just another symptom of weakness in the kidney and spleen and stomach, the physiological monthly release of female blood is impaired to the point of being blocked completely. Menstruation is, after all, yet another outwardly visible manifestation of the free flow, management, and discharge of fluids in the body. If Water Qì was the primary condition, successfully treating that, by restoring healthy and balanced kidney and spleen/stomach function, will cause the menstrual problem to resolve on its own. This is the water aspect that according to Qí is easy to treat.

More serious and difficult to treat is swelling that is a disease of the blood aspect, in which case Qí Zhòngfǔ identifies the impaired flow of blood due to the invasion of wind and cold as the key etiology. In this context, Qí's statement that "blood amasses to become Water" is an interesting way to conceptualize the swelling that can arise when menstruation fails to flow freely.

We can glean additional insight into this dynamic from the indications for the following formula for Jiāorén Wán. The drastic nature of this formula speaks volumes about the perceived severity of the condition. In addition, the indications include the symptom "stopped urination" and moreover explain that "water transforms to form blood, and when blood fails to flow through, it forms Water." What becomes apparent here is that in that context, and therefore in the context above, the first "water" refers to fluids, while the second "Water" actually refers to the disease called "Water Qì." In other words, when blood fails to flow and gathers into masses because menstruation is blocked or stopped, this can lead to the condition of Water Qì, with the accompanying symptom of stopped urination. Thus, I suggest that we interpret the final statement by Qí on blood-aspect Water swelling as "blood amasses to become [the disease of] Water Qì."

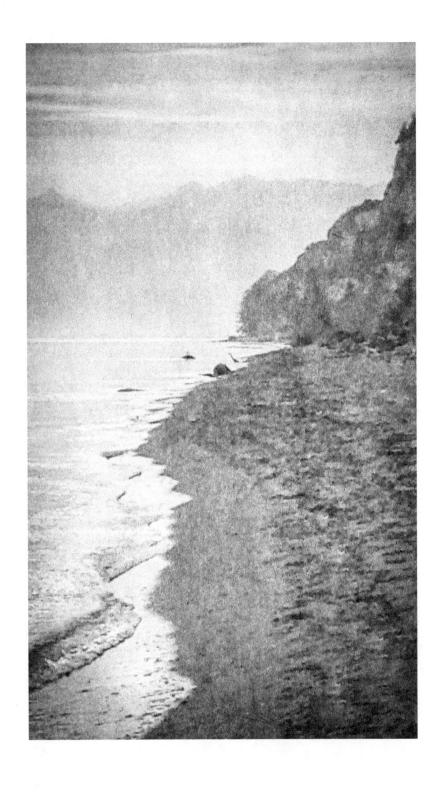

椒仁丸

治因經水斷絕，後致四肢面目浮腫，小便不通，名
曰血分。水化為血，血不通則為水矣。

五靈脂	
吳茱萸(湯洗七次，醋浸，炒)	
玄胡索	各半兩
芫花(醋浸一宿，炒焦)	一分
椒仁	
甘遂(炒黃)	
續隨子	
鬱李仁(去皮研)	
牽牛(炒熟)	各半兩
信砒(研)	一錢
石膏(煅通赤研細)	一分
附子(炮熟)	半兩
木香	半兩
膽礬	一錢

上為細末，麵糊為丸，如綠豆大。橘皮湯下一丸。
臨臥未通空心加一丸。腹未通日午再一服。

Jiāorén Wán
(Sìchuán Peppercorn Pill)

A treatment for superficial swelling in the four limbs, face, and eyes, with stopped urination, in cases when these arise consequently and subsequently to interrupted menstruation. This is called "blood aspect." Water transforms into blood, and when blood fails to flow through, it forms Water [Qì]!

wǔlíngzhī	
wúzhūyú (wash in hot water seven times, steep in vinegar, and stir-fry)	
xuánhúsuǒ	0.5 *liǎng* each
yuánhuā (steep in vinegar over night and scorch-fry	1 *fēn* each
jiāorén	
gānsuì (stir-fry until yellow)	
xùsuízǐ	
yùlǐrén (remove the skin and grind)	
qiānniú (stir-fry thoroughly)	0.5 *liǎng* each
xìnpī (grind)	1 *qián*
shígāo (calcine until red throughout and grind finely	1 *fēn*
fùzǐ (blast-fry thoroughly)	0.5 *liǎng*
mùxiāng	0.5 *liǎng*
dǎnfán	1 *qián*

Process the ingredients above into a fine power and mix with a paste of flour and water to form pills the size of mung beans. Drink down 1 pill [per dose] in a decoction of tangerine peel. Right before going to bed, if menstruation still fails to flow through, on an empty stomach, take an additional pill. If there is still no through-flow in the abdomen on the next day, take another pill at noon.

Formula Note

Potentially shedding some light on the indications and intended effect of this formula, Qí Zhòngfǔ's possible source can be found in a formula collection from the early twelfth century called *Quánshēng zhǐmí fang* 《全生指迷方》 (Formulas for All of Life that Point out Confusion). Before presenting this formula with the same ingredients and almost literally identical preparation method, the text mentions in its list of indications that this condition is also called Deep-Lying Beam disease:

> 若身體及髀股 皆腫，環臍而痛，不可動。動之為水。亦名伏梁。椒
> 仁丸主之。

> If both the trunk of the body and the thighs are swollen and the area around the umbilicus is painful, you cannot move it. If you move it, it forms Water [Qì]. It is also called Deep-Lying Beam. Jiāorén Wán rules this condition.

The disease of Deep-Lying Beam (伏梁 *fúliáng*) is a disease name mentioned already in the Hàn period classics. Most relevant to the context here, *Sùwèn* Chapter Forty ("Discourse on the Abdomen and Center") describes it as a life-threatening chronic condition marked by "exuberance" in the lesser abdomen with "roots above and below and to the left and to the right" and then subsequently as swelling in both trunk and thighs with periumbilical pain. Having "wind roots," it originates below the umbilicus and "if you move it, it forms Water [Qì]. It is a disease of inhibited urination."

Whether identified in a non-gendered context as Deep-Lying Beam, or when preceded by stopped menstruation as Water Qì, this disease was thus seen a dangerous condition that required a drastic intervention with the present formula.

To the best of my knowledge, the name-giving ingredient in this formula, 椒仁 jiāorén, must be read in its literal translation "seed of Sìchuān peppercorn," and is therefore simply an alternate name for the more common term chuānjiāo.

Lastly, I have chosen to translate the phrase 橘皮湯 literally as "decoction of tangerine peel" and to leave it in lower case, rather than marking it off as a formula name of Júpí Tāng, for a number of reasons: Most importantly, the written record contains several recipes for Júpí Tāng already by Qí Zhòngfǔ's times, and it seems unlikely that he would not have been more specific had he meant a particular one. Thus, it is most likely that the term here simply meant tangerine peels decocted in hot water. It could, however, also have suggested to his medically literate readers some additional ingredients. Most notably, it could be a reference to the formula for Júpí Tāng in the *Jīnguì yàolüè*, where it is a treatment indicated for "dry retching and hiccup with Reversal in the hands and feet," and consists of a decoction of 8 *liǎng* of gānjiāng with 4 *liǎng* of júpí.

葶藶丸

治因小便不利後，身面浮腫，致經水不通，名曰水分。其餘逆順，並同水氣。

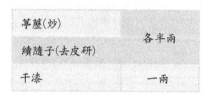

葶藶(炒)	各半兩
續隨子(去皮研)	
干漆	一兩

上為末，棗肉和丸，桐子大。煎扁竹湯下七丸。如大便利者，減葶藶續隨子各一分，加白术半兩。

Tínglì Wán
(Lepidium Pill)

A treatment for inhibited urination that subsequently causes superficial swelling in the body and face and then leads to failure of the menstrual fluids to flow through. This is called "blood aspect." Its remainder moves counter-current to the proper flow direction and combines with Water Qì.

tínglì (stir-fry)	0.5 *liǎng* each
xùsuízǐ (remove peel and grind)	
gānqī	1 *liǎng*

Process the above into a powder and combine with jujube meat into pills the size of *wútóng* seeds. Drink down 7 pills in a decoction of simmered shègān decoction. If defecation is not inhibited, reduce the tínglì and xùsuízǐ by 1 *fēn* each and add 0.5 *liǎng* of báizhú instead.

FORMULA NOTE

While the term 扁竹 biǎnzhú (or in an alternate version 萹竹) can sometimes also refer to 萹蓄 biǎnxù (Polygonum aviculare), which is the medicinal name for the whole plant we commonly call "knotgrass," I identify it here with the medicinal shègān (射干, belamcanda rhizome), for which it is also an accepted synonym, for two reasons: First, shègān is a good match for the intended effect of this formula since it is also indicated for counter-current movement in the abdomen, inhibited urination and defecation, accumulation of water, and blocked menstruation because it disperses bound Qì. Second, when the name biǎnzhú is used in the meaning of 萹蓄 biǎnxù (Polygonum aviculare), it is usually given as 扁竹草 biǎnzhúcǎo ("whole plant of biǎnzhú).

第三十三問

心腹痛，或又有小腹痛者，何也？

答曰：經云：五臟猝痛，何氣使然。岐伯對曰：寒氣稽留於脈外，故猝然而痛也。《舉痛論》中所載痛病，共有一十七証，皆由寒氣之所致也。

巢氏云：痛是臟虛受風冷，邪氣乘心也。其痛發有死者，有不死成疹者。心為諸臟主而藏神，其正經不可傷。傷之而痛者，名為真心痛，朝發夕死，夕發朝死。

若腑臟虛弱，風邪客於其間，痛隨氣之上下，或上攻於心則心痛，下攻於腹則腹痛。上下相攻則心腹俱痛。

或宿有風冷搏於血，血氣停結，小腹痛也。

QUESTION THIRTY-THREE

What is the Reason for Heart and Abdominal Pain, Possibly Accompanied by Lesser Abdominal Pain as Well?

ANSWER: According to the Classic, what kind of Qì is it that causes sudden pain in the five *zàng* organs? Qí Bó answered that when cold Qì slows down [the flow] and lodges outside the vessels, this is the reason for sudden pain. There are a total of seventeen patterns of pain conditions recorded in the "Treatise on Lifting Pain." All of these are caused by cold Qì.

According to Cháo Yuánfāng, [this] pain means that the *zàng* organs are vacuous and have contracted wind cold, and that this evil Qì has overwhelmed the heart. When this pain erupts, some patients die, and some do not die but suffer from papules. The heart is the ruler of all the *zàng* organs and stores the Shén. Its direct channel must not be damaged. If there is damage to it and subsequent pain, this is called true heart pain. If it erupts in the morning, the patient is dead by the evening, and if it erupts in the evening, the patient is dead by the next morning.

If the *fǔ* and *zàng* organs are weakened, wind evil intrudes into their space and the pain follows the upward and downward movement of Qì. Rising up and attacking the heart, this results in heart pain; descending and attacking the abdomen, it results in abdominal pain; attacking both above and below, it results in both heart and abdominal pain.

If there is an abiding presence of wind cold that has assaulted the blood, this causes blood and Qì to collect and bind. This means lesser abdominal pain.

DISCUSSION

This answer references the classic source for understanding pain in traditional Chinese medicine, the famous "Treatise on Lifting Pain" (《舉痛論》 *Jǔtòng lùn*), which is also known as *Sùwèn* Chapter Thirty-Nine. So that you may appreciate the poetic licence Qí Zhòngfǔ has taken in his quotation above, here is the full section in its original form:

帝曰：願聞人之五臟卒痛，何氣使然？

岐伯對曰：經脈流行不止，環周不休，寒氣入經而稽遲，泣而不行，客於脈外則血少，客於脈中則氣不通，故卒然而痛。

帝曰：其痛或卒然而止者，或痛甚不休者，或痛甚不可按者，或按之而痛止者，或按之無益者，或喘動應手者，或心與背相引而痛者，或脅肋與少腹相引而痛者，或腹痛引陰股者，或痛宿昔而成積者，或卒然痛死不知人，有少間復生者，或痛而嘔者，或腹痛而後泄者，或痛而閉不通者，凡此諸痛，各不同形，別之奈何？

The Emperor said: "I would like to hear what kind of Qì it is that causes sudden pain [in] a person's five *zàng* organs?"

Qí Bó answered: "The flow in the channels and vessels runs ceaselessly and circulates throughout the body without rest. When cold Qì enters the channels, it delays [this flow], slows it down to a trickle, and then stops it altogether. Taking up residence on the outside of the vessels, it results in scantiness of blood; taking up residence on the inside of the vessels, it results in stoppage of Qì. For this reason, all of a sudden there is pain.

The Emperor said: "This kind of pain might be sudden and then stop; or it might be severe and relentless; or it might be so severe that you must not press down on it; or it might be relieved by pressure; or it might not show any benefit from pressure; or it might manifest in a panting movement that responds to [the pressure of] the hand; or the pain may result from pulling between the heart and back or between the rib-sides and the lesser abdomen; or it may be abdominal pain pulling towards the inner thighs; or the pain may lodge chronically and form Gatherings; or there may be sudden pain and death or failure to recognize people but then return [of Qì] and subsequent revival after a short while; or there may be pain followed by vomiting; or there may be abdominal pain followed by diarrhea; or there may be pain followed by blockage and complete stoppage. All these various kinds of pain each manifest in different ways…"

As we can see, Qí has altered the original text slightly, associating the condition of slowed flow only with the presence of cold Qì outside the vessels. Why he felt the need to alter the original in this way, other than perhaps to abbreviate the citation, is unclear to me. The key point that he wanted to impress on his readers, though, was undoubtedly the fact that suddenly arising pain is caused by the presence and retention of cold Qì.

The remainder of Qí Zhòngfǔ's answer above consists of almost literal citations from Cháo Yuánfāng's Zhūbìng yuánhòu lùn. First, we can turn to the first essay on "Heart Pain" in Volume Sixteen on the "Various Signs of Heart Pain Disease." The source for Qí's quote is found at the very beginning and is almost literally identical with Qí's citation. It serves here to reiterate the fact that pain is caused by the presence of the "evil Qì of wind cold" but then emphasizes further how serious the condition is when it affects the heart as the ruler of the zàng organs. Especially in the most serious case of "true heart pain," the patient is said to die within twelve hours, and it is thus essential for any physician to correctly diagnose this disease and take the relevant measures.

When we then turn to Volume Thirty-Seven, which is one of the volumes on the "Various Diseases of Women," the chapters on "Heart Pain," "Heart and Abdominal Pain," and "Lesser Abdominal Pain," are again almost literally identical to the same quotation in Volume Sixteen and to Qí's version cited here, while adding some more details. We can see here how Sòng dynasty authors like Qí Zhòngfǔ used Cháo Yuánfāng's masterpiece as a reference text to refer to specific conditions and how the entries in Cháo's text frequently overlapped and repeated themselves.

In this context, it is significant that there is no gender-specific information in any of these presentations and no substantive difference between the description of these conditions in the general section of Cháo's text and the gynecological section towards the end of his book. Thus, we must ask ourselves why the conditions of heart pain, abdominal pain, and lesser abdominal pain were viewed as gendered and in need of inclusion both Cháo's and Qí's books.

Given the importance of blood and its movement and periodic discharge as menstruation as the key to women's health in Qí's work, the answer is undoubtedly related to the role of the heart in being the ruler of the *zàng* organs and managing the flow of the vessels. In addition, women's association with Yīn and their perceived openness and exhaustion as the result of their reproductive processes, both during and after menstruation and, to an even greater degree and in particular, during and after childbirth, clearly made them more vulnerable to the invasion of the "evil Qì of wind-cold." This view of the female body is a perspective that would strike most modern women, and Western feminists in particular, as strange or outdated, if not even offensive, but may be worth remembering as you diagnose and consult your female patients in clinic. The connection of this type of pain to the aftereffects of childbirth is mentioned in the indications for the following formula.

醋煎散

治婦人血氣腹脅刺痛，及產後敗血，兒枕急痛。

高良薑	一兩
當歸	
肉桂	
白芍	各半兩
橘紅	
烏藥	

上為細末，每服三錢。水醋各半盞，煎七分，通口
服，不拘時。

Cù Jiān Sǎn
(Vinegar-Simmered Powder)

A treatment for women's stabbing pain in the abdomen and
rib-sides from blood and Qì, as well as for decayed blood
after childbirth and acute Child's-Pillow Pain.

gāoliángjiāng	1 *liǎng*
dāngguī	
ròuguì	
báisháo	0.5 *liǎng* each
júhóng	
wūyào	

Process the ingredients above into a fine powder and take 3
qián per dose. Simmer in 0.5 cup each of water and vinegar
until reduced to 70 percent and ingest orally. Do not restrict
the timing.

FORMULA NOTE

Most medical histories credit the *Fùrén dàquán liángfāng* 《婦人大全良方》 (Compendium of Excellent Formulas for Women) by Chén Zìmíng 陳自明 as the earliest source for the term Child's Pillow Pain. However, given its publication date of 1237, which is seventeen years later than the *Nǔke bǎiwèn*, we must give due credit to Qí Zhòngfǔ. Nevertheless, the fact that he only mentions the term in passing and does not see a need to explain it shows that it was obviously a disease term well-known to gynecologists at this time and that earlier texts that mention it have simply not survived. Since it is not found in Cháo Yuánfāng's or Sūn Sīmiǎo's writings, though, we can be fairly certain that it was invented and popularized at some point between the eighth and thirteenth centuries. What is correct, however, is that Chén Zìmíng's essay, which I quote below at full, is our earliest extant description of this condition. Also suggesting that Child's Pillow was already a common term during Qí's and Chén's time is the fact that Chén Zìming cites a now lost text, the *Jīngyàn fùrén fāng* 《經驗婦人方》 (Proven Formulas for Women) as the source for one of his treatments for "postpartum Child's Pillow abdominal pain." Here is Chén Zìmíng's explanation of Child's Pillow Pain, found in Volume Twenty, Chapter Seven, titled "Discourse and Formulas for Postpartum Child's Pillow Stabbing Pain in the Heart and Abdomen."

夫兒枕者，由母胎中宿有血塊，因產時其血破散與兒俱下，則無患也。若產婦臟腑風冷，使血凝滯，在於小腹不能流通，則令結聚疼痛，名曰兒枕也。

《產寶》論產後心腹痛者，由產後氣血俱虛，遇風寒乘之，與血氣相搏，隨氣上衝於心；或下攻於腹，故令心腹痛。若久痛不止，則變成疝瘕也。

Child's Pillow is due to the abiding presence of blood clots in the mother's womb. When the mother's blood at the time of childbirth is broken up and scattered, and descends completely along with the child, there will be no trouble as a result. If the *zàng* and *fǔ* organs of a woman in childbirth contract wind-cold, this causes the blood to congeal and stagnate, so that it is unable to flow in the lesser abdomen. As a result, this causes bound and gathering [blood] and pain, which is called Child's Pillow.

In the discussion of postpartum heart and abdominal pain in the *Chǎnbǎo*, it is [said to be] caused by dual vacuity of Qì and blood after childbirth and a subsequent encounter of wind-cold that exploits this condition. Battling with the Qì and blood, [the wind-cold] follows the Qì upward to rush against the heart or downward to attack the abdomen. This causes heart and abdominal pain. If there is long-term pain that does not stop, [the condition] transforms into *shàn* Mounding and Conglomerations.

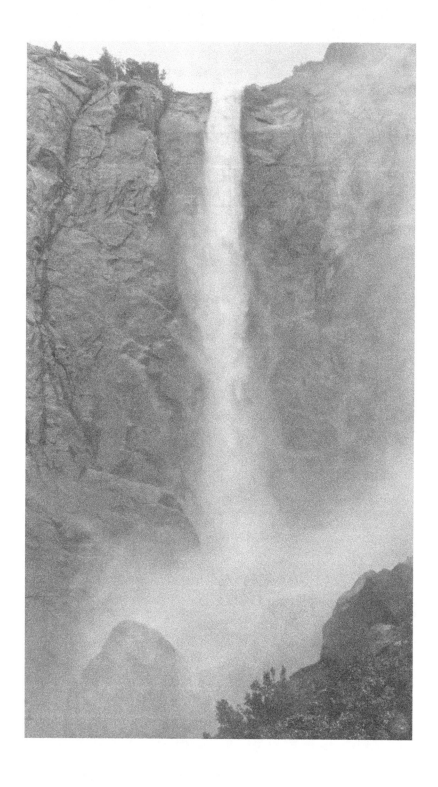

木香通氣丸

治氣刺疼痛。

京三棱		木香	
莪朮	各四兩	檳榔	各一兩
芫花	各一兩	大腹子	

上將米醋三斤同煮，令醋盡。獨去芫花。炒令乾，
餘五味切片子，焙為末，白麵糊和丸，如豌豆大。
橘皮湯下三十九，以止為度。

Mùxiāng Tōng Qì Wán
(Costusroot Qì-Flow-Promoting Pill)

A treatment for stabbing Qì pain.

jīngsānléng	*4 liǎng*	mùxiāng	
ézhú	*each*	bīnláng	*1 liǎng*
yuánhuā	*1 liǎng*	dàfùzǐ	*each*

Simmer the ingredients above all together in 3 *jīn* of rice
vinegar until the vinegar has evaporated. Only remove the
yuánhuā. Stir-fry [the herb mixture] until dry, then take the
remaining five ingredients and chop them into flakes. Roast
and pulverize them, mix with a white flour and water paste
into pills the size of peas. Drink down 30 pills [per dose] in
a decoction of tangerine peel and take as your measurement
when [the pain] stops.

玉抱肚

治停寒瘤冷疾，心腹刺痛。常系於臍腹間甚妙。

鄭主簿傳一方，用針砂如上法炒訖，止入硇砂半兩，並不用餘藥。

針砂 (鐵銚內炒，用柳條或小竹不住手攪煙出為度，放冷)	一兩
白礬	各二錢
粉霜	
硇砂	半兩

上件，白礬等三味同研為細末，與針砂拌和作一服。以水數點洒，用匙拌擁令濃，皮紙為貼，闊二寸以上，長四五寸，貼之。外以帕子系疼處，或常系臍下。如覺太熱，即以衣襯之。

若藥力過，再洒水如前，拌，用。其熱如初，可用四五次。藥力退，則將針砂再炒過，別入餘藥，仍可用。

Yù Bào Dù
(Jade Wrapping the Belly)

A treatment for urgent conditions of cold collecting and intractable coolness with stabbing pain in the heart and abdomen. It is most marvelous if you constantly tie it around the area of the umbilicus.

Assistant Magistrate Zhèng transmitted one recipe that uses the zhēnshā as in the method below but when finished stir-frying it, stops there and adds only 0.5 *liǎng* of náoshā but does not use any of the other medicinals.

zhēnshā (stir-fry in an iron kettle, using a willow branch or small bamboo stick to stir it continuously until it starts smoking, then let it cool down)	1 *liǎng*
báifán	2 *qián* each
fěnshuāng	
náoshā	0.5 *liǎng*

Of the ingredients above, grind the three ingredients from the báifán on together into a fine powder and combine with the zhēnshā to make one dose. Sprinkle several drops of water [on the mixture] and stir and gather it together with a spoon until it is a thick consistency. Make a plaster with packaging paper that is more than 2 *cùn* wide and 4-5 *cùn* long. Stick it on and tie it with a handkerchief on the outside, to the painful location. Or tie it to wear it all the time below the umbilicus. If you feel that it is too hot, line it with cloth.

If the strength of the medicinals has expired, sprinkle more water on it, as in the method above, mix it, and use. Its heat will be as strong as in the beginning. You can use it four or five times. When the strength of the medicinals has declined, take the zhēnshā and stir-fry it again, but do not add the other medicinals. You can still use it like that.

五香拈痛丸

木香	
官桂	
丁香	
乳香	各半兩
藿香葉	
沉香	
斑蝥	七枚
巴豆(去油)	三粒

上八味為細末，白麵糊丸，梧桐子大。每服五十丸，薑湯送下。

Wǔ Xiāng Niān Tòng Wán
(Five Fragrances Pain-Plucking Pill)

mùxiāng	
guān'guì	
dīngxiāng	
rŭxiang	0.5 *liǎng* each
huòxiāngyè	
chénxiāng	
bānmáo	7 specimens
bādòu (remove the oil)	3 seeds

Process the eight ingredients above into a fine powder and mix with white flour and water paste to form pills the size of *wútóng* seeds. Take 50 pills per dose and drink them down in a decoction of ginger.

第三十四問

下利經水反斷者，何也？

答曰：穀入於胃，脈道乃行；水入於經，其血乃成。胃，水穀之海也。

腸胃虛弱，為風邪冷熱之氣所乘，不能腐化穀食，先泄後變成利也。受熱則赤，虛寒則白。穀氣內虛，津液耗減，所以下利而經水反斷也。

經云：利止經當自下，故宜先治利也。

QUESTION THIRTY-FOUR

What is the Reason for Disinhibition Below but With a Paradoxical Interruption in the Flow of the Menstrual Fluids?

ANSWER: When grain enters the stomach, the vessel pathways flow. When water enters the channels, their blood is completed. The stomach is the Sea of Water and Grain.

In a situation where the intestines and stomach are weak, they get overwhelmed by the Qì of wind evil, coolness, and heat, so that they are unable to decompose food. First there is leakage, then this transforms into disinhibition below. Contraction of heat results in red coloration, vacuity cold in white coloration. Because of the internal depletion of grain Qì and diminishment of fluids, there is disinhibition below but then a paradoxical interruption in the flow of the menstrual fluids.

The Classic states: When the disinhibition stops, menstruation must descend again on its own accord. For this reason, you should first treat the disinhibition.

Discussion

Any reader who knows a bit of classical medical Chinese will wonder why I have chosen the awkward term "disinhibition" instead of the more common "diarrhea," to translate the Chinese term 利 *lì*, or here sometimes in the compound 下利 *xià lì* "disinhibition below," in this question. My reason is the need to show the conundrum that is posed in this question by the paradoxical symptoms of diarrhea and interrupted menstruation. From a biomedical perspective and for most clinical practitioners, loose bowels are simply a fairly common side effect of menstruation. It is only when we look at both of these processes, diarrhea and interrupted menstruation, as pathological manifestations of two similar forms of necessary and physiological downward and outward movements of substances in the body, which in the first case is pathologically disinhibited but in the second case pathologically inhibited, that we understand the paradoxical nature of this question. Once you have grasped this essential connection, feel free to replace "disinhibition" in the translation of the question and answer, and in the following formulas, with "diarrhea."

The stomach is the "Sea of Water and Grain," or in other words, the container that must hold solid and liquid foods and process them by decomposition. As the result of this process, grain Qì and fluids are extracted, to nourish the body and, among many other important processes, provide fuel and moisture for the formation of the blood. When the external evils of wind, cold, or heat impede this process so that the ingested substances leak or drain out instead of being processed and absorbed, blood lacks its basic building blocks, and its flow is interrupted as a result.

The "Classic" referred to in the last line most likely refers to the *Màijīng*, which contains the following passage in an almost literal quotation. The only addition is the explanation that stopped diarrhea means that the fluids have a chance to recover, as a result of which the menstrual flow returns on its own accord:

問曰：婦人病下利，而經水反斷者，何也？

師曰：但當止利，經自當下。勿怪。所以利不止而血斷者，但下利亡
津液，故經斷。利止，津液複，經當自下。

Question: Why is it that women fall ill with disinhibition below but
with a paradoxical interruption in the flow of the menstrual fluids?

The teacher answered: You must only stop the disinhibition, and
menstruation must descend again on its own accord. Do not consider
this strange. The reason why disinhibition that is not stopped leads to
interruption in [the flow of] blood is merely that disinhibition below
collapses the fluids, and therefore the menstrual period is interrupted.
When the disinhibition is stopped, the fluids recover, and the menstrual
period must descend again on its own accord.

For treatment, the take-away here is that while traditional Chinese gynecology places great emphasis on restoring the free flow of menstrual fluid,
it is essential to diagnose carefully what the cause of the interruption is
and to treat that cause, rather than just prescribing medicinal or manual
treatments that restore the bleeding. In the present case, prescribing
drastic formulas to "break the blood" or "free the flow," known in Chinese
as 通經藥 tōngjīngyào ("medicinals to free the menstrual flow," or emme-
nagogues in biomedical terminology), would be a tempting approach for
a mediocre medical practitioner who only sees the stopped menstruation and misses the root condition of weakness in the digestive system
compounded by the presence of external evils. Such a treatment might
succeed in temporarily restoring the menses and thus perhaps even satisfy
an unsuspecting patient, but at what price? These drastic medicinals would
surely aggravate the weakness in the stomach and intestines and further
deprive the body of the fluids that it needs for its healthy functioning. And
without additional treatment of the root condition, the problem of the
interrupted menses would surely return in the following month. If such
a patient originally consulted the practitioner because of fertility issues,
a harsh treatment of forcibly restoring the menstrual flow would have
the opposite long-term effect of only further weakening this patient's
digestive system and worsening the collapse of fluids.

大斷下丸

治下利不止。

附子	二兩
細辛(去蘆)	一兩半
乾薑	三兩
高良薑	五兩
肉豆蔻	
訶子皮	各二兩
龍骨	
赤石脂	各三兩
牡蠣(醋紙泥固濟火)	二兩
酸石榴皮(去穰,醋炙黑,心存性)	二兩
白礬(火飛)	二兩
陽起石(火燒赤,醋淬,別研)	三兩

上為細末,麵糊丸,梧桐子大。每服五十丸,米飲空心下。

Dà Duàn Xià Wán
(Major Interrupting-Downward-Flow Pill)

A treatment for incessant disinhibition below.

fùzǐ	2 *liǎng*
xìxīn (remove shoots)	1.5 *liǎng*
gānjiāng	3 *liǎng*
gāoliángjiāng	5 *liǎng*
ròudòukòu	
hēzǐpí	2 *liǎng* each
lónggǔ	
chìshízhī	3 *liǎng* each
mǔlì (seal it with mud in paper sprinkled with vinegar and [expose this to] fire)	2 *liǎng*
suānshíliúpí (remove the pith and mix-fry in vinegar until blackened [on the outside] with the core left uncharred)	2 *liǎng*
báifán (sublime by fire)	2 *liǎng*
yángqǐshí (burn over a flame until red, quench in vinegar, and grind separately)	3 *liǎng*

Process the ingredients above into a fine powder and form pills with a flour and water paste, the size of *wútóng* seeds. Take 50 pills per dose, drinking them down on an empty stomach in thin rice gruel.

滲濕湯

治濕勝濡泄。

白朮	一兩半
蒼朮(炒)	半兩
濃朴	
肉桂	
丁香	各一兩
乾薑	
陳皮	
細辛	各一兩
白茯苓	
肉豆蔻	半兩
砂仁	二兩
附子(同薑炒令赤，去薑，先炮切片)	二隻八錢者

上為粗末，每服四錢，水盞半，薑五片，棗二枚，煎一盞。食前熱服。

Shèn Shī Tāng
(Dampness-Percolating Decoction)

A treatment for dampness prevailing and soggy diarrhea.

báizhú	1.5 *liǎng*
cāngzhú (stir-fry)	0.5 *liǎng*
nóngpò	
ròuguì	1 *liǎng* each
dīngxiāng	
gānjiāng	
chénpí	
xìxīn	1 *liǎng* each
báifúlíng	
ròudòukòu	0.5 *liǎng*
shārén	2 *liǎng*
fùzǐ (stir-fry together with the gānjiāng until red and then remove the gānjiāng. First blast-fry and cut into slices)	2 pieces, 8 *qián*

Process the ingredients above into a fine powder and take 4 *qián* per dose, simmering it in 1.5 cups of water with five ginger slices and two jujubes until reduced to 1 cup. Take hot before meals.

第三十五問

婦人晝則明了，暮則譫語，如見鬼狀者，何也？

答曰：此婦人因傷寒之病，熱入於血室也。

何以明之？室者，屋室也，謂可以停止之處。人身之血室者，營血停止之所，經脈留會之處，即衝脈也。

衝為血海，王冰云「陰靜海滿而去血」，內經云「任脈通，太衝脈盛，月事以時下」者，是也。

若經水適來，感其寒邪之所搏，則熱入血室。其証晝則明了，暮則譫語，如見鬼狀者，此為熱入血室也。

若施治其病者，當無犯胃氣及上二焦，必自愈。

QUESTION THIRTY-FIVE

What Is the Reason for Women Being Lucid during the Day but Speaking Deliriously When the Sun Sets, as If They Were Seeing Ghosts?

ANSWER: This is a gynecological disease caused by cold damage and by heat entering the Blood Chamber.

How do we know this? Chamber means a house, referring to a place where you can stop moving and stay. The Blood Chamber in the human body is the place where *yíng* Provisioning and blood stop and where the channels come together. Thus, it is precisely the Chōngmài.

The Chōngmài is the Sea of Blood. This is what Wáng Bīng's statement, "when Yīn is still and the Sea is filled, the [menstrual] blood leaves," and the *Nèijīng* statement, "the flow in the Rènmài goes through, the flow in the Great Chōngmài is exuberant, and the monthly period therefore descends in time," are referring to.

If [the woman] suffers an assault by cold evil right at the moment when her menstrual fluids arrive, heat enters the Blood Chamber as a result. The evidence for this situation of heat entering the Blood Chamber is precisely lucidity during the day but delirious speaking when the sun sets, as if she were seeing ghosts.

If you carry out a treatment of this condition, you must not assail stomach Qì and the Middle and Upper Jiāo. In that case, she will invariably recover on her own accord.

DISCUSSION

For a discussion of the concept of the Blood Chamber, see *Channeling the Moon, Part One*, pp. 141-144. While the precise identity of this term is still being debated by scholars and practitioners of Chinese medicine today, from the uterus to the Chōngmài to the liver and heart, I suggest that we follow Nie Huimin, as cited in Guohui Liu's *Discussion of Cold Damage*, p. 423:

> After carefully reviewing all interpretations about this issue, everyone has their own explanation. But if one studies it carefully based on [Chinese medicine] theory, it would be appropriate to consider the blood chamber as the womb. Concerning the term "invasion of the blood chamber by heat," one must understand that it is based on clinical practice. This term does not only refer to the location of the disease but also to the cause of the disease, indicating that the condition of the womb during menstruation is relevant to the onset of the disease. However, the occurrence of the disease is not limited to the womb, as the human being is a network and the womb is not isolated from other organs. For example, the liver stores and regulates blood; its channel circulates through the lower abdomen and goes around the genital organs, while the chong channel starts at the womb. Obviously the chong channel has a close relation to the womb; therefore, the invasion of the blood chamber by heat cannot be located only in the womb...

As such, this condition must involve not only the womb but also the liver channel as the organ that stores the blood, the Chōngmài as the Sea of Blood, and even the heart, both because of its involvement with the flow of blood in the vessels and because it is connected to the Chōngmài. Heat that rises from the womb along the Chōngmài up to the heart can therefore affect the Shén, which resides in the heart, and thereby cause delirious speech.

The passages cited above by Wáng Bīng and from the *Nèijīng* both refer the reader back to the famous account of female development in multiples of seven that is found in *Sùwèn* Chapter One, the "Treatise on Heavenly

Perfection in the Ancient Past" 《上古天真論》. Wáng Bīng is the famous editor and commentator on the *Sùwèn* who lived from 710 to 805 CE. The *Sùwèn* passage referred to in the two quotations above is cited, translated and discussed in Question Four of the *Hundred Questions on Gynecology* (found in *Channeling the Moon, Part One*, pp. 100-107). Both citations explain the physiological process by which a woman's menstrual period begins flowing at the age of two times seven.

While Qí Zhòngfǔ's answer cites the *Sùwèn* and Wáng Bīng's commentary on that text as his sources, a solid practitioner of classical Chinese medicine will immediately recognize this whole answer as derived from the section on Tàiyáng disease in the *Shānghánlùn*《傷寒論》 (Treatise on Cold Damage) by Zhāng Zhòngjǐng 張仲景:

> 婦人中風發熱惡寒，經水適來，得之七八日，熱除而脈遲身涼，胸脅下滿如結胸狀，譫語者，此為熱入血室也，當刺期門，隨其實而瀉之。

> 婦人中風七八日，續得寒熱，發作有時，經水適斷者，此為熱入血室，其血必結，故使如瘧狀，發作有時，小柴胡湯主之。

> 婦人傷寒發熱，經水適來，晝日明了，暮則譫語，如見鬼狀者，此為熱入血室。無犯胃氣及上二焦，必自愈。

When a woman experiences wind strike with heat effusion and aversion to cold right when the menstrual fluids arrive, and after seven or eight days the heat [effusion] is eliminated, the pulse becomes slow, and the body cool, and she has fullness in the chest and below the rib-sides as in a chest bind, with delirious speech, this means heat has entered the Blood Chamber. Needle Qīmén (LV-14), following the repletion and draining it.

When a woman continues to suffer from intermittent eruptions of [aversion to] cold and heat [effusion] seven or eight days after a wind strike and the menstrual fluids are interrupted right at that moment, this means that heat has entered the Blood Chamber. Her blood is invariably bound, hence causing a presentation like malaria with intermittent eruptions. Xiǎo Cháihú Tāng rules this.

When a woman suffers from cold damage with heat effusion right when the menstrual fluids arrive, with lucidity during the day but delirious speech as if she were seeing ghosts when the sun sets, this is heat entering the Blood Chamber. You must not assault stomach Qì and the Middle and Upper Jiāo, and she will invariably recover on her own accord.

The parallels to Qí Zhòngfǔ's answer above are striking and would surely have been recognized by any educated reader of his times. This connection is also reinforced below by the fact that Qí lists a variation of Xiǎo Cháihú Tāng as the treatment for this condition.

The key point to take away from this question and answer is that delirious speech, when occurring in women and only at night, must not be treated directly in the upper part of the body as a Shén disturbance! Instead, we must recognize it as rooted in wind strike and cold damage and as involving menstruation, the uterus, the Chōngmài, and the liver. When treatment addresses this root condition, her mental instability will resolve on its own.

地黃湯

治熱入血室。

生地	三兩
柴胡	八兩
人參	
黃芩	各二兩
甘草(炙)	
半夏(湯炮七次)	二兩半

上為粗末，每服五錢，水二盞，薑五片，棗一枚，煎一盞，去滓溫服。

Dìhuáng Tāng
(Rehmannia Decoction)

A treatment for heat entering the Blood Chamber.

shēngdìhuáng	3 *liǎng*
cháihú	8 *liǎng*
rénshēn	
huángqín	2 *liǎng* each
gāncǎo (mix-fry)	
bànxià (bring to a rapid boil in hot water 7 times)	2.5 *liǎng*

Process the ingredients above into a fine powder and take 5 *qián* per dose. Simmer in 2 cups of water with 5 slices of ginger and 1 jujube until reduced to 1 bowl, remove the dregs and take warm.

龍齒琥珀散

治產前產後血虛，心神恍惚，語言失度，睡臥不安。

茯神	一兩
人參	
龍齒	
琥珀	
赤芍	各三分
黃芪	
牛膝(去蘆)	
麥門冬(去心)	各一兩半zi
生地	
當歸	半兩

上為粗末，每服三錢，水盞半，煎六分，去滓溫服。不拘時。

Lóngchǐ Hǔpò Sǎn
(Dragon Tooth and Amber Powder)

A treatment for blood vacuity before or after childbirth, with severe confusion in the Shén, unrestrained speech, and restless sleep.

fúshén	1 *liǎng*
rénshēn	
lóngchǐ	
hǔpò	3 *fēn* each
chìsháo	
huángqí	
niúxī (remove shoots)	
màiméndōng (remove the core)	1.5 *liǎng* each
shēngdìhuáng	
dāngguī	0.5 *liǎng*

Process the ingredients above into a fine powder and take 3 *qián* per dose. Simmer down to 60 percent in 1.5 cups of water, remove the dregs and take warm. Do not restrict the timing.

小柴胡加地黃湯

治傷寒發熱，或發寒熱，經水適來或適斷，畫則明了，夜則譫語，如見鬼神。亦治產後惡露方來，忽然斷絕。

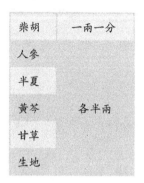

柴胡	一兩一分
人參	
半夏	
黃芩	各半兩
甘草	
生地	

上咀片，每服五錢，水二盞，薑三片，棗二枚，煎八分，去滓溫服。

Xiǎo Cháihú Jiā Dìhuáng Táng
(Minor Bupleurum Plus Rehmannia Decoction)

A treatment for cold damage with heat effusion or with cold and heat effusion, right when the menstrual flow has just arrived or been interrupted, with lucidity during the day but with delirious speech at night, as if seeing ghosts and spirits. It also treats sudden interruption in the flow of lochia postpartum when it has just arrived.

cháihú	1 *liǎng* 1 *fēn*
rénshēn	
bànxià	
huángqín	0.5 *liǎng* each
gāncǎo	
shēngdìhuáng	

Mince and slice the ingredients above and take 5 *qián* per dose. Simmer in 2 cups of water with 3 slices of ginger and 2 jujubes until reduced to 80 percent. Remove the dregs and take warm.

來復丹

亦名正一丹，此藥配類二氣，均調陰陽，奪天地沖和之氣，乃水火既濟之方。可冷可熱，可緩可急。善治營衛不交養，心腎不升降，上實下虛，氣閉痰厥，心腹冷痛，臟腑虛滑，但有胃氣，無不獲安。

硫黃(舶上，透明者)	一兩
硝石(同硫黃，並為細末，入定鍋內，微火炒，用木篦子不住手攪，令陰陽氣相入，不可火太過，恐藥力竭，再研細，名二氣末)	一兩
太陰玄精石(研水飛)	二兩
五靈脂(須五台山者，水澄去砂日乾研)	
陳皮(去白)	各二兩
青皮(去白)	

上用五靈脂二橘皮為細末，次入玄精石末，及前二藥末拌勻。好醋打糊為丸，豌豆大，每服三十粒，鹽湯下。甚者五十粒。

Lái Fù Dān
(Arriving and Returning Elixir)

Also called Zhèng Yī Dān ("Righting the One Elixir"), this medicine matches up the two Qì in all categories, fine-tunes the balance of Yīn and Yáng, and captures the amiably flow-ing Qì of heaven and earth, in a formula represented by *Jìjì*, the Consummation of Water and Fire. It is permissible for coolness or heat, for relaxation or urgency. It is excellent at treating a failure of *yíng* Provisioning and *wèi* Defense to interact with and nurture each other, a failure of the heart and kidney to upbear and downbear, repletion above and vacuity below, Qì blockage and phlegm Reversal, cold pain in the heart and abdomen, and vacuity and slippery outflow from the *zàng* and *fǔ* organs. If only the stomach Qì is still present, you cannot but obtain calm.

liúhuáng (the imported transparent kind)	1 *liǎng*
xiāoshí (process together with the liúhuáng into a fine powder, place in a stable pot, and stir-fry over a gentle flame, stirring it constantly with a wooden strainer to thoroughly mix the Qì of Yīn and Yáng. Do not allow the flame to get too strong, out of concern that it will exhaust the force of the medicine. Grind it again finely. This is called "Two Qì Powder.")	1 *liǎng*
tàiyīnxuánjīng shí (water-grind it)	2 *liǎng*
wǔlíngzhī (must be from Wǔtái Mountain, let it settle in water, remove the sand, dry it in the sun, and grind it)	2 *liǎng* each
chénpí (remove the white parts)	
qīngpí (remove the white parts)	

Of the ingredients above, process the wǔlíngzhī and the two kinds of citrus peel into a fine powder, next add the powdered xuánjīngshí and then blend this evenly with the last two medicinals. Mix it with high-quality vinegar into a paste and form into pills the size of peas. Take 30 pills per dose and down them in hot salty water. In serious cases, take 50 [pills per dose].

FORMULA NOTE

The indications section of this formula requires some explanations. First off, a reader knowledgeable in the history of Daoism will immediately recognize the phrase 正一 zhèngyī in the alternate name for this formula, 正一丹 Zhèng Yī Dān, which I have translated as "Righting the One Elixir." The term zhèngyī is famous for being the name of a major branch of Daoism and is usually translated as "Orthodox Unity" in that context. I have intentionally chosen a different translation here to alert the reader that this formula most likely had nothing to do with Daoist practices. While contemporary accounts of the school of Zhèngyī Daoism correctly situate its origin in the Hàn dynasty, it was known at that time as the "Way of the Celestial Masters" (天師道 Tiānshī Dào), and only its teachings were known as "orthodox unity" zhèngyī. It would thus be historically incorrect to introduce this association with Daoism and its struggles over orthodoxy into the name of a medical formula that aims at harmonizing the two Qì to produce a harmonious state of calm oneness.

Another issue in need of clarification is the phrase "consummation of Water and Fire" (水火既濟 shuǐhuǒ jìjì), which is clearly a reference to the name of the second to last hexagram 既濟 Jìjì ("Consummation") in the Yijīng, a combination of water on top of fire ䷾. In its perfectly balanced alternation of solid and broken, Yīn and Yáng lines, this hexagram visually represents the harmony between Yīn and Yáng Qì that this formula aims to achieve.

The balanced and balancing nature of the formula is emphasized in the following description: 可冷可熱，可緩可急 kělěng kěrè, kěhuǎn kějí. Translated literally word for word, it means "can cool, can warm, can relax/slow/moderate, can tense/rapid/critical." It is unclear from the context here and, I believe, left intentionally ambiguous by the author, whether this description refers to the pathologies that this formula is able to address, the therapeutic effects of the formula, or both. In literary Chinese, the same character can function as a verb or adjective and can be active or passive. Thus, the first part of this phrase can be read as "can be cooling or warming," or as "is permissible in cases of coolness or warmth," or even as "can be ingested cool or warm." The second half of the phrase is even more ambiguous, due to the broad range of meanings of the terms 緩 and 急. As a pair of opposites, they can mean "to relax and to tense" or "to slow down and speed up," or "slack and tense," "slow and quick," "moderate and urgent," or even "mild and acute" in reference to the nature of a patient's condition. I have tried to replicate this ambiguity as much as that is possible in modern English.

Regarding the reference to imported sulfur, the origin of this product must have been Japan, since sulfur was, next to gold and timber, one of its main commodities for export to China already at this period.[4]

---

4 Richard von Glahn, "The Ningbo-Hakata Merchant Network and the Reorientation of East Asian Maritime Trade, 1150-1350," p. 269.

第三十六問

顛狂之病，何以別之？

答曰：入並於陰則為顛，入並於陽則為狂。皆由風邪之所致也。

顛者，猝然僕地，嘔吐涎沫，口喎目急，手足撩戾，無所覺知，良久乃蘇。狂者，或言語不避親疏，或因自高賢，或棄衣踰走，亦有自定之時。又在有胎之時，其母猝大驚，亦令子氣發癇。

其顛有五：一曰陽顛，二曰陰顛，三曰風顛，四曰濕顛，五曰勞顛。此皆隨其感病之由而命名也。又有牛馬豬狗顛，以其顛發之時，聲形狀似於牛馬等，故以為名也。

俗云：病顛之人，忌食六畜肉，顛發之狀，悉皆象之。

Question Thirty-Six

How Do We Differentiate Between the Diseases of *Diān* Insanity and *Kuáng* Mania?

ANSWER: When [the disease] enters into Yīn, it results in *diān* insanity; when it enters into Yáng, it results in *kuáng* mania. Both of these diseases are caused by wind evil.

Diān insanity is characterized by suddenly falling to the ground, vomiting up saliva and foam, deviated mouth and rapidly moving eyes, arms and legs jerking uncontrollably, loss of consciousness, and recovery after a good long while. *Kuáng* mania is characterized possibly by unrestrained speech with no distinction between relatives and strangers, or by self-aggrandizement, or by running about naked, and also by having times when it settles down on its own accord. It also happens that a mother, when carrying a fetus, suddenly experiences great panic, which can also cause the Qì of the child to suffer from seizures.

There are five types of *diān* insanity: The first is called Yáng insanity, the second Yīn insanity, the third wind insanity, the fourth dampness insanity, and the fifth taxation insanity. These are all named in accordance with the cause from which they contracted the disease. In addition, there are [the types of] cow, horse, pig, or dog insanity, which are named according to the sounds and appearance of the patient during an episode resembling those of a cow, horse, etc.

It is commonly said that a person sick with *diān* insanity must avoid eating the meat of the six domestic animals [given the fact that] the appearance of a *diān* episode will completely resemble them.

Discussion

The translation of the term 顛 *diān* (or in the more common and perhaps more accurate form with the disease radical as 癲) is a conundrum that has plagued me for years. During my work on Sūn Sīmiǎo's writings on pediatrics, where this term makes a frequent appearance, I decided that Nigel Wiseman's translation as "withdrawal," while creating a nice contrast to 狂 *kuáng* (translated as "mania"), is not strong enough to adequately reflect the meaning of this disease in classical Chinese medicine. Coming at it from a very different angle and giving you a sense of the broad range of the term, *diān* is often translated as "epilepsy" in contemporary writings. This is certainly an important aspect of its pathology, but again, I don't find the overlap close enough to be acceptable in the context of historical sources, based on the different etiologies and associated signs and symptoms. As with its Yáng counterpart 狂 ("*kuáng* mania"), I have thus chosen to keep the English term for this Yīn type of mental derangement in pīnyīn, as *diān* insanity.

To better understand what this term meant for the original authors and readers of the classical literature, let us once again consult Cháo Yuánfāng's *Zhūbìng yuánhòu lùn* from 610 CE. My justification for so frequently referring back to this text is that it is obvious that Qí Zhòngfǔ himself used it as one of his main sources, as the numerous citations throughout the *Hundred Questions* prove. In Volume Thirty-Seven in the section on gynecological disorders, we find an almost literal quotation of the entire answer above, including a few helpful additional words to indicate, for example, that a person afflicted by this disease may not eat the meat of the domestic animals because if they do, the manifestation of the *diān* outbreak will then resemble that of the animal they have consumed.

In the second volume of the *Zhūbìng yuánhòu lùn*, which is dedicated to a discussion of wind disorders, we find three entries that discuss *diān* and *kuáng* as forms of mental derangement caused by wind with a bit more detail than the gynecology passage. I quote them at length to give the reader an impression of the relationship between these two texts and a bit more clinical information. One notable difference is that the passage below lists the fifth type of *diān* insanity as "horse insanity," while both Qí Zhòngfǔ and Cháo Yuánfāng in the gynecological section list it as "taxation insanity."

風癲候

風癲者，由血氣虛，邪入於陰經故也。人有血氣少，則心虛而精神離散，魂魄妄行，因為風邪所傷，故邪入於陰，則為癲疾。又人在胎，其母卒大驚，精氣並居，令子發癲。其發則仆地，吐涎沫，無所覺是也。…

THE SIGNS OF WIND DIĀN

Wind *diān* is caused by vacuity of blood and Qì and by evil entering the Yīn channels. When a person has a shortage of blood and Qì, the heart becomes vacuous, the Jīngshén gets scattered, and the *hún* and *pò* souls move frenetically. Because of damage from wind evil, the evil enters Yīn and causes the disease of *diān* insanity. Moreover, when a person is still in the womb and their mother suddenly experiences great panic, her Essence and Qì combine [with the evil Qì] and lodge there [in the womb], causing the child to suffer from eruptions of *diān* insanity. Eruptions of this disease result in falling to the ground, vomiting up saliva and foam, and loss of consciousness. …

五癲病候

五癲者，一曰陽癲，發如死人，遺尿，食頃乃解；二曰陰癲，初生小時，臍瘡未愈，數洗浴，因此得之；三曰風癲，發時眼目相引，牽縱反強，羊鳴，食頃方解。由熱作汗出當風，因房室過度，醉飲，令心意逼迫，短氣脈悸得之；四曰濕癲，眉頭痛，身重。坐熱沐頭，濕結，腦沸未止得之；五曰馬癲，發作時時，反目口噤，手足相引，身體皆熱。…

The five types of *diān* insanity are as follows: First, Yáng *diān* manifests with episodes [that cause the patient] to resemble a dead person and urinate involuntarily and that resolve shortly in the time it takes to eat a meal. Second, Yīn *diān* is contracted by newborns and small children because they have umbilical sores that have not healed and are washed repeatedly. Third, wind *diān* manifests with eyes that are rolled in towards each other, convulsions, arched-back rigidity, and bleating like a goat or sheep, all of which resolve shortly in the time it takes to eat a meal. It is contracted from exposure to wind when heat that has made the person sweat, from excessive sexual intercourse, and from drinking alcohol, causing emotional distress, shortness of breath, and palpitations in the pulse. Fourth, dampness *diān* causes pain between the eyebrows and generalized heaviness. It is contracted from heat [while] washing the head and dampness in the topknot, resulting in incessant boiling in the brain. Fifth, horse *diān* [is characterized by] constant outbreaks with rolled-back eyes, clenched mouth, convulsions in the arms and legs, and heat all over the body....

四十五、風狂病候

狂病者，由風邪入並受於陽所為也。風邪入血，使人陰陽二氣虛實不調，若一實一虛，則令血氣相並。氣並受於陽，則為狂發，或欲走，或自高賢，稱神聖是也。又肝藏魂，悲哀動中則傷魂，魂傷則狂忘不精明，不敢正當人，陰縮而攣筋，兩脅骨不舉，毛瘁色夭，死於秋。皆由血氣虛，受風邪，致令陰陽氣相並所致，故名風狂。

The Signs of Wind Kuáng Disease

Kuáng mania is caused by wind evil entering and aligning itself with [the patient's] Yáng. Wind evil enters the blood and causes an imbalance of vacuity and repletion between the two Qì of Yīn and Yáng. A state of repletion in one and vacuity in the other causes blood and Qì to combine [with the evil]. If the combined Qì is received in Yáng, *kuáng* mania erupts, possibly with wanting to run, or with self-aggrandizement, calling oneself a god or sage. Furthermore, the liver stores the *hún* souls, and when grief stirs up the center, this damages the *hún*. Damage to the *hún* souls results in mania, forgetfulness, and mental confusion, not daring to face others straight on, retracted genitals and convulsed sinews, inability to raise the ribs, brittle hair and a dark withered complexion, and death in autumn. All of these signs are caused by vacuity in the blood and Qì and contraction of wind evil, which has caused the Qì of Yīn and Yáng to both combine with it. Therefore it is called wind *kuáng* mania.

大聖一粒金丹

治諸風驚癇。

大川烏頭	
黑附子	各二兩
白附子	
白蒺藜 (炒，去刺)	各一兩
五靈脂	
沒藥 (別研)	半兩
白礬(枯，別研)	半兩
白殭蠶 (去絲，炒)	一兩
麝香 (淨肉)	半兩
細香墨 (別研)	半兩
朱砂 (別研)	半兩
金箔 (為衣)	二百片

上將前六味同為細末，後四味研細，合和。用井華水一盞，研墨盡為度，將墨汁搜和，杵臼內搗五百下。丸如彈子大，金箔為衣陰乾。

每服一粒，食後臨臥，生姜自然汁磨化，入熱酒服，再以熱酒隨意多少飲之。應無風暖處臥，衣被蓋覆，汗出即瘥。

病小者，每粒分作二服。忌發風物。孕婦不可服。

Dà Shèng Yī Lì Jīn Dān
(Great Sage Single Pill Gold Elixir)

A treatment for all sorts of wind panic seizures.

large chuānwūtóu	
hēifùzǐ	2 *liǎng* each
báifùzǐ	
báijílí (stir-fry and remove spines)	1 *liǎng* each
wǔlíngzhī	
mòyào (grind separately)	0.5 *liǎng*
báifán (dried, grind separately)	0.5 *liǎng*
báijiāngcán (remove silk and stir-fry)	1 *liǎng*
shèxiāng (clean the meat)	0.5 *liǎng*
xìxiāngmò (grind separately)	0.5 *liǎng*
zhūshā (grind separately)	0.5 *liǎng*
jīnbó (make a coating)	200 flakes

Of the ingredients above, process the first six together into a
fine powder. Grind the following four ingredients finely and
blend them well. Use a cup of well-flower water[1] to rub the
ink stick in an ink stone until it is completely dissolved as
your measure. Use the liquid ink to make everything come
together harmoniously and pound in a mortar with a pestle
500 times. Shape into pellet-sized pills, coat with the gold
leaf, and dry in the shade.

Take one pill per dose. After a meal, when [the patient] is
about to lie down, grind it up in pure juice [extracted] from

---

1 For an explanation on the significance of "well-flower water," see my Formula
Note for Sūhéxiāng Wán (Storax Pill) in Question Twenty-One above.

fresh ginger and then make her ingest it by adding it to heated rice wine. In addition, have her drink as much heated rice wine as she feels like. She should lie down in a place that is warm and not exposed to wind and cover herself with clothes and blankets. When she sweats, it means recovery.

If the disease is minor, each pill can be divided into two doses. Avoid substances that bring wind to the surface. Pregnant women must not take this medicine.

FORMULA NOTE

After much thought, I have decided that the only way to make sense of the instructions for this formula is by changing the order of ingredients and placing the zhūshā ahead of the xìxiāngmò, which literally just means "fine fragrant ink." Other citations of this formula, whether in various editions of the *Nǚkē bǎiwèn* or in the slightly earlier *Tàipíng Huìmín Héjìjú fāng* 《太平惠民和劑局方》 (Tàipíng Formulary from the Imperial Grace Pharmacy) 1078, where it is listed as a formula for wind strike in both men and women, maintain the same order and instructions and are therefore not helpful in solving this conundrum. If we place the ink (listed as xìxiāngmò in the table above) below the zhūshā, however, it becomes possible to follow the instructions for this formula: Process the first six ingredients into a fine powder and then grind the next four ingredients, including the zhūshā, separately first, before blending all these pulverized ingredients with each other. Next process the ink by grinding it with the well-flower water until completely dissolved, and pour this liquid over the powdered ingredients, pounding everything thoroughly until you create a smooth paste that can be shaped into pills.

A slightly different version of the formula found in another Sòng dynasty text called *Chuánxìn shìyòng fāng* 《傳信適用方》 (Trusted Transmitted Formulas for Clinical Application) from 1180, supports this reading: After first listing the same first six ingredients and instructing to pulverize them, that text then lists báifán, zhūshā, mòyào, shèxiāng, rǔxiāng, and quánxiē, each to be ground or crushed separately. All of these are combined with each other. Next, the text instructs us to grind ink with well-flower water and then drip this over the powdered ingredients until the mixture can be shaped into round pills the size of pellets. The rest of the instructions is similar to what Qí Zhòngfǔ details above.

While the research for this formula has proven to be a frustrating and time-consuming exercise, it is still interesting to see how inaccurate and careless instructions were copied literally from one text to the next, without any thought given to the actual practical application of the instructions in the clinic. If nothing else, this formula quotation shows that already by the Sòng dynasty, formulas were copied and pasted without careful editing in the compilation of voluminous collections for specialized purposes. This leaves me wondering about how involved Qí Zhòngfǔ himself might have actually been in the production and clinical application of the medicines in his text. On the other hand, it is possible, if less likely in my mind, that these formulas were so well-known, and their preparation so obvious, that he was able to recreate them without consulting his own book and therefore did not notice the mistakes found in the instructions.

Lastly, a note is in order concerning the second to last sentence in the instructions, namely to "Avoid substances that bring wind to the surface." This is a literal translation of the Chinese sentence 忌發風物. Given the location in the formula and the context here, it is likely that this is a warning against consuming any substances that would literally "bring wind to the surface," or in other words, cause another outbreak of mental derangement by stirring up the internal wind that is at the root of this condition.

黃牛丸

治風狂，喜怒不常，或欲狂走。

白龍骨（燒）	
鐵粉（研）	
茯神	
人參	
黃連	各一兩
鉛霜	
犀角（屑）	
防風	
朱砂（研）	
牛黃（研）	一錢
遠志（去心）	一兩
龍腦（研）	一錢
甘草（炙）	半兩
麥門冬（去心）	一兩半

上為細末，如桐子大。每服二十丸，熟水送下，不拘時服。

Huángniú Wán
(Bovine Bezoar Pill)

A treatment for wind *kuáng* mania, abnormal emotions, and possibly a desire to run around manically.

white lónggǔ (burn)	
tiěfěn (grind)	
fúshén	
rénshēn	
huánglián	1 *liǎng* each
qiānshuāng	
xījiǎo (flake)	
fángfēng	
zhūshā (grind)	
niúhuáng (grind)	1 *qián*
yuǎnzhì (remove the core)	1 *liǎng*
lóngnǎo (grind)	1 *qián*
gāncǎo (mix-fry)	0.5 *liǎng*
màiméndōng (remove the core)	1.5 *liǎng*

Process the ingredients above into a fine powder and [form into] pills the size of *wútóng* seeds. Take 20 pills per dose and chase them down in boiled water. Do not restrict the timing.

Formula Note

Translating the name of this formula has proven challenging: As my most likely conclusion, I read 黃牛 *huángniú* as a typographical error that has resulted in a reversal of the characters for 牛黃 *niúhuáng* (bovine bezoar), one of the ingredients of this formula. I have therefore translated the formula title as "Bovine Bezoar Pill." Besides the absence of a strong argument for any other readings, this interpretation is supported by two facts: Most importantly, *niúhuáng* is not only one of the ingredients in this formula, but a very crucial one, given that the formula addresses *kuáng* mania. As the *Shénnóng běncǎo jīng* states, *niúhuáng* is indicated for these conditions:

治驚癇，寒熱，熱盛，狂痙，除邪，逐鬼。

It treats fright seizures, cold and heat, exuberant heat, *kuáng* mania and tetany; expels evil, and drives out ghosts.

A second argument in support of reading Huángniú Wán as an error for Niúhuáng Wán is that the historical medical literature contains numerous variations of Niúhuáng Wán, including some formulas that are quite similar in indications and ingredients to the present formula from texts predating Qí Zhòngfǔ's work, but no other example of formula called Huángniú Wán that does not turn out to be a copy derived from the present text.

As two potential, but unlikely, alternatives, 黃牛 is the name of the domesticated cattle (Bos taurus), which was introduced to China's central plains around 2500-1900 BCE from the Near East. But what would be the significance of naming this formula "Cattle Pill" when it does not even contain any beef as an ingredient? Could it be a reference to the specific type of *diān* insanity that is mentioned in Qí's answer above as one of the five types associated with the five domesticated animals, depending on the manifestation of the insanity and the similarity of the patient's behavior and emitted sounds to those of cattle during an episode of 牛癲 *niúdiān* ("bovine *diān* insanity")? This seems too farfetched to me.

Lastly, could this name possibly be referring in an abbreviated form, as does happen in formula names, to the two ingredients huánglián and niúhuáng, in which case it should be translated as "Coptis and Bovine Bezoar Pill"? Again, this strikes me as a much less likely explanation of the formula title.

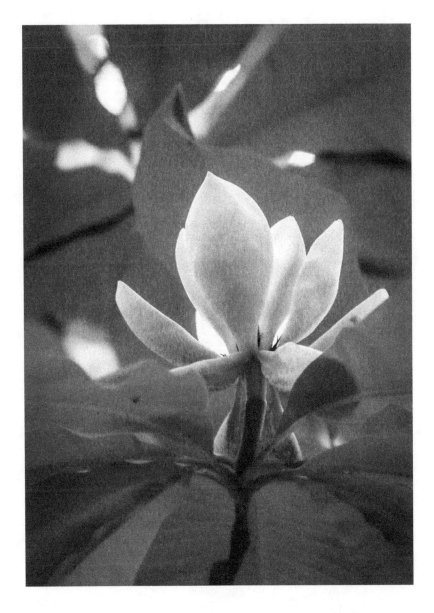

祛邪散

治顛邪惡候。

白礬(生，研)	三兩
黃丹	半兩

上為研細。用桑柴於瓦中燒一伏時。服半錢以乳香湯下。不拘時。

Qū Xié Sǎn
(Evil-Dispelling Powder)

A treatment for *diān* insanity with signs of evil.

báifán (use unprocessed, grind)	3 *liǎng*
huángdān	0.5 *liǎng*

Process the ingredients above by grinding them finely. Use mulberry kindling to burn them inside an earthen pot for twenty-four hours. Take 0.5 *qián* per dose and down it in a decoction of frankincense (*rǔxiāng tang*). Do not restrict the timing.

小柴胡加地黃湯

方見三十五問。每服五錢，水二盞，姜五片，棗二枚，煎八分，去滓溫服。

Xiǎo Cháihú Jiā Dìhuáng Tāng
(Minor Bupleurum Plus Rehmannia Decoction)

For the formula, see Question Thirty-Five above. Take 5 *qián* per dose and simmer it in 2 cups of water with 5 slices of ginger and 2 jujubes until reduced to 80 percent. Remove the dregs and take it warm.

來復丹

治產後熱入血室，如見鬼神狂語者。方見三十五問。以醋湯下十來服。

Lái Fù Dān
(Arriving and Returning Elixir)

A treatment for heat entering the Blood Chamber after childbirth, manifesting with an appearance as if she were seeing ghosts and with manic speech. For the formula, see Question Thirty-Five. Down about ten doses in a vinegar decoction.

第三十七問

病有一臂痛，有兩臂俱痛，何也？

答曰：臂痛有數證。有因寒而得之者，或因伏痰者，有形寒飲冷傷肺者，有汗出傷阻者。

夫肝主諸筋，肝經虛弱，風寒入傷，與氣血相搏，筋寒則急，上連兩臂俱痛。宜服醒風湯、理氣湯主之。

若或左或右，痛不能舉臂者，此由伏痰在內，中腕停滯，脾氣不能流行，止與氣搏。流伏於左則左痛，在右則右痛。

若右臂痛深連於骨，如斧搥，其氣自嗌已下至臍，左右氣不相通徹，其痛發時，氣上奔急，令人悶絕，肌肉日消，漿粥不下，心中煩悶，此由形寒飲冷，肺被寒結留滯於右邊。

若無故一臂無力，痛不能舉，襲襲，似汗偏阻，一邊肌肉時復掣痛，或有不仁，手不能近頭，久成偏枯，宜服百風湯主之。

QUESTION THIRTY-SEVEN

What Is the Reason for Conditions of Pain in One Arm or in Both Arms?

ANSWER: Arm pain has numerous [different] patterns: There are cases of contracting it because of cold, or it can be caused by deep-lying phlegm. There are cases where cold in the physical body or drinking cold fluids have damaged the lung, and there are cases where sweat exiting [has led to] damage and obstruction.

Now, the liver rules all the sinews. When the liver channel is vacuous, wind and cold can enter and cause damage, battling with the Qì and the blood. When the sinews [contract] cold, they tense up. Connecting upwards into the arms, they are both painful. [The patient] should take Xǐng Fēng Tāng (Wind-Rousing Decoction) or Lǐ Qì Tāng (Qì-Patterning Decoction) to rule this [condition].

If it is a case of [the pain] being either on the right or on the left, with pain preventing [the patient] from raising the arm, this is caused by deep-lying phlegm located inside, stagnating in the central stomach duct and preventing spleen Qì from flowing. Stopping and assaulting the Qì, when [the phlegm] streams and hides deep down in the left, pain in the left [arm] results; when it is located in the right, pain in the right [arm] results.

There are cases where there is pain in the right arm so deep as to connect to the bone [and the patient feels] as if being struck by an axe. This Qì reaches from the throat down to the umbilicus, but the Qì on the right side and the Qì on the left fail to flow through to each other. During outbreaks of the pain, the Qì ascends with bolting urgency, causing oppression and expiry in the person. Her flesh melts away with each passing day and she is unable to ingest even thick liquids or porridge and suffers from vexation and oppression in the heart. This condition is caused by cold in the physical body or by drinking cold fluids. The lung is afflicted by the cold, which binds and stagnates on the right side.

Lastly, there are cases where for no apparent reason one arm is without strength and [the patient experiences] pain and inability to raise the arm, a gentle warmth and a feeling as if sweat were unilaterally obstructed, recurring tugging pain in the flesh on one side, possibly with numbness, and inability to reach with the hand close to the head. Over a long period of time, this condition turns into unilateral withering. [The patient] should take Bǎi Fēng Tāng (Hundred-Winds Decoction) to rule this.

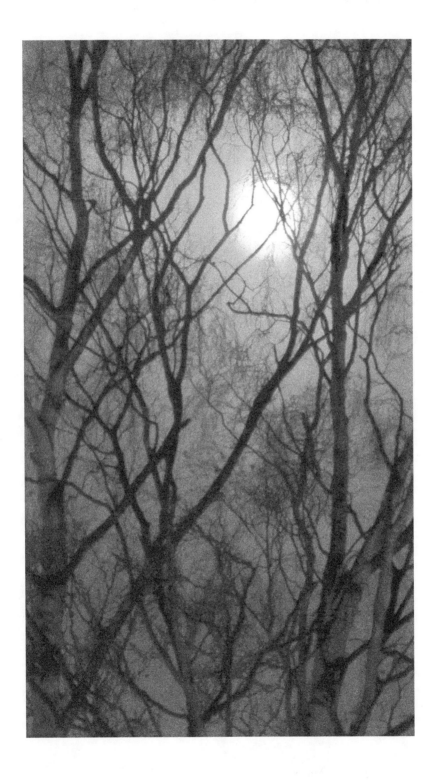

百風湯

治四肢垂曳，骨節疼痛。又名省風湯。

獨活	三錢
芎藭	
防風	
當歸	
桂心	各二兩
茯苓	
附子	
細辛	
天麻	一兩
干蠍（炒）	
甘草	一兩

上為㕮咀，每服三錢。水一盞半，姜五片，煎七分，去滓，食前稍熱服。

Bǎi Fēng Tāng
(Hundred Winds Decoction)

A treatment for drooping and dragging limbs and pain in the bones and joints. It is also called Shěng Fēng Tāng (Wind-Diminishing Decoction).

dúhuó	3 *qián*
xiōngqióng	
fángfēng	
dāngguī	
guìxīn	2 *liǎng* each
fúlíng	
fùzǐ	
xìxīn	
tiānmá	1 *liǎng*
gānxiē (stir-fry)	
gāncǎo	1 *liǎng*

Pound the ingredients above and take 3 *qián* per dose. Simmer in 1.5 cups of water with 5 slices of ginger until reduced to 70 percent. Remove the dregs and take it slightly heated before meals.

Formula Note

Unfortunately, the exact amounts of some of the ingredients are unclear from the way the formula is presented above and in other published editions. Most likely, we are simply missing the character 各 gè, which means "each," after the instruction to use 1 liǎng for tiānmá. How to dose the gānxiē (dried scorpion) is a bit trickier, since the following ingredient is also used in the amount of 1 liǎng. This would suggest that the amount of gānxiē is different. Due to the fact that the amount of gānxiē in classical Chinese formulas is often given as a number of specimens, it is possible or even likely that the amount used here is missing or at least differs from the 1 liǎng that is specified for the ingredients listed before and after it.

茯苓丸

治伏痰臂痛。

茯苓	一兩
半夏	二兩
枳殼 (去穰麩，炒)	半兩
風化樸硝	一分

上為細末，姜汁煮，糊為丸，如桐子大。每服三十丸，食前姜湯下。

Fúlíng Wán
(Poria Pill)

A treatment for arm pain [related to] deep-lying phlegm.

fúlíng	1 *liǎng*
bànxià	2 *liǎng*
zhǐké (remove the pith and bran-fry)	0.5 *liǎng*
fēnghuàpòxiāo	1 *fēn*

Process the ingredients above into a fine powder and boil with ginger juice. Make a paste and form into pills the size of *wútóng* seeds. Take 30 pills per dose and down them in ginger decoction before meals.

理氣湯

治痰飲臂痛。

半夏（湯洗）	二兩
桔梗	一兩
官桂	二兩
人參	一兩
橘皮（洗，乾）	二兩
甘草	半兩

上為麤末。每服五錢，水二盞，姜五片，煎一盞。
去滓，食前服。

Lǐ Qì Tāng
(Qì-Patterning Decoction)

A treatment for arm pain related to phlegm-rheum.

bànxià (wash in hot water)	2 *liǎng*
jiégěng	1 *liǎng*
guānguì	2 *liǎng*
rénshēn	1 *liǎng*
júpí (wash and dry)	2 *liǎng*
gāncǎo	0.5 *liǎng*

Process the ingredients above into a coarse powder. Take 5 *qián* per dose and simmer in 2 cups of water and 5 ginger slices until reduced to 1 cup. Remove the dregs and take before meals.

第三十八問

婦人渴病，與三消之病同異？

答曰：夫渴之為病一也，推其受病之源，所得各
異。

《指迷方》論消渴之病，自來有二：多緣嗜慾太甚，
自為虛寒，服五石湯丸，猛烈燥藥，積之在臟，遂
至精血枯涸。又久飲酒者，酒性酷熱，熏蒸於臟
肺，是致津液耗竭，渴乃生焉。

婦人之渴，多因損血，血虛則熱，熱則能消飲。所
以多渴，故與男子之病有異也。

QUESTION THIRTY-EIGHT

Is the Disease of Thirst in Women the Same or Different from the Three Diseases of Dissipation?

ANSWER: Thirst, as a disease, is a single disease. Extrapolating from the source for the contraction of the disease, what each patient suffers from is different.

The discussion of the disease Dissipation Thirst in the *Zhĭmí fāng* originally recognizes two kinds. In the majority of cases, it is caused by excessive passion and addictions leading to self-inflicted vacuity cold and ingestion of Five Stones decoctions and pills. These violently drying medicinals accumulate in the *zàng* organs and subsequently cause the Essence and blood to dry up. Additionally, there are patients who have been drinking alcohol for a long time. Alcohol is extremely hot by nature and fumigates the *zàng* organs and the lung. This causes the fluids to get exhausted and used up, and the thirst is generated from this.

Women's thirst is predominantly due to injury to the blood. Blood vacuity results in heat, and heat may then result in the dissipation of what the person drinks. For this reason, there is increased thirst. And thus there are differences to the disease in men.

DISCUSSION

The text referred to above as *Zhǐmí fāng* is a reference to the *Quánshēng zhǐmí fāng* 《全生指迷方》 (Formulas for All of Life that Point out Confusion), authored by Wáng Kuàng 王貺 in the early twelfth century. In this text, we find an essay on the "Disease of Dissipation Thirst" that clearly establishes that text as the source for Qí Zhòngfǔ's writing and is helpful for understanding Qí Zhòngfǔ's explanation above.

論曰：消渴之病，其來有二：或少服五石湯丸，恣欲不節，不待年高氣血衰耗，石性獨存，火烈焦槁，精血涸竭，其狀渴而肌肉消。

又有積久飲酒，酒性酷熱，熏蒸五臟，津液枯燥而血澀，其狀渴而肉不消。

如解五石毒者，宜罌粟湯。欲止渴者，宜菟絲子丸。大渴而加煩熱者，宜馬通散、栝蔞粉。

Essay: The disease of Dissipation Thirst originally has two sources: Sometimes patients in their younger years have taken Five Stones decoctions or pills and given free rein to their desires without restraint, as a result of which their Qì and blood have become exhausted before they reach old age. It is the nature of stones to prevail in solitude without offspring, and their fire ravenously scorches and withers, so that Essence and blood are all dried up. The patient presents with thirst that is accompanied by dissipation of the flesh.

In other cases, there are patients who have been drinking alcohol for a long period of time. Alcohol is extremely hot by nature and fumigates the five *zàng* organs. The fluids get scorched and the blood flow becomes rough. The patient presents with thirst but the flesh is not dissipated.

For resolving the Five Stones poison, Yīngsù Tāng (Opium Poppy Decoction) is appropriate. If you want to stop thirst, Tùsīzǐ Wán (Dodder Pill) is appropriate. For great thirst with complicating vexation and heat, Mǎtōng Sǎn (Horse Manure Powder) or guālóufěn (trichosanthes root) are appropriate.

The reference to 五石 wǔ shí (Five Stones) in the context of a powder or decoction, and later as "Five Stones poison," must indicate what was more commonly known as Hán Shí Sǎn 寒食散 ("Cold Food Powder"), an addictive and poisonous psychoactive drug popular among the elite in the early medieval period. While the exact composition of this formula varied, it was based on five minerals that most commonly included cinnabar, realgar, magnetite, alum, fluorite, quartz, stalactite, or sulfur. The name "cold food" is derived from its extreme heating effect, which caused people who took it to throw themselves in cold water or consume cold substances. In spite of the much appreciated and addictive euphoric state of mind that it produced, "Five Stones Powder" was declared illegal in the Táng. While originally of a much stronger alchemical nature, these extremely potent mineral preparations were considered licentious and immoral by the Sòng period, but most likely continued to be taken under different names and with gentler, less harmful ingredients in medicinal preparations that included five minerals but mitigated their extreme effect with herbal ingredients. Given the toxic and addictive nature of the drug, it makes sense in the quote above that the disease of thirst with dissipation of the flesh links Five Stones preparations with "giving free rein to their desires without restraint" as the cause of this disease, especially since passions and desires are also associated with fire and thus heat in Chinese medicine.

It is interesting that Qí Zhòngfǔ turns around this original association of the disease with the pathological heat from addiction to toxic Five Stones preparations and seems to imply that patients were taking medicinal Five Stones preparations to counteract or treat a pre-existing state of vacuity cold. Most likely, this reflects a change in the meaning of Five Stones preparations, from toxic mineral-based psychoactive drugs to much milder, balanced medicinal formulas that included smaller doses of "five minerals" for their therapeutic heating effect.

Lastly, it is worth contemplating why the detrimental effects of taking strong psychoactive mineral drugs, only recorded as an issue affecting male members of the elite, is mentioned in a book on gynecology. There could be two reasons for this: First, Qí Zhòngfū tends to start his answers by quoting the most important textual sources for any condition he discusses. So he may have cited the *Zhǐmí fāng* here simply for completeness' sake, to present background information on the disease of Dissipation Thirst before discussing its particular relevance and manifestations in the context of gynecology.

Second, it is possible that women were also taking Five Stones drugs and suffering from their aftereffects, and that this issue was simply never recorded in the literature still mostly produced by and for men. As such, they would have been affected by the disease of Dissipation Thirst as the result of Five Stones consumption just like their male counterparts, and it would have been important for any gynecologist to be able to properly diagnose the signs of this harmful addiction. In that case, this omission serves as yet another useful reminder of how our understanding of Chinese history is made deficient by the lack of women's voices.

As a last question, we need to consider the meaning of the "Disease of the Three Dissipations" mentioned in the title question. While this is not a standard TCM term that has survived the times, it is featured in a slightly later text appropriately titled 《三消論》 *Sānxiāolùn* ("A Discussion of the Three Dissipations"), composed by Liú Wánsù 劉完素 in the twelfth century. Here we find an explanation that can shed additional light on the meaning of the term 消 *xiāo* "dissipation" or "to dissipate," in the context of pathology for Qí Zhòngfū and his contemporaries:

故《濟眾》云：三消渴者，皆由久嗜鹹物，恣食炙，飲酒過度。亦有年少服金石丸散，積久石熱結於胸中，下焦虛熱，血氣不能 制石，熱燥甚於胃，故渴而引飲。

若飲水多而小便多者，名曰消渴。若飲食多而不甚飢，小便數而漸瘦者，名曰消中。若渴而飲水不絕，腿消瘦而小便有脂液者，名曰腎消。如此三消者，其燥熱一也，但有微甚耳。

Thus the (now lost) text *Jizhòng* ("Rescuing the Masses") states: The three kinds of Dissipation Thirst are all due to long-term craving of salty substances, indulgence in eating roasted meat, and the excessive consumption of alcohol. There is also the case of people who consumed mineral-based pills and powders in their youth. Accumulating over a long time, the heat of the stones has bound in the center of the chest. Due to vacuity heat in the Lower Jiāo, blood and Qì are unable to control the stones, and the heat and dryness become severe in the stomach. Thus we see thirst with drinking of fluids.

If the patient drinks a lot of water and urinates a lot, this is called Dissipation Thirst. If the patient drinks and eats a lot but is not greatly hungry, urinates a lot but gradually becomes emaciated, this is called Dissipation of the Center. If the patient experiences thirst and drinks fluids incessantly but the legs become emaciated and the urine has greasy fluid in it, this is called kidney Dissipation. In the case of these Three Dissipations, the dryness and heat are one but there is extreme subtlety here.

The author then complains how the standard formularies don't understand the root of this condition and mostly offer a single treatment, which is precisely what Qí Zhòngfú does below. While the details of Liú's criticism, and his suggested correction of these errors, transcend the framework of this book on gynecology, his explanation of the standard understanding of Dissipation Thirst might help the reader appreciate Qí Zhòngfú's response above. According to Liú Wánsù, the standard texts treat all three Dissipation Thirst conditions in the same way, on the basis of the patient's increased dissipation of water and grain (i.e., solid and liquid foods) in combination with a tendency to thirst. They explain it as repletion heat above, causing vexing thirst and increased fluid consumption, and vacuity cold below, which causes excessive urination. The root is a vacuity of kidney Water, which leads to a failure to control heart Fire in the Upper Jiāo. Thus, ultimately the condition is based on a lack of Water, which is the source of life and the root of human health. In terms of therapy, if you give warming medicinals to gently supplement the original Qì and make kidney Water replete in the lower body, the Water is then able to reduce heart Fire above, and the thirst will stop on its own accord, urination will return to normal, and the patient will recover. Without getting into the details of Liù's criticism of this view, this reckless lack of differentiation, and assumption that all Dissipation conditions are a case of vacuity cold in the Lower Jiāo, is to be blamed for countless deaths! In his eyes, it is essential to differentiate cases where wind heat is causing dryness and stagnation all over the body, with panting above and wilting and *bì* Impediment below, as well as cases of internal damp heat, which is preventing physiological passage and transformation from taking place, and thus resulting in water swelling and abdominal distention. No matter what, "Dissipation Thirst means increased fluid intake with frequent urination; Dissipation of the Center means increased eating with frequent urination; and kidney Dissipation means emaciation of the flesh and greasy fluid in the urine."

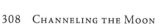

CLINICAL COMMENTARY BY SHARON WEIZENBAUM

DISSIPATION THIRST 消渴

Dissipation Thirst is a strange term to a Western ear. In my early education, I did not have any grasp on what this term meant. It is used to describe a condition for which certain formulas are prescribed such as Wūméi Wán (Mume Pill) and Wŭ Líng Săn (Poria Five Powder). In Guohui Liu's Discussion of Cold Damage: Commentaries and Clinical Applications, it is translated as "excessive thirst." In this text, three other terms are also translated in the same or a similar way: 烦渴 fánkě, 大烦渴 dà fánkě and 大渴 dàkě. These are translated as "vexation and thirst that is difficult to quench," "severe thirst that is difficult to quench and vexation," and "severe thirst," respectively. Altogether, from this, it is difficult to be clear on just what 消渴 xiāokě means. In this text, 消渴 is described this way,

The term Xiao Ke 消渴, in Chinese medicine bears two meanings: one refers to a disease that partially corresponds to type one diabetes mellitus in allopathic medicine with severe thirst, strong hunger and a large amount of urine, which is discussed in Chapter 13 of Essentials and Formula Discussions from the Golden Cabinet; and the other meaning just denotes a symptom, as in this line.

In my early education, I learned about Dissipation Thirst as in the first meaning stated above. I was under the impression that, unless I saw someone with untreated type 1 diabetes mellitus, which in itself is highly unlikely given the availability of insulin, it would be extremely unlikely I would ever see the symptom Dissipation Thirst.

However, as my understanding of the deeper meanings of Chinese medicine has matured, I've come to realize that I see Dissipation Thirst on a daily basis in my clinic. Not only that, it is an extremely important issue to be able to recognize and treat.

In the present chapter, Liú Wánsù 劉完素 is quoted from his *Sānxiāolùn* 《三消論》 ("A Discussion of the Three Dissipations") where he describes this Dissipation Thirst according to my understanding:

If the patient drinks a lot of water and urinates a lot, this is called Dissipation Thirst.

For me, this just about nails it, although I have one caveat. From my experience, we can also expand this definition to include pooling of fluids in the lower body in addition to urinating a lot. In fact, in the clinic, there is often the combination of pooling of fluids in the lower body with frequent urination. These two symptoms can arise together.

What is going on here that leads to the symptoms of thirst combined with frequent urination or pooling fluids below? The crux of what is happening is that fluids taken into the body are not absorbed as they pass through the digestive tract. These fluids end up pouring out below as frequent urination or pooling below as accumulated fluids.

Thirst and Urination Must Be Seen Together

When asking patients about thirst, it is important to consider this. Questions about urination must be asked and considered in relation to thirst. I often ask my patients, "do you feel that water runs right through you?" and often get clear answers in this way. Many patients have inhibited urination during the day and frequent night urination.

Fluids Pooling Below

When I ask about urination as a way to ascertain whether fluids are pooling below or not, I ask them "how is your urination?" To this question, most often I get the answer, "fine." I encourage you not to stop there but to ask more detailed questions, giving them options of pathology to choose from. For example, I often ask: "When you go to pee, do you ever have to wait before the flow starts?" "Does the flow ever stop and start or seem hesitant?" "Do you ever feel incomplete after peeing or feel you need to go again to finish soon after voiding?" When you ask this way, you will receive many affirmative answers. All of these symptoms indicate that fluids have pooled below. Keep in mind that, when fluids are pooling below, this can cause both inhibited urine as just described, as well as frequent urination or even incontinence. In other words, there are symptoms in which urine is coming out too much and not enough at the same time. One mustn't get confused by this, as both dynamics are from the same source.

Asking About Thirst

It can be very tricky to ask patients about thirst because, in my clinic, most patients have all kinds of ideas about how much they should be drinking. A common answer to my question, "how is your thirst?" is "Oh, I don't drink enough." In my experience, most people believe they should be drinking more than their bodies tell them to drink. They often are forcing fluids when they are not thirsty and therefore have no idea how thirsty they actually are! To get to the root of whether they are thirsty or not, I will ask them to take a week only drinking when they are compelled to drink. At the same time, I ask them to notice how they are getting other fluids, as through their tea, fruit, vegetables, soup etc. This way I can get a more accurate assessment about their thirst. Many people are actually waterlogged from over-drinking.

I also consider a dry mouth to be thirst. Even if patients only want to sip all day, this is still considered thirst. Even very chapped lips indicate a fluid deficiency of the middle.

What To Do About Dissipation Thirst

Having described my ideas about what Dissipation Thirst is, what needs to be done so that fluids are absorbed properly? In my opinion, Dr. Qí Zhòngfǔ's formula, Bǎizǐrén Tāng (Arborvitae Seed Decoction) reflects some, but not all, of the primary principles for treating Dissipation Thirst.

The principles reflected in Bǎizǐrén Tāng are as follows. He uses sweet gāncǎo, translucent sweet fluid-enriching herbs such as rénshēn, tiānméndōng, and màiméndōng, along with greasy herbs such as bǎizǐrén and shúdìhuáng to replenish fluids. To this — and for me, this is very key to restoring not just the fluids, but the body's ability to absorb fluids — he adds the chalky guālóugēn and fúlíng. The chalky quality of these herbs increases the absorptive capacity of the digestive tract. A nod is given to clearing the heat that may be giving rise to the Dissipation Thirst, as strong heat often damages the body's ability to absorb fluids, with the cold and bitter guālóugēn, tiānméndōng, and màiméndōng.

Looking at this text's next formula, Chénshā Jù Bǎo Dān (Chénzhōu Cinnabar Treasures-Gathering Elixir), we can see that he uses the method of clearing Yángmíng heat with huánglián and zhīmǔ, replenishing fluids with rénshēn, and increasing the body's absorptive function with the chalky guālóugēn and báibiǎndòu.

Of course, there are other methods, and these vary according to the presentation. The Wūméi Wán presentation uses very hot pungent herbs in combination with greasy, sweet and sour herbs to start a moisture-rich steaming up process from below. At the same time, it opens up Yángmíng with bitter, cold herbs so that the heat is no longer accumulating and damaging fluids above. This method does not require chalky herbs. The Wŭ Líng Săn method uses warm pungent and sweet guìzhī with chalky herbs to help the body absorb and drain properly. When fluids are properly absorbed, they don't leak or pool below but rather are steamed up to relieve thirst.

Hence, I would agree with Liú Wánsù that Dissipation Thirst cannot always be treated the same way.

When the questions are asked carefully, I find lots of Dissipation Thirst in my practice. The inability to absorb fluids properly can lead to many different kinds of serious health issues. Without fluids, muscles and tendons can dry up leading to serious pain issues, and blood is not produced properly leading to insufficient and dry blood. This can be the root of many fertility and menstrual issues. Nursing can be difficult as can general postpartum recovery.

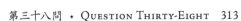

柏子仁湯

滋養營衛，調心順氣。亦治上焦虛熱，煩燥口苦，四肢倦怠，津液內燥。服之效。

新羅參	
黃芪	
茯神	
瓜蔞根	各一兩
天門冬（去心）	
麥門冬（去心）	
甘草	
北五味（炒）	半兩
柏子仁	
熟地	二兩

上為粗末。每服五錢，水一盞半，姜三片，棗三枚，煎七分。去滓溫服，不拘時。

Bǎizǐrén Tāng
(Arborvitae Seed Decoction)

[A formula] to saturate and nourish *yíng* Provisioning and *wèi* Defense, to attune the heart, and to restore the proper direction of the Qì flow. It also treats vacuity heat in the Upper Jiāo, vexing dryness and a bitter taste in the mouth, fatigue in the four limbs, and internal drying out of the fluids. Taking this is efficacious.

Silla (i.e., Korean) rénshēn	
huángqí	
fúshén	
guālóugēn	1 *liǎng* each
tiānméndōng (remove the core)	
màiméndōng (remove the core)	
gāncǎo	
Northern wǔwèizǐ (stir-fry)	0.5 *liǎng*
bǎizǐrén	
shúdì	2 *liǎng*

Process the ingredients above into a coarse powder. Take 5 *qián* per dose and simmer it in 1.5 cups of water with 3 slices of ginger and 3 jujubes until reduced to 70 percent. Remove the dregs and take it warm, with no restrictions on the timing.

辰砂聚寶丹

治心肺積蘊虛熱，口苦舌乾面赤，大便滲泄，肌肉瘦瘁，四肢少力，精神恍惚。又治消渴，消中，消腎，三焦留熱。

鐵粉	三錢半
牡蠣	三錢半
辰砂	半兩
瓜蔞根	半兩
黃連	二錢半
金銀箔（為衣）	各五十片
知母	三錢半
新蘿參	半兩
白扁豆（湯浸，去皮，取末）	半兩

上件瓜蔞根末等五味，同前藥末。

用生瓜蔞根，去皮，取汁一盞，白沙蜜一小盞，同銀器中煉七八沸，候冷，和藥為丸，如梧桐子大。每服三十九。煎麥門冬湯放冷送下，食後，一日之間三服。

Chénshā Jù Bǎo Dān
(Chénzhōu Cinnabar Treasures-Gathering Elixir)

A treatment for latently smoldering vacuity heat in the heart and lung, with bitter taste in the mouth, dry tongue, and red face; fecal incontinence; emaciated and withered flesh; reduced strength in the four limbs; and severe mental confusion. It also treats Dissipation Thirst, Dissipation of the Center, and Dissipation of the kidney, with abiding heat in the Sānjiāo.

tiěfěn	3.5 *qián*
mǔlì	3.5 *qián*
chénshā	0.5 *liǎng*
guālóugēn	0.5 *liǎng*
huánglián	2.5 *qián*
jīnyínbó (for coating)	50 leaves each
zhīmǔ	3.5 *qián*
Silla (i.e., Korean) rénshēn	0.5 *liǎng*
báibiǎndòu (soak in hot water, remove the skin and use it powdered)	0.5 *liǎng*

Of the ingredients above, pulverize the five ingredients following the guālóugēn, and combine with the powder made from the preceding medicinals.

Use fresh guālóugēn, remove the peel, and take 1 cup of its juice. Combine it with a small cup of honey, and melt [the two ingredients] together in a silver pot, bringing them to a boil 7 or 8 times. Wait until [the mixture] is cool and blend with the [other] medicinals to form pills the size of *wútóng* seeds. Take 30 pills per dose. Boil màiméndōng decoction, let it cool, and use that to down the pills, after meals, three doses in the space of a single day.

第三十九問

腰痛如折者，何也？

答曰：腰者，腎之外候，足太陽經之所流注。

若痛連小腹，不得俯仰，短氣，此由腎氣虛弱，勞傷過度，風冷乘之，有所不榮，故腰痛也。

內經云：「腰者，腎之府，轉搖不能，腎將憊矣。」

若妊娠腰痛者，其胎必墮也。

QUESTION THIRTY-NINE

What is the Meaning of Excruciating Lumbar Pain?

ANSWER: The lumbus is the external sign of the kidney and the location where the Foot Tàiyáng Channel pours in.

If the pain connects to the lower abdomen and is accompanied by an inability to bend the head forward and backward and shortness of breath, this is caused by a weakness of kidney Qì and by excessive taxation damage, which has been exploited by wind cold. There are locations that lack *yíng* Provisioning, and thus there is lumbar pain.

According to the *Nèijīng*, "the lumbus, it is the palace of the kidney. When the person is unable to twist and shake, the kidney shall be exhausted."

If you see lumbar pain during pregnancy, this means that her fetus will invariably drop.

Discussion

The quote from the *Nèijīng* mentioned above is indeed a literal citation from *Sùwèn* Chapter Seventeen, 《脈要精微論》 *Mài yào jīngwēi lùn* (Discourse on the Crucial and Essential Subtleties of the Flow in the Vessels):

夫五臟者，身之強也，頭者精明之府，頭傾視深，精神將奪矣。背者胸中之府，背曲肩隨，府將壞矣。腰者腎之府，轉搖不能，腎將憊矣。膝者筋之府，屈伸不能，行則僂附，筋將憊矣。骨者髓之府，不能久立，行則振掉，骨將憊矣。得強則生，失強則死。

Now the five *zàng* organs are what make the body strong. First the head, it is the palace of luminous astuteness. When the head leans to the side and the eyes are sunken, the Jīngshén shall be seized. Next the back, it is the palace of the center of the chest. When the back is bent and the shoulders slumping, the *fǔ* organs shall be ruined. Next the lumbus, it is the palace of the kidney. When the person is unable to twist and shake, the kidney shall be exhausted. Next the knees, they are the palace of the sinews. When the person is unable to bend and stretch, and walks stooped over, the sinews shall be exhausted. Next the bones, they are the palace of the marrow. When the person is unable to stand for a long time and has an unstable gait with a tendency to fall, the bones shall be exhausted. Obtaining strength means life, losing strength means death.

There are several reasons why the condition of excruciating lumbar pain is of special significance for women. To begin with the last sentence of Qí Zhòngfǔ's answer, it is essential to diagnose and actively address lumbar pain during pregnancy because it is a key sign for a threatened miscarriage. Unfortunately, according to the statement here, by the time a pregnant woman experiences lumbar pain, it is really too late, and she will invariably lose her fetus.

In addition, based on what we have learned from Qí Zhòngfǔ about women's physiology and pathology, we can see now why lumbar pain is a condition that women are particularly prone to. It is, after all, a condition that combines the state of depletion in the kidney with the twin etiology of taxation damage and invasion of wind-cold. Due to women's reproductive cycles, the burden of regular monthly bleeding in menstruation is compounded by the possible, if not likely, taxation in women's adult lives from repeated experiences of pregnancy and then childbirth and breastfeeding or from abortion or miscarriage. While multiple rounds of pregnancy and childbearing are perhaps no longer as common as they used to be before the arrival of birth control, this freedom comes at a price, and birth control comes with its own challenges for the female body. As a result of all of these processes, the kidney as the organ in charge of reproduction can easily get exhausted. In addition, as is repeated over and over in all gynecological literature, women are more susceptible to an external invasion of wind and cold, due to weakness and exhaustion, the physical and energetic openness during menstruation and childbirth, and their constitutional affinity with cold.

It is interesting that contemporary TCM associates lumbar pain in women primarily with menstrual cramps (before, during, and after, or even mid-cycle) and treats it by restoring a healthy blood flow to "regulate menstruation," a treatment strategy that is not mentioned at all here. The first rule students learn in TCM gynecology is, after all that "where there is stoppage, there is pain" (不通則痛). This approach is also borne out by the following formulas, especially the second one for Dāngguī Wán. Including shuǐzhì and táorén, which are two very strong blood-moving ingredients, it surely seems to be aimed primarily at resolving stagnation or even "breaking the blood," rather than at addressing the root cause mentioned in Qí Zhòngfǔ's answer, namely kidney deficiency with wind cold. It is worth contemplating what Qí's reasons may have been for conceptualizing lumbar pain as weakness in the kidney instead of as blocked or stagnant menstrual flow, even though in terms of the recommended clinical treatment, he addressed the latter. Given the importance of attuning and restoring the monthly blood flow in both earlier gynecological formularies like Sūn Sīmiǎo's writings and in later texts, Qí's answer here strikes me as an important reminder that, at least in theory, it behooves us to remember the state of the kidney as a potential underlying root cause, instead of just focusing on restoring a free-flowing menstruation.

杜仲散

杜仲（去皮，杵爛，酒浸一宿，焙）	一兩
官桂	
牡丹皮	各一兩

上為細末，溫酒調二錢。不拘時服。

Dùzhòng Sǎn
(Eucommia Powder)

dùzhòng (remove the peel, pound to a pulp, steep in rice wine overnight, and roast)	1 *liǎng*
guāngùi	
mǔdānpí	1 *liǎng* each

Process the ingredients above into a fine powder. Stir two *qián* [per dose] into warm rice wine, and do not restrict the timing for taking it.

當歸丸

當歸 (切，洗)	三兩
水蛭 (炒)	三十枚
桃仁 (去皮，研)	三十粒

上為細末，酒煮糊丸，如桐子大。溫酒下十丸。未愈，加至三十丸。

Dāngguī Wán
(Chinese Angelica Pill)

dāngguī (slice and wash)	3 *liǎng*
shuǐzhì (stir-fry)	30 specimens
táorén (remove the skin and grind)	30 kernels

Process the ingredients above into a fine powder, [blend into] rice wine, simmer, and make a paste to form pills the size of *wútóng* seeds. Down ten pills [per dose] in warm rice wine. If she has not yet recovered, increase the dosage to as much as 30 pills.

腎著湯

治身體重，腰冷痺，如坐水中狀，反不渴，小便自利，飲食如故。病屬下焦，從身勞汗出，衣裡冷濕，久而得之。腰以下冷痛，腰重如帶五貫錢重者。

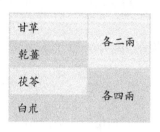

甘草	各二兩
乾薑	
茯苓	各四兩
白朮	

上為粗末，每服五錢，水二盞，去滓，溫服。不拘時。

Shèn Zhuó Tāng
(Kidney Clinging Decoction)

A treatment for heaviness of the body, cold *bì* Impediment in the lumbus, an appearance as if sitting in water, but contrary to one's expectations no thirst, spontaneous and free-flowing urination, and eating and drinking as usual. This condition belongs to the Lower Jiāo and is obtained from taxation of the body with sweating and then cold dampness inside the clothes that has gone on for a long time. [In such cases,] there is cold and pain below the lumbus and the lumbus feels heavy as if she were carrying the weight of five thousand-coins strings of cash.

gāncǎo	2 *liǎng* each
gānjiāng	
fúlíng	4 *liǎng* each
báizhú	

Process the ingredients above into a coarse powder and take 5 *qián* per dose in 2 cups of water. Get rid of the dregs and take it warm. Do not restrict the timing.

第四十問

婦人面多生黑䵟與黑子者，何也？

答曰：黑䵟黑子者，皆生於面上，本是二證也。

五臟六腑之經血華充於面。或痰飲漬臟，或腠理受風，致血氣不和，或澀或溫。不能榮於皮膚，故變生黑䵟。

若黑點凝聚，謂之黑子。若生而有之者，非藥可治也。

QUESTION FORTY

What is the Reason for the Profuse Formation of Dark Discolored Areas and Moles on a Woman's Face?

ANSWER: Dark discolored areas and moles both are created on the face and are originally two [distinct] patterns.

The channel blood from the five *zàng* and six *fǔ* organs shows its luster and fullness in the face. Whether phlegm-rheum has soaked into the *zàng* organs, or the interstices have contracted wind, this leads to disharmony of blood and Qì, possibly with rough flow or with warmth. [The blood and Qì] are unable to supply *yíng* Provisioning to the skin, therefore they transform and create dark discolored areas.

If black dots conglomerate, we call them moles. If the person already has them at birth, this is not something that can be treated with medicinals.

Discussion

The Chinese text uses two technical terms here to describe two kinds of dark pigmented lesions on the skin. I have intentionally avoided using modern biomedical terms like melanoma or congenital or dysplastic nevi, which carry etiological implications that may be too narrow or misleading to delineate the sense of the Chinese term. According to Qí Zhòngfǔ's answer, there is an important difference between them, beyond just the fact that the first one refers to a large area of discoloration and the second one to small spots. And this difference is of great significance for a doctor: In the case of small dark spots, these cannot be treated when the person has had them since birth. Even though Qí emphasizes that the large dis-colored areas known as 黑皯 hēigǎn and the smaller moles known as 黑子 hēizǐ are two distinct patterns, he only offers one etiology, with important pointers for treatment: In his eyes, the formation of pigmented lesions in the skin is due to the failure of channel blood to provide yíng Provisioning to the face, whether due to phlegm-rheum soaking into the zàng organs or to the invasion of wind through the interstices. Both of these are dangers that women are particularly prone to. To better appreciate and clinically apply Qí's insistence that we are indeed dealing with two distinct patterns, beyond the fact that lesions that exist since birth are untreatable, we must dig deeper into Qí's possible sources. As so often, his answer provides a summary of an earlier text that sometimes leaves out key aspects of the explanation in his source.

According to the *Shuōwén jiězì* dictionary from the second century, the character *gǎn* is defined as 「面黑氣」 *miàn hēi qì* "dark Qì in the face." But beyond this dictionary definition of the term, what are Qí Zhòngfǔ's medical sources in earlier technical writings? Without needing to look beyond the usual suspects, it is obvious that his answer is lifted almost lit-erally from Volume Thirty-Nine of Cháo Yuánfāng's gynecological section in the *Zhūbìng yuánhòu lùn*. In fact, we find the two patterns discussed in two essays directly following each other and providing some additional information that indeed helps us understand how and why we are dealing with two distinct patterns. Pay particular attention to the conclusion of the first essay!

Here is the full text of the first essay on the "Signs of Dark Discolored Areas in the Face":

面黑皯者，或臟腑有痰飲，或皮膚受風邪，皆令血氣不調，致生黑皯。五臟六腑十二經血，皆上受於面。夫血之行，俱榮表裡。人或痰飲漬臟，或腠理受風，致血氣不和，或澀或濁，不能榮於皮膚，故變生黑皯。若皮膚受風，外治則瘥，腑臟有飲，內療方愈也。

Regarding dark discolored areas in the face, either the presence of phlegm-rheum in the *zāngfǔ* organs or the contraction of wind evil in the skin have caused a lack of attunement between blood and Qì, which in turn has led to the creation of black discolored areas on the face. The blood from all the twelve channels of the five *zàng* and six *fǔ* organs rises up to be received in the face. Now this movement of blood always supplies *yíng* Provisioning to the exterior and interior. In a person, whether phlegm-rheum has soaked into the *zàng* organs or the interstices have contracted wind, this leads to disharmony between blood and Qì, possibly with roughly-flowing movement or turbidity, and inability to supply *yíng* Provisioning to the skin. Therefore they transform and create dark discolored areas on the face. If the skin has received wind, external treatment leads to recovery. If there is rheum present in the *zàngfǔ* organs, a formula for an internal cure mean recovery!

This essay is followed by an essay on the "Signs of Moles on the Face":

面黑子者，風邪搏血氣，變化所生。夫人血氣充盛，則皮膚潤悅。若虛損，疵點變生。黑子者，是風邪變其血氣所生。若生而有之者，非藥可治也。

Moles in the face mean that wind evil has assaulted the blood and Qì and thereby created this pathological change. Now when a person's blood and Qì are abundant, the skin is moist and lustrous. If they are vacuous, the pathology of blemish spots develops. Moles are created by wind evil transforming the person's blood and Qì. If the person has them already at birth, it is impossible to treat it with medicinals.

On the basis of these two essays, we can now see how Qí Zhòngfǔ has conflated two different terms with two different patterns with important differences in treatment, but not in the way his answer suggests. Is it possible that treating women's discolorations on the face was perhaps not his greatest strength?

To summarize, Cháo Yuánfāng explains that there are two patterns that can give rise to the dark discolored areas on the face known as 皯 gǎn, and that these must be treated completely differently: An invasion of wind through the interstices is treated with an external facewash, presumably like the formula for Washing-Away-The-Wind Powder that is listed below here. In stark contrast, the presence of phlegm-rheum in the internal organs must be treated internally. Similar to the first pattern, the formation of moles as smaller spots, when these were not already present at birth, is caused by wind striking the blood and Qì, impeding the proper distribution of *yíng* Provisioning to the face and thus causing blemishes. By implication, these should also be treated with external face washes.

Lastly, many modern readers may be unaware of the traditional Chinese art of facial diagnosis, which has been an established aspect of Chinese medical practice throughout its history. Already mentioned by the Yellow Emperor and Sūn Sīmiǎo, it is alive and well today, as we can see from the success of Lillian Pearl Bridges' *Face Reading in Chinese Medicine*, one of the bestselling books about Chinese medicine on Amazon.

洗風散

治面上游風，或癮疹，或風刺，或黑皯。

茺蔚草	僵蠶
晚蠶沙	白附子
赤小豆	草烏頭
黑牽牛	白蘞
白芷	蔓荊子
藁本	

上件等分為末。每一錢澡面用之。

Xǐ Fēng Sǎn
(Washing-Away-the-Wind Powder)

A treatment for roaming wind on the face, perhaps manifesting as dormant papules or as wind stabbings, or as dark discolored areas.

chōngwèicǎo	jiāngcán
wǎncánshā	báifùzǐ
chìxiǎodòu	cǎowūtóu
hēiqiānniú	báiliǎn
báizhǐ	mànjīngzǐ
gǎoběn	

Process equal amounts of the ingredients above into a powder. For each dose, take 1 *qián* and use it to wash the face.

第四十一問

身目黃者，何也？

答曰：黃疸之病，皆屬於脾。脾屬土而色黃。濕勝則土氣不流，瘀熱鬱發，則真色見矣。

大抵黃疸本得之於濕，濕熱相搏，身必發黃。若先有流熱，後有濕氣者，先治其熱。栀子柏皮湯、茵陳五苓散主之。

或先感其濕，後加其熱者，先去其濕。五苓散、瓜蒂散主之。

亦有因冷氣痞結於脾陰，濕鬱而為黃。先瀉其痞，半夏瀉心湯、枳實理中湯主之。然後利其小便。

若病人一身面目悉黃，四肢微腫，胸滿不得臥，汗出如黃柏汁者，此由大汗出，猝入水中所致，謂之黃汗。宜苦酒湯。

若非濕熱所鬱，婦人面萎黃者，亡血之過也。宜服地黃散、滋陰養血丸（方見第三十問）。

QUESTION FORTY-ONE

What is the Meaning of Yellowing of the Body and Eyes?

ANSWER: The disease of jaundice is always associated with the spleen. The spleen belongs to Earth and its color is yellow. When dampness prevails, Earth Qì fails to flow, stagnant heat becomes constrained and erupts to the surface. As a result, the true color becomes visible.

Generally speaking, jaundice is originally contracted from dampness, and when dampness and heat assault each other, the body will invariably turn yellow. In cases where there is streaming heat first, later followed by dampness Qì, you first treat the patient's heat. Zhīzǐ Bǎipí Tāng (Gardenia and Phellodendron Decoction) or Yīnchén Wǔlíng Sǎn (Virgate Wormwood and Poria Five Powder) rule this condition.

Alternatively, if the patient first contracted dampness and this was subsequently complicated by heat, you first remove the patient's dampness. Wǔlíng Sǎn (Poria Five Powder) or Guādì Sǎn (Melon Stalk Powder) rule this condition.

There are also cases where yellowing is caused by cold Qì forming pǐ Glomus bind in spleen Yīn and oppressive constraint of dampness. [In such cases,] first drain the patient's pǐ Glomus. Bànxià Xiè Xīn Tāng (Pinellia Heart-Draining Decoction) or Zhǐshí Lǐ Zhōng Tāng (Unripe Bitter Orange Center-Patterning Decoction) rule this condition. And then afterwards, you disinhibit the patient's urine.

If the patient [presents with] complete yellowing all over the entire body, face, and eyes, mild swelling in the four limbs, fullness in the chest with inability to sleep, and discharge of sweat that looks like huángbǎi juice, this is caused by [the patient having experienced] great sweating and then having abruptly entered water. It is called Yellow Sweat and should be treated with Kǔ Jiǔ Tāng (Bitter Rice Wine Decoction).

If it is not a cause of oppressive constraint of damp-heat, and you have a woman [presenting with] a withered yellow face, this means the trespass of blood collapse. It should be treated with Dìhuáng Sǎn or Zī Yīn Yǎng Xùe Wán (For the latter formula, see Question Thirty).

DISCUSSION

Once again, it is interesting to consider why Qí Zhòngfǔ might have felt a need to include the topic of jaundice among his "hundred questions." With the exception of pregnancy and perhaps postpartum, jaundice is not a disease that we would ordinarily think of as a gynecological condition. The most obvious reason for its inclusion in this text is presented in the very last sentence, namely the diagnostic pearl that a withered yellow facial complexion can be the sign for the condition of blood collapse. Obviously, this is a completely different condition and requires a very different treatment than the yellow face, eyes, and body that we see in ordinary jaundice, as related to dampness and an impaired spleen function.

Following the lead of modern biomedicine, contemporary TCM often treats jaundice as a condition of the liver-gallbladder. This is even reflected in the current way of writing the traditional name of the disease: Instead of the traditional 黃疸 huángdǎn, it is now often written with different characters that have the same pronunciation, as 黃膽 huángdǎn (literally, yellow gallbladder). Unfortunately, it transcends the framework of this book to reconstruct the history of jaundice in Chinese medical history back to the moment where this disease became associated not just with the spleen-stomach but also with the liver-gallbladder. As a side note and good reminder of the need to consult printed, as opposed to digital, editions of our source texts, the digitized version of the Nǚkē bǎiwèn on ctext.org has the disease written as 黃膽 even though its manuscript source has it written in the historically correct way as 黃疸. It is so easy for our contemporary ways of looking at a disease, whether in modern China or in the West, to slip into historical literature in this innocuous way! This is one of the reasons why I am always cautious about consulting contemporary TCM information, whether in Western languages or in modern Chinese. What is important to remember about classical Chinese medicine is that jaundice is associated not with the liver-gallbladder, but with the spleen-stomach, through its function of managing dampness. You might want to modify your treatment plan and include the liver-gallbladder on the basis of the modern explanation of jaundice as caused by high bilirubin levels, yet the classical Chinese view also has obvious ramifications for treatment.

For a classical understanding of jaundice, Cháo Yuánfāng offers an entire volume on different conditions of "yellowing," including one on the disease of 黃疸 huángdǎn, which is worth quoting in full here:

黃疸之病，此由酒食過度，腑臟不和，水穀相并，積於脾胃，復為風濕所搏，瘀結不散，熱氣鬱蒸，故食已如飢，令身體面目及瓜甲及小便盡黃，而欲安臥。

若身體多赤黑多青皆見者，必寒熱身痛。面色微黃，齒垢黃，爪甲上黃，黃疸也。

渴而疸者，其病難治；疸而不渴，其病可治。發於陰部，其人必嘔；發於陽部，其人振寒而欲熱。

The disease of jaundice is caused by excessive consumption of alcohol and food and by disharmony in the *fǔ* and *zàng* organs, so that water and grain combine with each other and accumulate in the spleen and stomach. This condition is further complicated by an assault of wind-dampness, which stagnates and binds instead of dispersing. The Qì of heat steams oppressively, and [patients] therefore feel starving after they finish eating. This condition causes the body, face, and eyes, as well as the nails of the fingers and toes and the urine to turn thoroughly yellow, and it makes patients want to rest and sleep.

If the body is marked by an increased appearance of both black-red and blue-green, she must [suffer from] cold and heat and generalized pain. If the facial complexion is slightly yellow, the teeth are filthy yellow, and there is yellow on the nails of the fingers and toes, this means jaundice.

In cases of thirst with the jaundice, the condition is difficult to treat. If there is jaundice but no thirst, the condition can be treated. If it breaks out in the Yīn part, this person invariably suffers from retching. If it breaks out in the Yáng part, such a person will be shivering with cold and about to have heat effusion.

It is interesting that Qí Zhòngfǔ ignores a separate entry by Cháo Yuánfāng on "Women's Taxation Jaundice":

女勞疸之狀，身目皆黃，發熱惡寒，小腹滿急，小便難。由大勞大熱而交接，交接竟入水所致也。

The appearance of women's taxation jaundice is like this: Both the body and the eyes are yellow, and she has heat effusion and aversion to cold, fullness and tension in the lower abdomen, and difficult urination. It is caused by sexual intercourse after great taxation and great heat and by entering water after the sexual intercourse.

苦酒湯

黃耆	五兩
芍藥	三兩
官桂	

上為㕮咀，每服五錢，水盞半，苦酒半盞，煎一盞，去滓溫服。不拘時。

Kǔ Jiǔ Tāng
(Bitter Rice Wine Decoction)

huángqí	5 *liǎng*
sháoyào	3 *liǎng*
guānguì	

Pound the ingredients above and take 5 *qián* per dose. Simmer in 1.5 cups of water and 0.5 cups of bitter rice wine until reduced to 1 cup. Remove the dregs and take it warm. Do not restrict the timing.

地黃散

治婦人血少，氣多寒，面色青白。

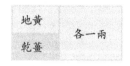

上為細末，每服二錢。溫酒調下，不拘時。

Dìhuáng Sǎn
(Rehmannia Powder)

A treatment for women's scantiness of blood with a profusion of cold in the Qì [aspect], with a greenish-white facial complexion.

dìhuáng	1 *liǎng* each
gānjiāng	

Process the ingredients above into a fine powder and take 2 *qián* per dose. Down it by mixing it into warm rice wine, and do not restrict the timing.

茵陳五苓散

豬苓(去皮)	
茯苓	
澤瀉	各一兩
白朮	
官桂(去皮)	五錢

上為細末，以茵陳一分，水一盞，煎七分，去滓調
服。加鹽點妙。

Yīnchén Wǔ Líng Sǎn
(Virgate Wormwood and Poria Five Powder)

zhūlíng (remove the skin)	
fúlíng	1 *liǎng* each
zéxiè	
báizhú	
guānguì (remove the skin)	5 *qián*

Process the ingredients above into a fine powder. Simmer
with 1 *fēn* of yīnchén in 1 cup of water until reduced to 70
percent. Remove the dregs, stir well, and take it. Adding
salt is excellent.

瓜蒂散

瓜蒂	
赤小豆	各一兩
秫米	

上為細末，粥飲調下半錢。以吐為度。

Guādì Sǎn
(Melon Stalk Powder)

guādì	
chìxiǎodòu	1 *liǎng* each
shúmǐ	

Process the ingredients above into a fine powder. Down 0.5 *qián* [per dose], blended into rice gruel liquid. Take vomiting as your measure [to stop taking more medicine].

柏皮湯

柏皮	三兩
梔子	二兩
甘草	一兩

上為粗末，每服五錢。水二盞，煎八分，去渣，溫
服。

Bǎipí Tāng
(Arborvitae Root Bark Decoction)

bǎipí	3 *liǎng*
zhīzǐ	2 *liǎng*
gāncǎo	1 *liǎng*

Process the ingredients above into a fine powder and take 5 *qián* per dose. Simmer in 2 cups of water until reduced to 80 percent, remove the dregs, and take it warm.

第四十二問

陰崩陽崩，何以別之？

答曰：夫血氣之行，外行經絡，內榮腑臟，皆衝任二脈之所主也。

倘若勞傷過度，致腑臟俱傷，衝任經虛，不能約制其血，故忽然暴下，謂之崩下。

經云：三焦絕經，名曰血崩。受熱而赤者，謂之陽崩；受冷而白者，謂之陰崩。

其白者形如涕，赤者形如絳，黃者形如爛瓜，青者形如藍色，黑者形如衄血。是謂五崩也。（當與第六問兼看）

QUESTION FORTY-TWO

How Do We Differentiate Between Yīn Landslide Collapse and Yáng Landslide Collapse?

ANSWER: Regarding the movement of blood and Qì, externally it flows in the channels and network vessels, and internally it supplies *yíng* Provisioning to the *fǔ* and *zàng* organs. It is always [a function] that is ruled by the two vessels Chōngmài and Rènmài.

Whenever a person suffers taxation damage that is excessive, this leads to damage to both the *fǔ* and the *zàng* organs and to vacuity in the Chōng and Rèn channels, so that they are unable to restrain the person's blood. For this reason, suddenly there is a Landslide Collapse downward. This is what is called "Landslide Collapse downward."

The Classic says: "When the channels are interrupted in the Sānjiāo, this is called 'blood Landslide Collapse'." In cases where the patient contracted heat and it is red, it is called Yáng Landslide Collapse; in cases where the patient contracted cold and it is white, it is called Yīn Landslide Collapse.

If it is white, it looks like nasal mucus; if it is red, it looks like the color of crimson; if it is yellow, it looks like overripe melon; if it is green-blue, it looks like the color of indigo; and if it is black, it looks like a nosebleed. These are what we call the "Five [Forms of] Landslide Collapse." (Also see Question Six.)

Discussion

Given the importance of discharge "below the belt" in classical Chinese gynecology and the life-threatening nature of the condition here, it is worth unpacking and contextualizing this answer on the basis of its historical predecessors. Here is the parallel passage from the *Zhūbìng yuánhòu lùn*, which once again is clearly at least a partial source for Qí Zhòngfǔ's answer and at the same time presents some additional information. The essay on the "Sign of Landslide Collapse of the Center in All of the Five Colors" is found in the second of the four volumes on women's miscellaneous conditions towards the end of this text:

崩中之病，是傷損衝任之脈。衝任之脈皆起受於胞內，為經脈之海。勞傷過度，衝任氣虛，不能統制經血，故忽然崩下，謂之崩中。

五臟皆禀血氣，五臟之色，隨臟不同。傷損之人，五臟皆虛者，故五色隨崩俱下。其狀：白崩形如涕，赤崩形如紅汁，黃崩形如爛瓜汁，青崩形如藍色，黑崩形如乾血色。

The disease of Landslide Collapse of the center means damage to the Chōngmài and Rènmài. The Chōngmài and Rènmài all begin inside the womb and constitute the sea of the channels. Taxation damage that is excessive means that the Qì in the Chōngmài and Rènmài is vacuous and that they are unable to restrain the blood in the channels. For this reason, suddenly there is a movement like a landslide downward. This is what is called "Landslide Collapse of the center."

The five *zàng* organs are all endowed with blood and Qì, and the color of the five *zàng* organs differs from one organ to the next. If the person who has been injured suffers from vacuity in all the five *zàng* organs, the five colors consequently are all discharged along with the Landslide Collapse. Their appearance is as follows: White Landslide Collapse resembles nasal mucus, red Landslide Collapse resembles red juice, yellow Landslide Collapse resembles overripe melon juice, green-blue

Landslide Collapse resembles indigo in color, and black Landslide Collapse resembles the color of dry blood.

We must note here that the condition 崩中 *bēngzhōng* "Landslide Collapse of the center," does not exist in isolation, but as the most severe and critical variety among other types of women's pathological discharge from the vagina. Most importantly, it is related to, and sometimes accompanied by, the more chronic form known as 漏下 *lòuxià* "spotting (or literally "leaking") below." Both of these conditions are seen as varieties of vaginal discharge, which is referred to in Chinese medical literature as 帶下 *dàixià*, literally "below the belt," and introduced by Cháo Yuánfāng in the beginning of the same volume.

It is important to keep in mind that for the authors of classical gynecological literature, discharge "below the belt" did not just include the white or colorless variety emitted from the vagina that we tend to think of today, but also discharge in the other four colors, depending on the *zàng* organ involved. In addition to the connection of the color to the *zàng* organ, red and white discharge in particular are not just seen as stemming from vacuity in the heart and lung respectively, but also from a preponderance of either heat or cold. Both of these diagnostic models also appear in Qí Zhòngfǔ's answer above, with the added piece that drastic voluminous red discharge is now called Yáng Landslide Collapse, and white discharge Yīn Landslide Collapse.

As the *Zhūbìng yuánhòu lùn* explains in the section immediately preceding the quote on Landslide Collapse above, the condition of *lòuxià* also manifests in discharge in the five colors depending on the *zàng* organ that is affected by vacuity, i.e., green-blue for the liver, yellow for the spleen, red for the heart, white for the lung, and black for the kidney. While clearly related to Landslide Collapse, the more chronic pathology of spotting below is explained in slightly different terms from the condition of Landslide Collapse, adding an important etiological piece to the puzzle:

漏下者，由勞傷血氣，衝任之脈虛損故也。衝脈、任脈為十二經脈之海，皆起受於胞內。而手太陽小腸之經也，手少陰心之經也，此二經主上為乳汁，下為月水。

婦人經脈調適，則月水以時，若勞傷者，以衝任之氣虛損，不能制其經脈，故血非時而下，淋瀝不斷，謂之漏。

Spotting below is caused by taxation damage to the blood and Qì and vacuity detriment in the Chōngmài and Rènmài. The Chōngmài and Rènmài are the sea of the twelve channels and both arise inside the womb. In addition, the Hand Tàiyáng Small Intestine Channel and the Hand Shàoyīn Heart Channel, these two channels rule what constitutes breast milk above and menstrual fluids below.

When women's channels are well-attuned, the menstrual fluids flow in their proper time, but if there is taxation damage, which has caused vacuity detriment to the Qì of the Chōngmài and Rènmài, so that they are unable to control the channels, the blood consequently descends when it is not its proper time, dribbling and dripping uninterruptedly. This is called spotting.

Thus we can see that any discharge "below the belt," whether as chronic "spotting below" or as critical "landslide collapse," is strictly a gynecological condition and has an important dimension through its connection to female bleeding and menstrual flow, even if not mentioned explicitly in Qí Zhòngfǔ's answer above. Some of the following formulas make this connection explicit in the indications.

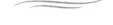

CLINICAL COMMENTARY BY SHARON WEIZENBAUM

What is the difference between heavy bleeding and Landslide Collapse?

What is the difference between heavy uterine bleeding and bēng, Landslide Collapse? Women know the difference and can tell you if you ask the right questions. A heavy menstruation can feel exhausting and messy, but when there is Landslide Collapse, a woman will feel that all ability to consolidate her lower body is gone. It's a feeling as if a plug of control has been removed. It is an out-of-control feeling and it's scary! Ask your patients if they feel that the bottom has fallen out or if it feels as if there is absolutely no restraint. Ask if it feels alarming. If they say yes, then this is Landslide Collapse.

A word about the color of the blood in relation to diagnosis.

We learn that when there is bleeding, if the blood is bright red, this means that the bleeding is due to heat. This always confused me since blood itself is bright red! In this passage, Qí Zhòngfǔ clarifies by saying "if it is red, it looks like crimson." Yes, crimson is more accurate. What happens to the blood if it gets heated up? It actually gets cooked and thickens just like a soup will thicken if it is exposed to heat over time. The color becomes a deep red or crimson. In addition, the "bright" of the bright red actually means shiny. Normal blood is bright red but of a rather matte finish. If the blood gets cooked with heat, it not only becomes deep red and thicker, it also develops more of a reflective sheen. If we see bright red blood as heat, we will misdiagnose in many cases. To diagnose heat, from looking at the blood, look for the deep crimson with a sheen and you won't make an error.

As for white-colored blood, again Qí Zhòngfǔ clarifies by saying "If it is white, it looks like nasal mucus." Now, what do we do with this diagnostically? I learned that pale-colored menstruate means blood deficiency. I would like to challenge this idea as it does not play out in the clinic. This also relates to the idea of white-colored blood. If we see pale-colored blood, this means that the blood is diluted with fluid. In turn, this means that there is both blood and there is leukorrhea mixing with the blood. This is true if we are seeing something that looks like nasal mucus as well. This is leukorrhea mixing with the blood. If the blood is pale-colored, then the leukorrhea is watery. If you see a mucus-like substance with the blood, then the leukorrhea is a bit thicker. Either way, it is very important to recognize that both of these are pathological fluids flowing out. The cause will either be deficiency, which means that the body's physiological fluids are not being stored properly, or excess, which means that there is an abundance of dampness in the lower body. If it is deficiency, it is important to determine where the deficiency lies. If there is excessive dampness, the root of the dampness must be determined. One mustn't jump to conclusions about the cause of the damp as it can be due to blood stasis, in which case the fluids of the blood leave the blood because of stasis, deficiency of the spleen, or deficiency of the kidney.

One may think that you would never see something like "white-colored blood." It sounds strange. I hope this discussion shows that it actually shows up in clinic quite regularly.

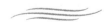

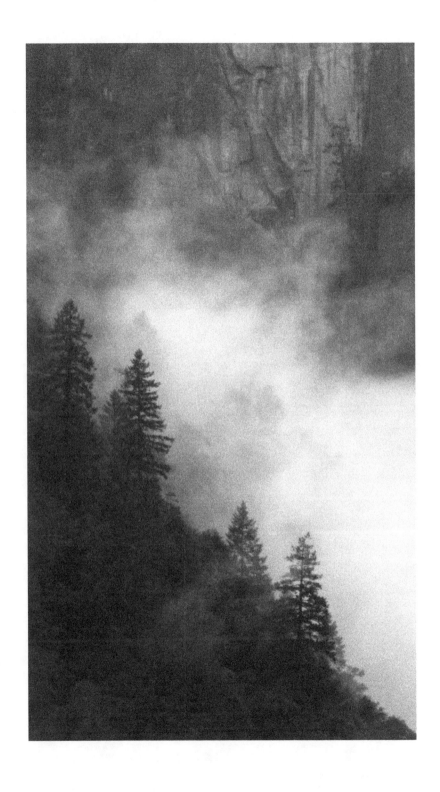

陽崩膠艾湯

治婦勞傷血氣，衝任虛損，月水過多，淋漓漏下，
連夕不斷，臍腹疼痛。

阿膠(炒)	
川芎	各二兩
甘草	
艾葉	各三兩
當歸	
白芍	各四兩
熟地	

上為飲子，每服三錢，水一盞，煎六分，去滓熱
服，空心食前。

甚者連夜並服之。

Yáng Bēng Jiāo Ài Tāng
(Yáng Landslide Collapse Donkey Hide Glue and Mugwort Decoction)

A treatment for women's taxation damage to blood and Qì, vacuity detriment to the Chōngmài and Rènmài, excessive menstrual fluids, dribbling and dripping and spotting below, continuing without interruption night after night, with pain in the umbilical area.

ējiāo (stir-fry)	
chuanxiong	2 *liǎng* each
gāncǎo	
àiyè	3 *liǎng* each
dāngguī	
báisháo	4 *liǎng* each
shúdì	

Make a drink with the ingredients above. Take 3 *qián* per dose and simmer in 1 cup of water until reduced to 60 percent. Remove the dregs and take warm on an empty stomach before meals.

In severe cases, take it continuously also throughout the night.

黃芩散

治崩中下血。

黃芩為末，每服一錢，燒秤錘酒調下。

崩中多是止血藥。此法治乘陰，經所謂天暑地熱，
經水沸溢者也。

Huángqín Sǎn
(Scutellaria Powder)

A treatment for Landslide Collapse of the center and bleeding from the lower body.

Process huángqín into a powder and take 1 *qián* per dose. Drink it down mixed into rice wine that has been warmed up by tossing in steelyard weights that had been heated in the fire.

Landslide Collapse of the center is most commonly [treated with] medicinals that stop bleeding. The present method treats overwhelmed Yīn, [a condition like] what the Classic refers to as "When there is summer-heat in heaven and the earth is hot, the river channels boil over."

FORMULA NOTE

The "Classic" mentioned above refers to *Sùwèn* Chapter Twenty-Seven, which contains this beautiful passage in Qí Bó's answer to the Yellow Emperor's question about the significance of the number nine and the manifestations of evil Qì being present in the channels:

夫聖人之起度數，必應於天地，故天有宿度，地有經水，人有經脈。
天地溫和，則經水安靜；天寒地凍，則經水凝泣；天暑地熱，則經
水沸溢；卒風暴起，則經水波湧而隴起。

> The sage's measurements and numbers must resonate with heaven and earth. As such, heaven has constellations, earth has river channels, and humans have vessel channels. When heaven and earth are harmonious, the river channels are calm. When there is winter-cold in heaven and the earth is frozen, the river channels become congealed and stagnant. When there is summer-heat in heaven and the earth is hot, the river channels boil over. When a windstorm arises suddenly, the river channels billow turbulently and rise in big swells.

Unlike most less educated modern readers perhaps, Qí Zhòngfǔ's contemporaries would have immediately recognized the source of his citation and been familiar with its context. Therefore they would have known that the term 經水 *jīngshuǐ* (literally "channel water") in the original context of the quote in *Sùwèn* Twenty-Seven has the meaning of the major rivers that structure the earth in the same way that the constellations structure heaven above. Much more commonly, however, the phrase is used in medical literature, especially in the context of gynecology and throughout the *Hundred Questions*, to mean "menstrual fluids." Unfortunately for readers of any translated version of the text, there is no way in English to replicate Qí Zhòngfǔ's witty use of the phrase here in a formula for Landslide Collapse in such a way that it reflects this dual meaning and still incorporates the context of the quote from *Sùwèn* Twenty-Seven. The dramatic image of a body of water roiling and boiling over and leaving its proper channels because of abnormal heat in the environment is the perfect metaphor for the critical condition addressed by this formula.

陰崩固經丸

治婦人衝任虛弱，月候不調，來多不斷，淋漓不
止。

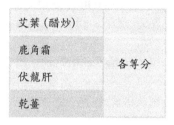

艾葉（醋炒）	
鹿角霜	各等分
伏龍肝	
乾薑	

上為末，溶鹿角膠，和藥乘熱丸，梧桐子大，食前
淡醋湯下五十丸。

Yīn Bēng Gù Jīng Wán
(Yīn Landslide Collapse Menses-Securing Pill)

A treatment for vacuity in the Chōngmài and Rènmài in
women, with the menstrual signs being unattuned, [menses]
arriving often and [flowing] uninterruptedly, and with dribbling and dripping without stopping.

àiyè (stir-fry in vinegar)	
lùjiǎoshuāng	equal amounts of each
fúlónggān	
gānjiāng	

Process the ingredients above into a powder. Dissolve the
lùjiǎoshuāng, mix all the medicinals together and, with the
help of heat, form into pills the size of *wútóng* seeds. Down
50 pills per dose before meals in a mild vinegar decoction.

赤龍丹

治崩漏不止，餘血作痛。

禹餘糧（煅）	乾薑
·烏賊骨	當歸
鹿茸（酒炙）	石燕子（煅）
龍骨	阿膠（炒）

上等分為末，酒醋糊丸，桐子大。每服五十丸，溫酒下，艾醋湯亦得。

Chì Lóng Dān
(Red Dragon Elixir)

A treatment for Landslide Collapse and spotting that will not stop, and for [the presence of] residual blood causing pain.

yǔyúliáng (calcine)	gānjiāng
wūzéigǔ	dāngguī
lùróng (mix-fry in rice wine)	shíyànzǐ (calcine)
lónggǔ	ējiāo (stir-fry)

Process equal amounts of the ingredients above into a powder and form flour pills with rice wine or vinegar, the size of *wútóng* seeds. Take 50 pills per dose, drinking them down in warm rice wine. Mugwort vinegar decoction is also permissible [for drinking them down with].

Formula Note

The name of the formula seems to suggest to the reader that we are dealing with an alchemical recipe from the Daoist tradition. First of all, the formula is called 丹 *dān*, or in other words, an "elixir." In addition, the term "red dragon" is a technical term used in literature on female inner alchemy (女丹 *nǚdān*) to refer to menstruation, especially in the phrase "slaying the red dragon" (斬龍 *zhǎnlóng* or 斷龍 *duànlóng*). Referring to the intentional cessation of menstruation, this is the first step in Daoist cultivation for women, in the process of refining the body in the pursuit of longevity and immortality through meditation, massage, Qi-circulation, and similar practices. Obviously, it far transcends the limitations of the present book to give an overview of the history or content of these practices, but we also need to keep in mind that female inner alchemy emerged in the written literature only many centuries after the publication of the present text. Interested readers are referred to Elena Valussi's excellent article "Blood, Tigers, Dragons: The Physiology of Transcendence in Women." As Valussi emphasizes, while medical and Daoist texts share a view of women as ruled by blood, they are aimed at two very different goals: health in the case of medical literature, and transcendence in the case of religious texts. According to Valussi, the phrase "slaying the red dragon" first appears in a text compiled in 1310, so less than a hundred years after the publication of the *Hundred Questions of Gynecology*.

Regardless of when Daoist cultivation practices might have begun to concern themselves with women's menstrual cycles, the present formula does not have anything to do with the Daoist cultivation practices aimed at intentionally manipulating women's physiological functions and stopping menstruation in the pursuit of immortality. In the present context, "red dragon" is used simply as a reference to female bleeding from the vagina, both in critical cases of Landslide Collapse and in the chronic form of spotting below. The last indication of "residual blood causing pain" most likely refers to blood that is left over in the uterus after childbirth, or in other words, the dreaded pathological substance of 惡露 *èlù* "Malign Dew." While not specifically mentioned here or in the later questions on postpartum conditions, the incomplete elimination of blood and other substances being left behind in the uterus after childbirth (lochia in biomedicine) are a key cause in traditional Chinese gynecology for all sorts of problems in later years, from infertility to pain to irregular and excessive or inadequate menstrual bleeding. The condition of Landslide Collapse in particular was a term also associated with the life-threatening hemorrhaging that sometimes occurs during and after delivery.

第四十三問

眠臥多汗者，何也？

答曰：盜汗者因眠臥而身體流汗也。

此由陽虛所致。久不已令人羸瘦，心虛不足，亡津液故也。

診其脈虛弱細微，皆盜汗脈也。

QUESTION FORTY-THREE

What is the Meaning of Profuse Sweating During Sleep?

ANSWER: "Thief sweating" means streaming sweat all over the body during sleep.

This is caused by Yáng vacuity. If this persists for a long time, it causes the person [to suffer from] marked emaciation, heart vacuity and insufficiency, and collapse of the fluids.

When examining the pulse, if it is vacuous, weak, fine, or faint, all of these are pulses of "thief sweating."

DISCUSSION

Cháo discusses the condition of "vacuity taxation thief sweating" (虛勞盜汗 *xūláo dàohàn*) in Volume Three of the *Zhūbìng yuánhòu lùn* on "The Various Signs of Vacuity Taxation Diseases." Because his wording is virtually identical to the passage above, it is clear once again that this text was one of the main sources for Qí Zhòngfǔ's writings. The passage above is one of the more drastic examples where Qí has simply copied the entry from the general section of Cháo's book, without adding any information on how this condition might manifest or need to be treated differently in women.

For a more specific understanding of the condition as it affects the female body, we need to consult Volume Thirty-Seven, on "The Various Signs of Women's Miscellaneous Diseases." Here, Cháo Yuánfāng explains the condition of "vacuity sweating" (虛汗 *xūhàn*) in women:

> 人以水穀之精，化為血氣津液，津液行於腠理。若勞傷損動，陽氣外虛，腠理開，血氣衰弱，故津液泄越，令多汗也。其虛汗不止，則變短氣，柴瘦而羸瘠也。亦令血脈減損，經水痞澀，甚者閉斷不通也。

Humans take the essence of water and grain and transform it into blood and Qì and fluids, and the fluids move into the interstices. If taxation has caused injury and stirring, and Yáng Qì is vacuous on the outside, the interstices are open, and the blood and Qì are feeble, the fluids drain astray. This causes profuse sweating. If this vacuity sweating is not stopped, it transforms into shortness of breath and extreme emaciation like a stick. It also reduces the flow of blood in the vessels and makes the fluid in the channels blocked. In severe cases, it results in complete interruption of flow.

As is so often the case in traditional Chinese gynecology, the cause of night sweating is taxation damage resulting in vacuity of blood and Qì. And also typical for gynecology, the most serious effect of this condition is an impairment and eventual interruption of the flow of blood in the vessels.

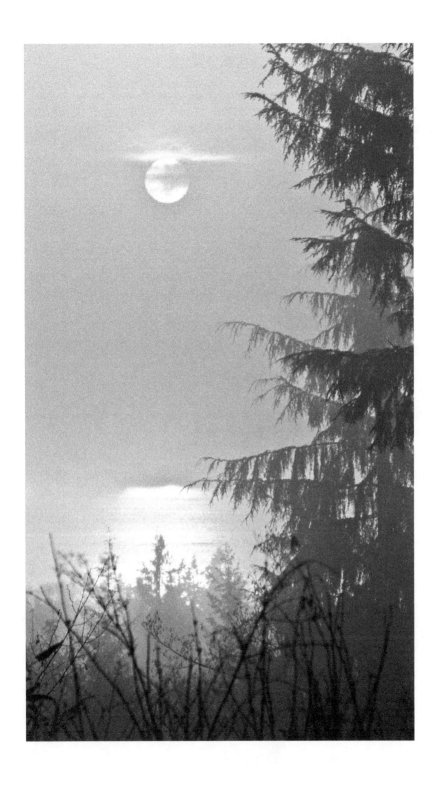

大建中湯

治熱自腹中，或從背脊，漸漸蒸熱，或寐而汗，日漸羸瘦。

白芍	六兩
黃芪	
遠志	
當歸	各三兩
澤瀉	
龍骨	
人參	各二兩
甘草（炙）	
吳朮	一分

上為粗末，每服五錢。水二盞，薑三片，棗一枚擘破，入飴少許，煎一盞。食前溫服。

Dà Jiàn Zhōng Tāng
(Major Center-Fortifying Decoction)

A treatment for heat from the center of the abdomen, or from the back and spine, gradual steaming, possibly sweating in one's sleep, and gradually increasing emaciation.

báisháo	6 *liǎng*
huángqí	
yuǎnzhì	
dāngguī	3 *liǎng* each
zéxiè	
lónggǔ	
rénshēn	2 *liǎng* each
gāncǎo (mix-fry)	
báizhú from the state of Wú[2]	1 *fēn*

Process the ingredients above into a coarse powder and take 5 *qián* per dose. Simmer in 2 cups of water with 3 slices of ginger, 1 jujube broken up into pieces, and a small amount of malt sugar, until reduced to 1 cup. Take warm before meals.

---

2 The ancient kingdom of Wū 吳 was located in the southeast of early China, around the mouth of the Yangtze river east of the kingdom of Chǔ 楚.

黃芪飲子

治婦人血氣不足，夜間虛乏，有汗倦怠者。

黃芪	
五味子	各半兩
當歸	
白茯苓	
白芍	
遠志	
麥子(一方用麥門冬)	各一分
人參	
吳朮	
甘草	三銖

上㕮咀，每服三錢。水盞半，薑三片，煎七分，去滓溫服，不拘時。神驗。

Huángqí Yǐnzi
(Astragalus Drink)

A treatment for women [suffering from] insufficiency of blood and Qì, with exhaustion at night, and sweating and fatigue.

huángqí	
wǔwèizǐ	0.5 *liǎng* each
dāngguī	
báifúlíng	
báisháo	
yuǎnzhì	
màizǐ (another formula uses màiméndōng)	1 *fēn* each
rénshēn	
báizhú from the state of Wū	
gāncǎo	3 *zhū*

Pound the ingredients above and take 3 *qián* per dose. Simmer in 1.5 cups of water with 3 slices of ginger until reduced to 70 percent, remove the dregs, and take warm, without restricting the timing. It is divinely effective.

加味理建湯

治男子婦人夜多盜汗並便濁者。此方昌國州方順齋傳到，經驗。

乾薑

吳朮

人參

黃芪

白芍

肉桂

甘草

牡蠣

浮麥

當歸

上件㕮咀，每服水二盞，薑五片，棗一枚，煎八分。食前熱服，渣再煎。

Jiā Wèi Lǐ Jiàn Tāng
(Augmented Patterning and Fortifying Decoction)

A treatment for men and women for increased night sweating in combination with turbid urine. This formula was transmitted by Fāng Shùnzhāi from Chāngguó Prefecture. It has proven efficacy.

gānjiāng
báizhú from the state of Wū
rénshēn
huángqí
báisháo
ròuguì
gāncǎo
mǔlì
fúmài
dāngguī

Pound the ingredients above. For each dose, simmer in 2 cups of water with 5 slices of ginger and 1 jujube until reduced to 80 percent. Take hot before meals, and reboil the dregs.

第四十四問

左脅痛如刀刺，不得喘息者，何也？

答曰：肝居脅之左，以藏血。

針經云：「邪在肝，兩脅痛。」

巢氏云：「左脅偏痛者，由經絡偏邪，客於旁之故也。人之經絡，旋環於身，左右表裡皆周遍。若血氣調和，不生虛實痛証。」

或偏者邪傷之也。其左脅痛如刀刺者，則知其邪偏客於左也。甚者不得喘息也。

QUESTION FORTY-FOUR

What Is the Reason for Pain in the Left Rib-Side [That Feels] Like Being Stabbed with a Knife, So That the Patient is Unable to Breathe?

ANSWER: The liver resides in the left rib-side, and stores the blood there.

According to the Needling Classic, "when the evil is in the liver, there is pain in both rib-sides."

According to Master Cháo, "Unilateral pain in the left rib-side is caused by unilateral evil in the channels and network vessels that has lodged on the side. A person's channels and network vessels circulate through the body and reach everywhere, to the left and the right and the exterior and the interior. If the blood and Qì are harmoniously attuned, they do not engender vacuity or repletion pain patterns."

If there happens to be some unilateral [imbalance], it means that evil has caused damage there. Because of the pain in the left rib-side as if being stabbed with a knife, we know that the evil in this case has lodged unilaterally on the left. If it is severe, the patient is unable to breathe.

Discussion

Qí Zhòngfǔ's answer to this question about severe unilateral pain in the left rib-side appears to be contradictory. On the one hand, the very first sentence suggests an important association of pain in the left rib-side with the liver by conflating two established facts of Chinese medicine theory: As the quotation from the "Needling Classic," which refers to *Língshū* Chapter Twenty on the "Five Evils" (五邪 *wǔ xié*), states:

邪在肝、則兩脇中痛。

When the evil is in the liver, the result is pain in both rib-sides.

Thus, a key area for pathologies in the liver (and gallbladder) to manifest is the rib-sides, or in other words, the upper part of the flanks from below the armpit to the side of the lowest rib.

In addition, we can further differentiate pain by the side of the body where it occurs. And this is precisely why Qí starts out his answer with the well-known theory of Chinese medicine here that the liver, which stores the blood, is associated with the left side of the body. As a result, it seems that a physician wanting to diagnose and treat any pain that predominantly affects the left upper flank of the body, especially in women, needs to take the state of the liver into consideration. This is suggested by authors like Cháo Yuánfāng who state clearly that "accumulations in the liver are called fat Qì and are located below the left rib-side."

Nevertheless, the two quotations from the classics that Qí Zhòngfǔ offers up to shed light on this question at the same time challenge this connection between the liver and unilateral pain in the left rib-side: In apparent contradiction to the previous statement about the liver being on the left, the *Zhēnjīng* quotation actually states that evil in the liver manifests in pain in both rib-sides, and not just the left. A related statement is found in the *Sùwèn* Chapter Sixty-Three, the "Discourse on Baffling Needling" (繆刺論 *miùcì lùn*):

邪客於足少陽之絡，令人脅痛不得息。

Evil that lodges in the network vessels of the Foot Shàoyáng causes the person to suffer from rib-side pain and inability to breathe.

The next quotation cited by Qí Zhòngfǔ is clearly derived from the entry on "Pain in the left rib-side that feels like being stabbed with a knife" in Volume Thirty-Nine on women's miscellaneous diseases in Cháo Yuánfāng's *Zhūbìng yuánhòu lùn*, even if Qí has taken a bit of poetic license to condense the entry:

左脅偏痛者，由經絡偏虛邪故也。人之經絡，循環於身，左右表裏皆周徧。

若氣血調和，不生虛實，邪不能傷。偏虛者，偏受風邪。

今此左脅痛者，左邊偏受病也。但風邪在於經絡，與血氣相乘，交爭衝擊，故痛發如刀刺。

Unilateral pain in the left rib-side is caused by unilateral vacuity evil in the channels and network vessels. A person's channels and network vessels circulate through the body and reach everywhere, to the left and the right and the exterior and the interior.

If the Qì and blood are harmoniously attuned, they do not engender vacuity or repletion, and evil is unable to cause damage. In the case of unilateral vacuity, the person has contracted wind evil unilaterally.

Now the present case of pain in the left rib-side means that the left side has unilaterally contracted disease. If wind evil is present in the channels and network vessels, overwhelming the blood and Qì, clashing with and assaulting them, for this reason the pain erupts as if getting stabbed with a knife.

In other words, pain on either side of the body is due to an underlying vacuity that allowed for contraction of a disease there. The severity of the pain indicates the presence of wind assaulting the Qì and blood. No mention is made of the role of liver here, whether in relation to the location of the pathology in the left side of the body or in the location of the pain in the rib-sides!

Qí Zhòngfǔ concludes his answer by reinforcing this sentiment that the location of the pain in the left rib-side merely indicates a vacuity in that area that allowed an external evil to intrude, with no relevance to any organs or channels located there. Thus he pointedly emphasizes the incidental nature of this location with the particle 或 *huò*, meaning "perhaps" or "possibly." In other words, this last paragraph suggests that stabbing pain in one rib-side or the other simply means that a pathogenic factor has taken up residence on that side but has nothing to do with the liver. This is, of course, significant both for diagnosis and treatment.

It is possible or perhaps even likely that Qí Zhòngfǔ's position that the location of pain in conditions on the left carried no special significance and did not indicate a problem with the liver was somewhat unorthodox, especially in the context of diagnosing and treating female patients, in whom the storage of blood was of great importance. Thus the *Zhèngzhì huìbǔ* 《證治彙補》 (Collected Supplements to Patterns and Treatments), a much later text by Lǐ Yòngcuì 李用粹 from 1687, explains:

> 脅痛宜分左右、辨虛實。左脅痛者，肝受邪也；右脅痛者，肝邪入肺也；左右脅痛者，氣滯也；。。。

> Pain in the rib-sides should be divided into left and right and differentiated as vacuity or repletion. Pain in the left rib-side means that the liver has contracted the evil. Pain in the right rib-side means that the evil from the liver has entered the lung. Pain in both the left and the right rib-sides means Qì stagnation...

The differentiation into the level of the Qì and blood, implied by the affected organs in this quote, namely the liver on the left side versus the lung on the right, is taken up in the following formula, which specifically mentions that it treats both Qì and blood pain.

醋煎散

治婦人血氣腹脅刺痛。

良薑	一兩
當歸	
肉桂	
白芍	各半兩
陳皮	
烏藥	

上為細末，每服三錢。水醋各半盞，煎七分。通口
服。

Cù Jiān Sǎn
(Vinegar-Simmered Powder)

A treatment for women's stabbing blood-pain and Qì-pain
in the abdomen and rib-sides.

liángjiāng	1 *liǎng*
dāngguī	
ròuguì	
báisháo	0.5 *liǎng* each
chénpí	
wūyào	

Process the ingredients above into a fine powder and take 3
qián per dose. Simmer in half a cup each of water and vinegar
until reduced to 70 percent. Take it by oral ingestion.

趁痛散

治血氣刺痛，起於一邊，或左或右，行環上下，或在肌肉之間，如錐刀所刺，其氣不得息。

莪朮	各一兩
官桂	
檳榔	半兩
芫花(醋炙)	各一兩
附子	
細辛	半兩

上為飲子，每服三錢，水盞半。煎七分，去滓溫服。薑棗同煎。

Chèn Tòng Sǎn
(Pain-Alleviating Powder)

A treatment for stabbing blood-pain and Qì-pain, arising on one side, whether the left or the right, moving in a circle up and down, possibly in the space of the flesh, as if being stabbed with an awl, [to the point where the patient is] unable to breathe.

ézhú	1 *liǎng* each
guānguì	
bīnláng	0.5 *liǎng*
yuánhuā (mix-fry with vinegar)	1 *liǎng* each
fùzǐ	
xìxīn	0.5 *liǎng*

Prepare the ingredients above into a drink, using 3 *qián* per dose in half a cup of water. Simmer until reduced to 70 percent, remove the dregs, and take warm. Simmer it with ginger and jujubes.

第四十五問

積聚之病，何以別之？

答曰：積聚者，由陰陽不和，腑臟虛弱，受其風邪，搏於腑臟之氣所為也。

積者，五臟所生；聚者，六腑所生。

然陽化氣，氣屬於六腑；陰成形，形主於五臟。

陽則動而不息，故聚者，始發無根本，上下無所留止，其痛無常處，故謂之聚也。

陰則定而守住，故積者，始發有常處，其痛不離其部，上下有所終始，左右有所窮處，乃謂之積也。

積脈陰沉而伏，象陰體之沉靜。聚脈陽浮而動，法陽性之浮高。

然積病有五，隨其五臟相傳而生焉。經云：在肝則曰肥氣，在心則曰伏梁，在脾則曰痞氣，在肺則曰息賁，在腎則曰奔豚。故曰積聚之病，此可別也。

QUESTION FORTY-FIVE

How do you Differentiate Between the Diseases of Accumulations and Gatherings?

ANSWER: Accumulations and Gatherings are caused by Yīn-Yáng disharmony, weakness of the *zàng* and *fǔ* organs, and contraction of wind evil there, which assaults the Qì in the *zàng* and *fǔ* organs.

Accumulations are engendered in the five *zàng* organs, while Gatherings are engendered in the six *fǔ* organs.

This being so, Yáng transforms Qì, and Qì belongs to the six *fǔ* organs. Yīn completes the material body, and the material body is ruled by the five *zàng* organs.

Yáng, then, moves and does not rest. For this reason, Gatherings start out without a root and rise and fall without a stopping place. Their pain does not have a constant location, and therefore they are called Gatherings.

Yin, then, is fixed and safeguards where it stays. For this reason, Accumulations start out with a constant location, and their pain does not leave this area. Above and below, they have a beginning and an end, and to the right and left, they have defined edges. Thus we call them Accumulations.

The pulse of Accumulations is Yīn, deep and latent, resembling the deep stillness of Yīn substance. The pulse of Gatherings is Yáng, floating and stirring, imitating the high floating nature of Yáng.

This being said, there are five kinds of Accumulation diseases, based on their formation in transmission from the five zàng organs. The Classic states: "Located in the liver, they are called Fat Qì; located in the heart, they are called Deep-Lying Beam; located in the spleen, they are called pǐ Glomus Qì; located in the lung, they are called Breath Bolting; and located in the kidney, they are called Bolting Piglet." Thus it is said that this is how you can differentiate diseases of Accumulations and Gatherings.

DISCUSSION

The first three sentences and the section on the five different types of accumulation disease are derived from the introductory essay of Volume Nineteen on "Accumulations and Gatherings" in Cháo Yuánfāng's *Zhūbìng yuánhòu lùn*. The rest of this answer is almost entirely copied from *Nànjīng*, Difficulty Fifty-Five, which discusses how to differentiate between Accumulations and Gatherings. Instead of the way in which Qí Zhòngfǔ presents the association of the conditions with Yīn and Yáng here, the *Nànjīng* simply states, "Accumulations are Yīn Qì; Gatherings are Yáng Qì," and explains that "Where the Qì accumulates is called Accumulations, and where the Qì gathers is called Gatherings." In other words, this classic, and many later authors following its lead, distinguish between Accumulations and Gatherings on the basis of the literal meaning of the characters: The character for Accumulations is 積 *jí*, which has the grain radical 禾 and literally means "to amass," "to pile/stack up grain." By contrast, the character for Gatherings is 聚 *jù*, which has the radical 众, a version of 眾, meaning "a crowd of people." In its original and most limited sense, it thus refers to a temporary gathering or assembly of people, with the important implication that it is transitory and not a permanent, immovable, strictly defined situation.

Abdominal masses are a recurring key concern in early gynecological texts, such as Cháo Yuánfāng's *Zhūbìng yuánhòu lùn*. After a literal repetition of the differentiation between Accumulations and Gatherings into Yīn and Yáng that was introduced in the non-gendered Volume Nineteen, the entry on this topic in the gynecological section of this text includes the following information:

> 婦人病積經久,則令無子,亦令月水不通。所以然者,積聚起受於冷氣,結入子臟,故令無子;若冷氣入於胞絡,冷搏受於血,血冷則澀結,故令月水不通。

When women suffer from Accumulations for a long time, this causes infertility, as well as a failure of the menstrual fluids to flow through. The reason for this is that Accumulations and Gatherings arise due to contraction of cool Qì, which binds and enters the uterus. Hence it causes infertility. If the cool Qì enters the uterine network vessels, the cold assaults the blood, the blood becomes cool, and consequently flows haltingly and binds. Hence it causes a failure of the menstrual fluids to flow through.

Abdominal masses of all kinds, movable or fixed, hard or soft, palpable or not, painful to the touch or not so tender, with clearly marked boundaries or diffused in size, are an important factor in gynecological literature, seen as the result of impeded menstrual flow and contraction of cold, and as a key causative factor in infertility. Given this context, it is puzzling to me that Qí Zhòngfǔ chose to omit any reference to female anatomy or physiology, or to the role of blood in his explanation on these conditions. My best guess is that this association was so obvious to, and so well-accepted by his contemporary clinically educated readers that he saw no need to repeat it, instead emphasizing the non-gendered aspect of this condition and the importance of diagnostic differentiation on the basis of Yīn and Yáng.

Throughout the centuries, Chinese medical authors have made many attempts to distinguish between the various terms for masses of Qì and blood, such as Accumulations, Gatherings, Concretions, and Conglomerations. Apparently, they were almost as confused as modern students of TCM who don't read Chinese who suffer from one more layer of obfuscation because the various terms tend to be translated inconsistently into English. Contradicting Qí Zhòngfǔ's writings above and many other gynecological texts that frequently mention women suffering from Accumulations and Gatherings, Lǐ Chān 李梴, for example, argued in his *Yīxué rùmén* 《醫學入門》 (Fundamentals of Medicine, published in 1575) that Accumulations and Gatherings occur in male bodies while Concretions and Conglomerations are specifically female diseases. Introducing yet more terms and offering yet another explanation of their differences, Shěn Jīn'áo 沈金鰲 proposed in his *Zábìng yuánliú xīzhú* 《雜病源流犀燭》 (Illuminating the Origin and Development of Miscellaneous Diseases) of 1773 that these names indicated a different location in the body:

痞癖见于胸膈间，是上焦之病；痃积滞见于腹内，是中焦之病；癥瘕见于脐下，是下焦之病。…

故积聚痃癖痞，多生于男子，而女子偶患之；癥瘕多生于女子，而男子偶患之。

Pǐ Glomus and Aggregations manifest in the area of the chest and diaphragm and are diseases of the Upper Jiāo. *Xián* Strings, Accumulations, and stagnations manifest in the middle of the abdomen and are diseases of the Middle Jiāo. Concretions and Conglomerations manifest below the navel and are diseases of the Lower Jiāo…

For this reason, Accumulations, Gatherings, *xián* Strings, *pǐ* Glomus, and Aggregations are generated mostly in men, while women occasionally suffer from them. Concretions and Conglomerations are generated mostly in women, and men occasionally suffer from them.

In contrast to all of these attempts at differentiation, and perhaps more practically oriented, the illustrious Sòng emperor Huīzōng 宋徽宗 proposed in his *Shèngjì zǒnglù* 《聖濟總錄》 (Encyclopedia of Sagely Benefaction) from 1117:

癥瘕癖結者，積聚之異名也，症狀不一，原其病本大略相似。

Concretions and Conglomerations and Aggregations and Binds were alternate names for Accumulations and Gatherings, with differing patterns and symptoms, but originally the diseases were basically identical."

鱉甲丸

治小腹中積聚，大如七八寸，盤面，上下周旋，痛
不可忍。

鱉甲		蟅蟲	
官桂	各一兩半	乾薑	
蜂房	半兩	牡丹皮	
川椒		附子	
細辛		水蛭	
人參		皂角(一本牛白角腮)	各一兩
苦參		當歸	
丹參		赤芍	
沙參		甘草	
吳茱萸	各十八銖	防葵	
蟅蟲	二十枚		
大黃			
虻蟲			
玄參	十八銖		

上為細末，蜜丸桐子大。每服七丸，溫酒下，日三
服。加之，以效為度。

Biējiǎ Wán
(Turtle Shell Pill)

A treatment for Accumulations and Gatherings inside the lower abdomen, about 7 or 8 *cùn* in size and disc-shaped, moving up and down in circles, with unbearable pain.

biējiǎ		zhèchóng		
guāngù	1.5 *liǎng* each	gānjiāng		
fēngfáng	0.5 *liǎng*	mǔdānpí		
chuānjiāo		fùzǐ		
xìxīn		shuǐzhì		1 *liǎng* each
rénshēn		zàojiǎo (another edition has the white base of an oxen's horn instead)		
kǔshēn		dāngguī		
dānshēn		chìsháo		
shāshēn		gāncǎo		
wúzhūyú	18 *zhū* each	fángkuí		
qícǎo	20 specimens			
dàhuáng				
méngchóng				
xuánshēn	18 *zhū*			

Process the ingredients above into a fine powder and turn into honey pills the size of *wútóng* seeds. Take 7 pills per dose, downing them in warm rice wine, three doses a day. Increase this dosage [as needed], using efficacy as your measure.

沒藥散

治婦人一切血氣臍腹撮痛。

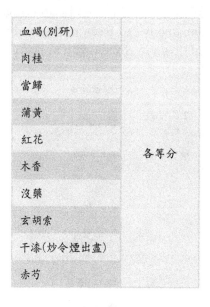

血竭(別研)	
肉桂	
當歸	
蒲黃	
紅花	各等分
木香	
沒藥	
玄胡索	
干漆(炒令煙出盡)	
赤芍	

上為細末，每服二錢。熱酒調下，食前。

Mòyào Sǎn
(Myrrh Powder)

A treatment for every kind of women's pinching blood-pain and Qì-pain in the navel and abdomen.

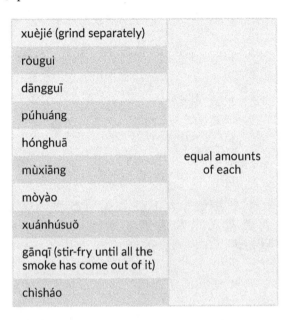

xuèjié (grind separately)	
ròuguì	
dāngguī	
púhuáng	
hónghuā	equal amounts of each
mùxiāng	
mòyào	
xuánhúsuǒ	
gānqī (stir-fry until all the smoke has come out of it)	
chìsháo	

Process the ingredients above into a fine powder and take 2 *qián* per dose. Down it mixed into hot rice wine before meals.

紫金散

治婦人血氣不和，血塊疼痛。常服暖子宮，通經絡。

橘紅	
枳殼	
肉桂	各一兩
玄胡索	
甘草(炙)	
紫金牛(一本紫金皮)	五兩
當歸(酒浸一宿，焙乾，銼)	各三兩
香附(炒，去毛)	
南木香 (生)	半兩

上為末。婦人室女月水不調，久閉羸瘦，蘇木煎湯調下，白雞冠花末煎酒調下亦得，每服一匙。常服，安胎養氣。

臨產橫逆，蔥白煎酒下。

血氣脹滿，催生下死胎，煎枳殼酒下，地榆末煎酒下亦得。

產後血運，頭旋中風口噤，惡證發動，虛腫，豆淋酒下。

產後惡血不止，血海衰敗，赤白帶下，胞漏，棕櫚灰酒下，綿灰亦得。

胎氣絞刺，肋脅腹肚疼痛，炒薑酒下。

心氣不足，陳皮湯下。

產後敗血停積，攻刺腰痛，無灰酒下。日午臨睡三服。 忌生冷淹藏毒魚。

Zǐjīn Sǎn
(Japanese Ardisia Powder)

A treatment for women's disharmony between Qì and blood, with blood lumping [and causing] pain. Taken constantly, it warms the uterus and frees the flow in the channels and network vessels.

júhóng	
zhǐké	
ròuguì	1 *liǎng* each
xuánhúsuǒ	
gāncǎo (mix-fry)	
zǐjīnniú (another edition uses zǐjīnpí)	5 *liǎng*
dāngguī (soak overnight in rice wine, then roast until dry and grate)	3 *liǎng* each
xiāngfù (stir-fry and remove the hairs)	
nánmùxiāng (fresh)	0.5 *liǎng*

Process the ingredients above into a powder. For married women and unmarried maidens who suffer from lack of attunement in the menstrual fluids, with chronic blockage and marked weakness and emaciation, down it mixed into a decoction of simmered sūmù. It is also possible to down it mixed into a decoction of simmered báijīguānhuā (white cockscomb) powder. Take 1 spoonfull per dose. Taken constantly, it calms the fetus and nurtures Qì.

For approaching childbirth and for breech and transverse position, down it [mixed into] rice wine simmered with cōngbái.

For blood and Qì distention and to hasten delivery and bring down a dead fetus, down it in rice wine simmered with zhǐké. You can also down it in rice wine simmered with powdered dìyú.

For postpartum blood dizziness with spinning head, wind strike, and clenched mouth, signs of malignity starting up, and vacuity swelling, down it in rice wine sprinkled over scorch-fried soybeans.

For incessant postpartum bleeding of malign blood, deterioration of the Sea of Blood, red and white vaginal discharge, and "leaking womb," down it in rice wine zōnglú ashes. Ashed silk floss can be substituted [for the zōnglú].

For fetal Qì twisting and stabbing, [causing] pain in the ribs, ribs-sides, abdomen, and belly, down it in rice wine with stir-fried ginger.

For insufficiency of heart Qì, down it in a decoction of chénpí.

For postpartum accumulation of decayed blood with aggressively piercing lumbar pain, down it in ash-free rice wine. Take two doses, at noon and before going to sleep. Avoid raw and cold foods, pickles, and poisonous fish.

Formula Note

I translate 胞漏 *bāolòu* literally as "leaking womb," rather than to follow Wiseman's terminology as "fetal spotting," because the condition in Chinese medicine does not only refer to the light bleeding that the English term "spotting" implies. Rather, it is a term that includes all types of bleeding during pregnancy, from occasional dripping to intermittent or even incessant bleeding, and is a key sign of threatened miscarriage. Some English authors, especially in a TCM context, even choose to translate it as "threatened miscarriage." In Chinese literature, the *Zhōngyī dà cídiǎn* 《中醫大辭典》 (Great Dictionary of Chinese Medicine) equates it with other terms like 妊娠下血 *rènshēn xià xuè* ("bleeding during pregnancy," *Jīnguì yàolüè*) or 胎漏 *tāilòu* ("fetal leaking," *Tàipíng shēnghuì fang* 《太平聖惠方》).

"Ash-free rice wine" does not just refer to plain rice wine that has not been adulterated with other medicinal substances to address a specific condition, but rather to rice wine that has been fermented without adding any ashed rice straw, a traditional method for adding lime to control the PH of the final product.

While the last line of the original text in all the editions I have available says to take "three doses" (三服) of the medicine, I have taken the liberty to change it in my translation to "two doses" and interpret the discrepancy as a typographical error. There is no way to make sense of the text otherwise.

第四十六問

身體常瘙癢者，何也？

答曰：身瘙癢者，是體虛受風，風入腠理，與血氣相搏而俱往來在皮膚之間，邪氣散而不能沖擊為痛也，故但瘙癢也。

仲景云：癢者名泄氣風，久久成痂癩，亦由體虛，受風邪之所致也。

QUESTION FORTY-SIX

What Is the Reason for Constant Eczema and Itching of the Body?

ANSWER: Eczema and itching of the body means that the body is vacuous and has contracted wind, which has entered the interstices and is battling with the blood and Qì, simultaneously coming and going in the area of the skin. Because the evil Qì has scattered and is unable to launch an attack and cause pain, there is only eczema and itching.

Zhāng Zhòngjǐng states: "Itching is called 'discharging Qì and wind' and, when persisting over a very long period, forms scabs and Lài disease." It is also caused by vacuity of the body and the contraction of wind evil.

DISCUSSION

As so often in this text, Qí Zhòngfǔ almost literally cites Cháo Yuánfāng's *Zhūbìng Yuánhòu lùn*. Thus, the entry on "Wind Itching" in Volume Two of this text states:

邪氣客於肌肉，則令肌肉虛，真氣散去，又被寒搏皮膚，外發腠理，
閉毫毛。淫邪與衛氣相搏，陽勝則熱，陰勝則寒。
寒則表虛，虛則邪氣往來，故肉癢也。
凡痺之類，逢熱則癢，逢寒則痛。

Evil Qì intrudes into the flesh, causing vacuity there and scattering genuine Qì. This situation is further complicated by cold striking the skin, from the outside launching into the interstices and blocking the fine body hair. This oozing evil battles with the *wèi* Defense Qì, resulting in heat if Yáng prevails, and in cold if Yīn prevails.

Cold results in vacuity in the exterior, and this vacuity results in evil Qì coming and going. Therefore there is itching in the flesh.

In all the categories of *bì* Impediment, chance encounters with heat result in itching, and chance encounters with cold in pain.

Adding to this explanation, a separate entry on "Wind Eczema and Itching" offers the following etiology:

此由游風在於皮膚，逢寒則身體疼痛，遇熱則瘡癢。

This is caused by roaming wind being present in the skin. A chance encounter with cold results in pain in the body, and a meeting with heat in eczema and itching.

Confirming Qí Zhòngfǔ's explanation above, we can thus conclude that eczema and itching is a wind condition at its core (hence its roaming, unpredictable, and intermittent nature), and a manifestation of external evil coming and going in the superficial layer of the skin. In this context, the presence of pain indicates cold while the presence of eczema and itching indicates heat. In all cases, a generalized vacuity of the physical body is the root of the condition, because it allowed for the initial invasion of wind.

Some good news about this condition is implied by Qí's observation that eczema and itching without pain means a coming and going of "scattered" evil Qì in the superficial layer, "unable to launch an attack" and enter the deeper layers of the body.

This interpretation of eczema itching as a superficial condition is also supported by the quotation from Zhāng Zhòngjǐng that itching means the discharge of the external pathogen. The quote in Qí Zhòngfǔ's answer comes from a line on "wind water" in Volume Fourteen on "Water Qì" of the *Jīnguì yàolüè*:

脈浮而洪，浮則為風，洪則為氣。風氣相搏，風強則為隱疹，身體為癢，癢為泄風，久為痂癩；氣強則為水，難以俯仰。風氣相擊，身體洪腫，汗出乃愈。

When the pulse is floating and surging, floating means wind and surging means Qì. Wind and Qì assault each other. If wind is stronger, the result is dormant papules and itching in the body. Itching means discharging wind. Over a long time, it forms scabs and Lài disease. If Qì is stronger, the result is water [disease] with difficulty bending and stretching. Wind and Qì assault each other, there is generalized swelling, and the emission of sweat means recovery.

The meaning of 痂癩 *jiā lài*, which I have translated as "scabs and Lài disease," requires a brief note. Most likely, here it means that when the itching continues for a long time without proper treatment, it can turn into a skin condition marked by scabs and a leprosy-like manifestation. The character 癩 *lài* is often translated as "leprosy" in modern TCM texts and equated with 癘風 *lìfēng* (which literally means "pestilential wind"), but can also refer to a much wider range of transmissible skin conditions marked by hair loss.

胡麻散

治脾肺風毒，攻沖遍身，皮膚瘙癢，或生瘡疥，或生癮疹，用手搔時，浸淫成瘡，久而不瘥，愈而復作，面上游風，或如蟲行，紫癜白癜頑麻等風，或腎臟風，攻注腳膝生瘡，並宜服之。

胡麻	三兩
苦參	二兩
何首烏(洗)	二兩
甘草(炙)	半兩
荊芥	三兩
威靈仙	一兩半

上為細末，每服二錢，薄荷湯茶點，食後服，或酒調蜜湯點亦得。服此後頻頻洗浴，得出汗而立效。

Húmá Sǎn
Black Sesame Powder

A treatment for spleen-lung wind poison, attacking all over the body, with eczema and itching in the skin, possibly forming scabby sores or dormant papules; when scratched with the hand, oozing and spreading to form sores; persisting for a long time without healing, or healing but erupting again; "roaming wind" sores on the face, possibly [with a sensation] like insects crawling; and Purple Patch, White Patch, stubborn numbness, and similar wind diseases. It is equally suitable to take this medicine if wind in the kidney *zàng* organ has attacked and poured into the lower legs and feet and engendered sores there.

húmá	3 *liǎng*
kǔshēn	2 *liǎng*
héshǒuwū (rinse)	2 *liǎng*
gāncǎo (mix-fry)	0.5 *liǎng*
jīngjiè	3 *liǎng*
wēilíngxiān	1.5 *liǎng*

Process the ingredients above into a fine powder and take 2 *qián* per dose, made into a tea by pouring boiling mint decoction over it. Take after meals. Alternatively, it is also possible to take it mixed into rice wine or by pouring boiling honey decoction over it. After taking this, bathe repeatedly. When [the patient] is able to emit sweat, this establishes recovery.

FORMULA NOTE

The famous encyclopedia *Yīzōng jīnjiàn* 《醫宗金鑒》 (Golden Mirror of the Orthodox Lineage of Medicine) from 1742 defines "face roaming wind" as follows:

此證生於面上，初發面目浮腫，癢若蟲行，肌膚乾燥，時起白屑，次後極癢，抓破，熱濕盛者津黃水，風燥盛者津血水，痛楚難堪。由平素血燥，過食辛辣厚味，以致陽明胃經濕熱受風而成。癢甚者，宜服消風散；痛甚者，宜服黃連消毒飲；外抹摩風膏緩緩取效。

This pattern forms on the face and manifests with puffy swelling in the face and eyes when it first erupts, itching as if from crawling insects, dry skin, and occasional white scales; followed by extreme itching [and sores that] break open when scratched, which if heat-damp is exuberant, ooze a yellow fluid, and if wind dryness is exuberant, ooze a bloody fluid; and with anguish that is difficult to bear. This disease forms due to chronic blood dryness and excessive consumption of acrid, spicy, and rich foods, which has led to damp heat and contraction of wind in the Yángmíng stomach channel. If the itching is severe, it is suitable to take Xiāo Fēng Sǎn (Wind-Dissipating Powder); if the pain is severe, it is suitable to take Huánglián Xiāo Dú Yǐn (Coptis Toxin-Dissipating Drink); and externally daub with Mó Fēng Gāo (Wind-Rubbing Ointment), and very slowly you will achieve results.

While we can read the two conditions of 紫癜 *zǐdiàn* and 白癜 *báidiàn* literally as "purple patch" and "white patch" in the sense of simply the manifestation of purple or white patches in the skin, the disease radical in the Chinese character indicates that we are dealing with actual disease names. In modern TCM literature, they therefore tend to be translated as purpura and vitiligo, respectively. Here it may be helpful for the reader to consult Wiseman and Feng's *Practical Dictionary of Chinese Medicine*, which does equate the disease of White Patch Wind with vitiligo and defines it in this way:

Also *White Patch*. White patches on the skin attributed to the disharmony of the blood arising when wind evil assails the exterior, causing the interstices to lose their tightness. White Patch Wind is most common in youth and the prime of life. It is characterized by creamy white macules of varying size, clearly distinguishable from the normal skin coloring. Any hair growing in the patches also turns white. Some of the patches have a brown or pale red papule in the center. The condition is associated with neither pain nor itching. It is of gradual onset, and often persist for a long period.

苦參丸

治心肺積熱,腎臟風毒,攻於皮膚,時生疥癩,瘙
癢難忍,時出黃水,及大風手足爛壞眉毛脫落。一
切風疾,並皆治之。

苦參	四兩
荊芥(去梗)	三兩

上為細末,水糊丸,如桐子大,每服二十丸,好茶
吞下,或荊芥湯,食後。

Kǔshēn Wán
(Flavescent Sophora Pill)

A treatment for accumulating heat in the heart and lung, and wind poison in the kidney *zàng* organ, attacking the skin and occasionally forming scabs and Lài disease, with eczema and itching that is difficult to bear, occasionally emitting yellow fluid; as well as great wind with erosion in the hands and feet and loss of eyebrows. [This formula] is able to equally treat every single kind of wind illness.

kǔshēn	4 *liǎng*
jīngjiè	3 *liǎng*

Process the ingredients above into a fine powder and mix with water into a paste to form pills the size of *wútóng* seeds. Take 20 pills per dose, swallowing them down in high-grade tea or in a decoction of jīngjiè, taken after meals.

FORMULA NOTE

The term "Great Wind" (大風 *dàfēng*) is an old synonym for "Numbing Wind" (麻風 *máféng*) or "Pestilential Wind" (癘風 *lìfēng*), all of which refer to a chronic skin disease characterized by contagiousness, numbness, and potentially spreading red patches. Also known as 癩 *lài*, which is in modern TCM literature equated with leprosy, this disease is, however, not limited to conditions defined as leprosy in biomedicine caused by bacteria Mycobacterium leprae. The "Discourse on Expanded Needling" (*Sùwèn* Chapter Fifty-Five) explains the disease of "Great Wind" in this way:

骨節重，須眉墮，名曰大風。

Heaviness in the bones and joints and the loss of facial hair and eyebrows is called Great Wind.

The "Discourse on Wind" (*Sùwèn* Chapter Forty-Two) offers additional information on "pestilential wind." Given the significance of wind as a pathogenic factor in Chinese medicine in general, and in gynecology in particular, it is worth quoting an excerpt from this chapter:

黃帝問曰：風之傷人也，或為寒熱，或為熱中，或為寒中，或為癘風，或為偏枯，或為風也。其病各異，其名不同，或內至五臟六腑，不知其解，願聞其說。

岐伯對曰：風氣藏於皮膚之間，內不得通，外不得泄，風者善行而數變。。。

。。。癘者，有榮氣熱胕，其氣不清，故使其鼻柱壞而色敗，皮膚瘍潰。風寒客於脈而不去，名曰癘風。。。

The Yellow Emperor asked: "When wind causes damage in a person, it may cause [alternating] cold and heat, or heat strike, or cold strike, or pestilential wind, or unilateral withering, or wind. These diseases each differ from each other and their names are not the same. [Wind] may reach the five *zàng* and six *fǔ* organs. Since I do not know how to understand this, I would like to hear your explanation."

Qí Bó answered: "Wind Qì hides out in the space of the skin, internally unable to penetrate, externally unable to discharge. Wind likes to move and transform in numerous ways…

…Pestilence means that the *yíng* Provisioning Qì is hot and decomposing and the patient's Qì is not clear. This causes the bridge of the nose to erode and the facial complexion to be ruined, and festering ulcers to form in the skin. When wind cold invades the vessels and does not leave, it is called "pestilential wind."

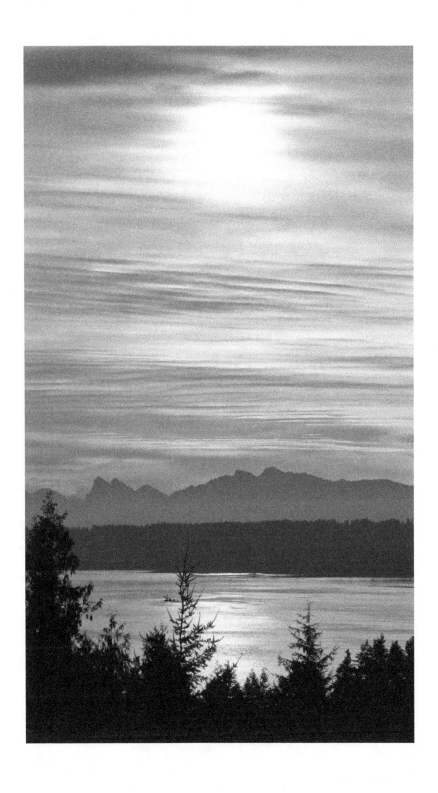

第四十七問

夜與鬼交者，何也？

答曰：人有五臟，臟有七神，臟氣盛則神強，外邪
鬼魅不能干犯。

若攝養失節，而血氣虛衰，鬼邪侵損，故婦人夢中
多與鬼魅交通。其狀不欲見人，如有對忤，並獨言
獨笑，或時悲泣者，是也。其脈來遲，或如鳥啄，
顏色不變，皆邪物病也。

說今宮中人，尼師，寡婦，曾夢中與鬼魅交通，邪
氣懷感，久作癥瘕，或成鬼胎，往往有之。

QUESTION FORTY-SEVEN

What Is the Reason for Having Intercourse with Ghosts at Night?

ANSWER: Humans have five *zàng* organs, and the *zàng* organs have seven Shén (spirits). When the Qì of the *zàng* organs is exuberant, the Shén is/are strong, and evil ghosts and demons from the outside are unable to violate or harass.

If they have been irregular in protecting and caring for their health and blood and Qì have become debilitated, ghosts and evils encroach and cause harm. For this reason, women in their dreams more frequently have intercourse with ghosts and demons. This manifests as refusing to be social, as if she were bearing grudges, and at the same time talking and laughing to herself, or sometimes crying and grieving. Her pulses arrive slowly and hidden, or like a bird pecking, but her facial complexion is unchanged. All of this means a disease [caused by] evil things.

Talking about today's women in the palace, Buddhist nuns, and widows, if they have ever in their dreams had intercourse with ghosts and demons and are harboring this evil Qì, over a long time this turns into Concretions and Conglomerations, or possibly the formation of a ghost fetus. These situations are very common.

DISCUSSION

The disease category of "intercourse with ghosts" (與鬼交 *yǔ guǐ jiāo*) or "dreaming of intercourse with ghosts" (夢與鬼交 *mèng yǔ guǐ jiāo*) is a rabbit hole that has tempted me for a long time, ever since I first came across it in Sūn Sīmiǎo's volumes on gynecology. For a broad range of treatment options that reflect various lay and professional medical ideas about this affliction, let us look at the *Ishimpō* (醫心方 "Formulas from the Heart of Medicine), a Japanese compendium of medieval Chinese medical texts that was compiled in 984. The section on "Prescriptions for Treating Women Having Intercourse with Ghosts" (治婦人鬼交方 *zhì fùrén guǐ jiāo fāng*) is tucked in between a section on "Prescriptions for Treating Women Desiring Men," which involves advice on repeatedly inserting a flour dildo that is soaked in soy sauce and wrapped in gauze into the vagina, and "Prescriptions for Treating Women Wanting to Interrupt Childbearing," or in other words, birth control. Given the fact that "intercourse with ghosts" is not a category most modern readers will be familiar with, I am quoting the entire section on this topic from the *Ishimpō* here.

This information may not only be of interest to clinical practitioners strange or creative or open-minded enough to treat this pathology as an actual condition or translate it into relevant modern language for their suffering patients. In addition, this fascinating topic also sheds light on the gender-specific vulnerabilities women were associated with by society at large and by the medical profession in particular in early China. As Hsiao-wen Cheng has pointed out in a fascinating article on "Manless Women and the Sex–Desire–Procreation Link in Song Medicine," "There is ample precedent in Chinese history and beyond for pathologizing women's heterosexual inactivity or explaining women's unconventional behavior as a medical disorder caused by their longing for men."

Qí Zhòngfǔ's text is clearly aimed at an educated audience of literate medical professionals, or at least medically inclined members of the elite who took their role as stewards for the women in their extended family seriously; in contrast, the Japanese *Ishimpō* offers an important glimpse into a broader range of more popular treatments that made it across the Sea of Japan and Korea Strait to be preserved in Japanese Buddhist temples when the original Chinese sources were destroyed in the centuries of civil war and foreign invasions in China itself. Note that in the second passage, it is actually unclear whether Péngzǔ's answer and the first and third treatments methods address a gendered condition that occurs in women alone, or whether the explanation and treatments are for both men and women. Only the second method specifies that it is meant for women. In contrast, some of the language, such as references to "leaking Essence" and "driving" (i.e., what we would now call "riding" the sexual partner) usually refers only to a man's sexual activity.

治婦人鬼交方第三十

SECTION THIRTY: PRESCRIPTIONS FOR TREATING WOMEN HAVING INTERCOURSE WITH GHOSTS

《病源論》云：婦人夢與鬼交通者，亦由腑臟氣弱，神守虛衰，致鬼靈因夢而交通也。

A quote from the *Zhūbìng yuánhòu lùn*: "This condition of women dreaming of having intercourse with ghosts is also due to weakness of Qì in the *zàngfǔ* organs and by a debilitated ability to safeguard the Shén, which allows ghosts and magical powers to have intercourse by taking advantage of her dreaming.

《玉房秘訣》云：採女曰：何以有鬼交之病。彭祖曰：由於陰陽不交，情欲深重，即鬼魅假像與之交通，與之交通之道，其有勝於人，久則迷惑，諱而隱之，不肯告人，自為佳，故至獨死而莫之知也。

治之法：但令女與男交而勿瀉精，晝夜勿息。困者，不過七日，必愈；若身體疲勞，不能獨御者，但深按勿動亦善。

又方：當以石硫黃數兩，燒以熏婦人陰下身體，並服鹿角末方寸匕，即愈矣。當息，鬼涕泣而去。

A quote from the *Yùfáng mìjué*: "Cǎinǚ asked why the disease of ghost intercourse exists, and Péngzǔ answered that it was caused by a lack of intercourse between Yīn and Yáng (i.e. lack of sexual intercourse), so that the desires [of such patients] become deep and serious. At this point, ghosts and demons disguise themselves [as human] and have intercourse with them. Their way of having intercourse is superior to that of humans, and over time leads to [the victims] becoming delusional. They will shun others and conceal this [situation], not willing to inform others. Regarding themselves as superior, they will consequently reach the point of dying alone, without anyone being aware of this."

Treatment methods: Merely make the woman have intercourse with the man but do not allow any leakage of Essence, day and night without rest. With worn-out patients, do not exceed seven days, and the patient is bound to recover. If the [patient's] body is so exhausted that they are unable to "drive" without assistance, it is also excellent if you merely massage them deeply without getting them aroused.

Another prescription: Take several *liǎng* of sulphur and burn it to fumigate the woman's body from below her genitals. At the same time, make her ingest a square-*cùn* spoonful of powdered lùjiǎo (deer antler), and she will immediately recover! [The condition] should stop, and the ghost will weep and cry and then depart."

《小品方》別離散治男女風邪，男夢見女，女夢見男，悲愁憂恚，怒喜無常，或半年，或數月，日複發者方：

楊上寄生（三兩）　朮（三兩）　桂肉（一兩一方三兩）　茵芋（一兩）天雄（一兩，炮）薊根　（一兩）菖蒲（一兩）　細辛（一兩）　附子（一兩，炮）　乾薑（一兩）

凡十物，合搗，下篩，酒服半方寸匕，日三。合藥勿令婦人，雞犬見之。又無令見病者，病者家人見合藥，知藥者，令邪氣不去，禁之，為驗。

From the *Xiǎopǐnfāng*, a formula for Separating-and-Leaving Powder, which treats men's and women's wind evil, men dreaming of seeing women and women dreaming of seeing men, abnormal sorrow and grief, worry and rage, anger and joy, possibly for half a year or for several months or days erupting repeatedly:

Willow jìshēng (mistletoe, 3 *liǎng*), báizhú (3 *liǎng*), ròuguì (1 *liǎng* or, in another edition, 3 *liǎng*), yīnyù (1 *liǎng*), tiānxiōng (1 *liǎng*, blast-fried), jìgēn (thistle root, 1 *liǎng*), chángpú (1 *liǎng*), xìxīn (1 *liǎng*), fùzǐ (1 *liǎng*, blast-fried), gānjiāng (1 *liǎng*)

Combine the total of ten ingredients and pound and sift them. Take a square-*cùn* spoonful in rice-wine, three doses a day. When compounding the medicine, do not let women, chickens, or dogs see it. Also do not let the patient or the patient's family see it. If they see you compounding the medicine and are aware of the medicine, this will allow the evil Qì to not depart. Keeping it secret will make it efficacious!

《千金方》治婦人忽與鬼交通方：

松脂（二兩）　雄黃（一兩）

二味，先烊松脂，乃納雄黃末，以虎爪絞令相得，藥成。取如雞子中黃，夜臥以著熏籠，中燒，令病患自升其上，以被自覆，唯出頭，勿令過熱，及令氣得泄也。

From the *Qiānjīnfāng* a formula to treat women suddenly having intercourse with ghosts

Sōngzhī (pine rosin, 2 *liǎng*), xiónghuáng (1 *liǎng*)

Of these two ingredients, first melt the pine rosin and then add the realgar, powdered. Use a tiger claw to stir it until blended well and the medicine is done. Take an amount the size of a chicken egg yolk and, at night, make the patient lie down next to an incense burner. Burn [the medicine] in it, making the patient herself climb on top of it, make her cover herself up with a blanket, with only her head sticking out. Do not let her get too hot, and allow the Qì to be able to get discharged.

《玄感傳尸方》主婦人患骨蒸者，多夢與鬼夫交接，為之方：

雄黃（一兩，破）　虎爪（一枚，末）　沉香（一兩，末）　青木香（一兩，末）　松脂（二兩，破）

凡五味，合，和以蜜丸，丸如彈丸，納火籠中，以熏陰，夜別一度，大良。

From the *Xuán'gǎn chuánshī fang*, a formula indicated for women suffering from bone steaming who dream more frequently of having intercourse with a ghost husband:

Xiōnghuáng (1 *liǎng*, broken up), tiger claw (1 claw, pulverized), chénxiāng (1 *liǎng*, pulverized), qīngmùxiāng (1 *liǎng*, pulverized), sōngzhī (1 *liǎng*, broken up)

Combine all the five ingredients to make honey pills the size of pellets. Place them in a brazier and use it to fumigate the genitals. Doing this once every other night is excellent.

The reason I have quoted this passage in its entirety is because I want to give the reader an idea of the various ways in which medical men in traditional China thought about this condition. Even though the *Ishimpō* is a practical text that does not spend much time on theoretical explanations, we can deduce etiological concepts from the various treatments proposed. The text does offer two explanations: "weakness of Qì in the *zàngfǔ* organs and a debilitated ability to safeguard the Shén" and "lack of intercourse between Yīn and Yáng (i.e. lack of sexual intercourse), so that the desires [of such patients] become deep and serious." Similarly, treatments range from the medical to the magical, from taking a medicinal powder aimed at eliminating evil Qì internally to making the victim of sexual infatuation with a ghost have intercourse with a real man for seven days straight, "day and night without rest," or fumigating her with exorcistic substances to force the demonic Qì out of her system.

In all of these passages, one question that remains unanswered is the patient's agency, with regard to both the invading ghost and then the treatment. In this context, the statement that "[Ghosts' and demons'] way of having intercourse is superior to that of humans" is tantalizing, as are references to women behaving abnormally, displaying emotions, laughing or talking to themselves, or "refusing to be social, as if she were bearing grudges." Especially in light of "[the victims] becoming delusional... shun others and conceal this [situation], not willing to inform others," who decided to label a female patient as suffering from this disease and thus in need of treatment?

Since ghosts tend to be invisible to outside observers, and the "victim" of a ghost invasion was known to become reticent and withdrawn, is it possible that this medical label of "dreams of intercourse with ghosts" as a pathology was used by men to address women's abnormal and deviant behavior when other methods failed? Is it possible, on the other hand, that "intercourse with ghosts" was a category used by women to cover up illicit sexual relations since it placed them in the role of a weak and blameless victim whose Shén was too debilitated to protect her from invasion by evil forces? For an elite husband concerned with marital fidelity and his family honor who was perhaps forced to spend extended periods of time away from home, labeling his wife's suspicious behavior and identifying a strange invader who might have been observed by a servant or neighbor as a ghost might have been a convenient way to avoid open conflict and the drastic consequences forced on him and his wife by a detected affair with a human actor?

Not directly addressed in the earlier sources is also the fact that by Sòng times this condition become associated not just with women's constitutional vulnerability, exacerbated by vacuity taxation. Qí Zhòngfǔ's reference to "today's women in the palace, Buddhist nuns, and widows" demonstrates an additional dimension: Starting in the Sòng dynasty, dreams of intercourse with ghosts was a pathology that was seen as particularly common in and dangerous for women who were not having regular inter-course with human men! Whether real or imagined, this link between dreams of intercourse with ghosts and the lives of women "protected" or prevented from regular interactions with men most likely reflects the increasingly restricted social sphere and more and more limited interaction with the outside world, especially in terms of contact with men who were not family members, for elite women from Sòng times and later.

A question in my mind, and one that appears to be answered by the material in the *Ishimpō*, is the concrete meaning of "intercourse" in this context. I have intentionally chosen an English word with the exact same ambiguous meaning that marks the Chinese term 交 *jiāo*. Along the lines of the implications of the Chinese character, which appears to depict a person with crossed legs 㚒, both the Chinese and the English terms can refer to sexual intercourse but can also simply mean interaction, commu-nication, or crossing paths. It is possible, but unlikely in my mind when I look at the totality of explanations and treatments presented here, that the Chinese phrase "intercourse with ghosts," as used in the context of traditional gynecological literature, could have referred also to a woman having more innocuous interactions with an invisible presence, including such signs as talking to herself and inexplicable (perhaps from a male perspective?) episodes of happiness or rage and loss of temper.

We might also want to think about this "pathology" from the angle of female possession, especially given the fact that female shamanism and spirit possession continue to thrive in some corners of Korea and Japan to this day. The notion that women have a special connection to the spirits is one that is not uncommon in traditional cultures throughout the world. It is fascinating to me how Chinese medical texts pathologized, explained, and treated this special connection between women and the spirits. At what point, for what reasons, and by whom was a woman's interaction with the spirit world not defined as shamanism, and hence as a sacred power investing her with special knowledge, powers, and skills, including healing, but instead as a disease in need of treatment?

For the prime example of the medicalization and pathologizing of this "situation," we can follow the *Ishimpō* and cite Cháo Yuánfāng's *Zhūbìng yuánhòu lùn*. In the section on gynecology there, the entry on "signs of dreaming of intercourse with ghosts" that is cited above is preceded by an entry on "signs of intercourse with ghosts," which offers this explanation:

人稟五行秀氣而生，承五臟神氣而養。若陰陽調和，則臟腑強盛，
風邪鬼魅不能傷之。

若攝衛失節，而血氣虛衰，則風邪乘其虛，鬼干其正。然婦人與鬼交
通者，臟腑虛，神守弱，故鬼氣得病之也。其狀，不欲見人，如有對
忤，獨言笑，或時悲泣是也。脈來遲伏，或如鳥啄，皆邪物病也。。。

People are born endowed with the flourishing Qì of the Five Agents. They are nourished by receiving the Shén Qì of the five *zàng* organs. When Yīn and Yáng are balanced and harmonized, the *zàngfǔ* organs are strong and abundant, and wind evil and ghosts and goblins are unable to hurt them.

When a person's health preservation has been irregular and their Qì and blood become debilitated, wind evil seizes their vacuity, and ghosts interfere with what is right. The present condition of women having intercourse with ghosts is a case of vacuity in the *zàngfǔ* organs and a weakened ability to safeguard the Shén. As a result, ghost Qì is able to make them sick. The condition manifests with refusing to be social, as if she were bearing grudges, talking and laughing to herself, or sometimes crying and grieving. Her pulses come slow and hidden, or like a bird pecking, which is always a disease [caused by] evil things...

To understand Cháo Yuánfāng's perspective on the relationship between physical exhaustion and sexual dreams not just in women but in a non-gendered context, Volume Four on "vacuity taxation" (虛勞 *xūláo*) in the general section of the *Zhūbìng yuánhòu lùn* offers some insights. The entry on "signs of vacuity taxation dreaming and discharging Essence" (虛勞夢泄 精候 *xūláo mèng xièjīng hòu*), or in other words, men's involuntary seminal emissions as the result of vacuity taxation," gives this explanation:

腎虛為邪所乘，邪客於陰，則夢交接。腎藏精，今腎虛不能製精，因
夢感動而泄也。

When kidney vacuity is exploited by evil and the evil intrudes into
the Yīn, [the person] dreams of having intercourse. The kidney stores
the Essence. In the present case, the kidney's vacuity and inability to
control Essence leads to arousal and subsequent discharge in one's
dreams.

The next entry on the "signs of vacuity taxation and tendency to dream"
(虛勞喜夢候 xūláo xǐmèng hòu) stands out for its length and detail in comparison with the surrounding entries. In addition to providing insight into
sexual dreams, it also offers a rare glimpse into traditional Chinese dream
analysis in a medicalized context.

夫虛勞之人，血氣衰損，臟腑虛弱，易傷於邪。邪從外集內，未有定
舍，反淫於臟，不得定處，與榮衛俱行，而與魂魄飛揚，使人臥不
得安，喜夢。氣淫於腑，則有餘於外，不足於內；氣淫於臟，則有
餘於內，不足於外。

若陰氣盛，則夢涉大水而恐懼；陽氣盛，則夢大火燔焫；陰陽俱盛，
則夢相殺。上盛則夢飛；下盛則夢墜。甚飽則夢行，甚飢則夢臥。肝
氣盛則夢怒；肺氣盛則夢恐懼哭泣飛揚；心氣盛則夢喜笑恐畏；脾
氣盛則夢歌樂，體重身不舉；腎氣盛則夢腰脊兩解不屬。凡此十二
盛者，至而瀉之立已。

厥氣客於心，則夢見山嶽燔火；客於肺，則夢飛揚，見金鐵之器奇
物；客於肝，則夢見山林樹木；客於脾，則夢見丘陵大澤，壞屋風
雨；客於腎，則夢見臨深，沒於水中；客於膀胱，則夢游行；客於胃，
則夢飲食；客於大腸，則夢田野；客於小腸，則夢游聚邑街衢；客於
膽，則夢鬬訟自割；客於陰，則夢接內；客於項，則夢多斬首；客於
脛，則夢行走而不能前，又居深地中；客於股肱，則夢禮節拜起；客
於胞，則夢溲便。凡此十五不足者，至而補之立已。尋其茲夢，以設
法治，則病無所逃矣。

In a person with vacuity vexation, Qì and blood are debilitated, the *zàng* and *fǔ* organs are vacuous and weak, and they are easily damaged by evil. Coming from the outside, the evil accumulates inside. Not yet having a fixed lodging place, it instead soaks into the *zàng* organs. Unable to find a fixed location, it moves around together with *yíng* Provisioning and *wèi* Defense, and takes off flying with the *hún* and *pò* souls. This causes the person to not find peace in their sleep and have a tendency to dream. If it soaks into the *fǔ* organs, there is excess outside and insufficiency inside. If it soaks into the *zàng* organs, there is excess inside and insufficiency inside.

Exuberance of Yīn Qì results in dreaming of fear and dread from crossing large bodies of water; exuberance of Yáng Qì results in dreaming of great fires burning and scorching; dual exuberance of Yīn and Yáng results in dreams of mutual killing. Exuberance above results in dreams of flying; exuberance below, in dreams of falling. Great overeating results in dreams of action; great hunger, in dreams of resting. Exuberance of liver Qì results in dreams of anger; exuberance of lung Qì, in dreams of great fear, crying, and flying; exuberance of heart Qì, in dreams of joyful laughter and fear; exuberance of spleen Qi, in dreams singing and music, and of a heavy body and inability to lift the body up; exuberance of kidney Qì, in separation and lack of connection between the lumbus and the backbone. All of these twelve cases of exuberance, if you arrive there and drain it, you can stop [the condition].

Intrusion of the evil Qì into the heart results in visions of lofty mountains and blazing fires in one's dreams; intrusion into the lung, in dreams of flying and visions of seeing gold and iron implements and unusual things in one's dreams; intrusion into the liver, in visions of mountain forests and trees in one's dreams; intrusion into the spleen, in visions of hills and large swamps, ruined houses and wind and rain in one's dreams; intrusion into the kidney, in visions of being near deep abysses and drowning in water in one's dreams; intrusion into the bladder, in dreams of traveling; intrusion into the stomach, in dreams of drinking and eating; intrusion into the large intestine, in dreams of open fields; intrusion into the small intestine, in dreams of roaming and gathering in city streets; intrusion into the gallbladder, in dreams of fighting and quarreling and cutting oneself; intrusion into the genitals, in dreams of linking up inside (i.e. sexual intercourse); intrusion into neck, in dreams of many beheadings; intrusion into the shins in dreams of walking without being able to move forward; intrusion into the womb in dreams of urination. All of these fifteen cases of insufficiency, if you arrive there and supplement it, you can stop [the condition].

By seeking out the specific dream and then setting up your treatment method accordingly, the disease will not have a place to flee to!

As we can see from this lengthy paragraph, dreams are seen as a disturbance of rest caused by vacuity taxation that has weakened the *zàngfǔ* organs and thereby allowed evil Qì to intrude. A careful and specific diagnosis of the content of pathological dreams offers important insights for treatment, whether you need to drain the excess or supplement the insufficiency, and also informs which location you may want to focus particular attention on. No mention is made of ghosts or sexual intercourse, beyond the fact that "intrusion into the genital" results in sexual dreams. The previous entry on seminal emissions in one's sleep, which seems like the closest andrological equivalent to the gynecological condition of "dreams of intercourse with ghosts," also does not mention any involvement of ghosts or demons and instead explains it clinically as related to "the kidney's vacuity and inability to control Essence." For more information on dreaming as a form of harmful sleep, see my discussion on Question Forty-Nine below.

We can thus see that the key element in this condition as a manifestation of female vulnerability is not so much the fact that the woman is having troubling dreams but rather that she is seen as more susceptible to "intercourse with ghosts." The obvious explanation for this link is that earthly ghosts and related demonic entities are Yīn, in comparison to celestial *shén* "spirits" being Yáng, just as women are also Yīn in relation to men being Yáng. In addition, the gynecological literature also emphasizes women's state of vacuity taxation as the result of her reproductive processes, which negatively affects their ability to safeguard the Shén.

As a minor side note to this fascinating topic, Qí Zhòngfǔ's answer above is the perfect demonstration for the reason why I hesitate to translate the Chinese term 神 shén as the English word "spirit," or its related counterparts in other Western languages, as most contemporary Western translations tend to do. I greatly appreciate that Elisabeth Rochat de la Vallée, to my knowledge the only major translator to do so, sometimes translates it in plural as "spirits." From the passage above, which discusses seven Shén, it is clear that this term was indeed conceived as a plurality of entities by the traditional medical authors, a fact with which most modern TCM practitioners in both China and the rest of world are uncomfortable. Given the fact that it is impossible to express the English singular "spirit" and plural "spirits" both at the same time, I use Shén consistently in my own translations, except for those contexts where we are clearly talking about a plural or singular Shén. Even if we use this pīnyīn term, we should still always bear in mind that even the "Shén" should be thought of as both singular and plural.

茯神散

治婦人風虛，鬼神交通，妄有所見聞，語言雜亂。

茯神	一兩半
茯苓	
人參	各一兩
菖蒲	
赤小豆	半兩

上㕮咀，每服三錢，水一盞半，煎六分。去滓，溫
服，食前。

Fúshén Sǎn
(Root Poria Powder)

A treatment for women's wind vacuity, [manifesting with]
having intercourse with ghosts and spirits, hallucinating
about seeing or hearing things, and chaotic and disordered
speech.

fúshén	1.5 *liǎng*
fúlíng	
rénshēn	1 *liǎng* each
shíchāngpú	
chìxiǎodòu	0.5 *liǎng*

Pound the ingredients above and take 3 *qián* per dose.
Simmer in 1.5 cups of water until reduced to 60 percent,
remove the dregs, and take warm before meals.

Unnamed Formula

治女人與鬼神交通，獨言獨笑，或悲或思，或謳謠恍惚。

松脂(炒)	三兩
雄黃(研末)	一兩

上二味，用虎爪攪勻，丸如彈大，夜內籠中燒之，令女裸坐籠上，彼急自蒙，唯出頭耳，過三熏即斷。

Unnamed Formula

A treatment for women having intercourse with ghosts and spirits, talking or laughing to themselves, possibly feeling grief or pensiveness, or singing and crooning by themselves, and severe mental confusion.

sōngzhī (stir-fry)	3 *liǎng*
xiónghuáng (grind into a powder)	1 *liǎng*

For the two ingredients above, use a tiger claw to stir them until evenly mixed and form pills the size of pellets. At night, place them in a brazier and burn them. Make the woman sit naked on top of the brazier and have others cover her up tightly, with only her head and ears sticking out. Making her go through three fumigations will interrupt [the condition or the connection to the ghost].

秦丞相灸法

狐魅神邪，及癲狂病，諸般醫治不瘥者。

以並兩手大拇指，用綠絲繩急縛之。灸三壯，艾著
四處，半在甲上，半在肉上，四處盡繞。一處不
燒，其疾不愈。神效不可量也。

小兒胎癇驚癇，一依此法灸之一壯，炷如小麥。妊
癇亦妙。

Qín Chéngxiàng Jiǔ Fǎ
(Moxibustion Method of the Grand Counsellor of Qín)

For fox demons and spectral evils, as well as *diān* insanity and *kuáng* mania, and all sorts of conditions that physicians are unable to treat successfully:

Line up both hands and thumbs with each other and use a green silk rope to tie them together tightly. Burn three cones of moxa [per location], placing the moxa on four different locations, half on the nail and half on the flesh. Burn the moxa completely down on all four locations. If a single location is not burned, the patient's disease will not be cured. Divine efficacy that is immeasurable!

To treat fetal seizures and panic seizures in small children, another [text] follows this method to burn a single stick-shaped cone of moxa the size of a grain of wheat. It is also marvelous for pregnancy seizures.

Formula Note

It is not clear to me whether this method for a moxibustion treatment refers all the way back to the most famous prime minister of the Qín dynasty, namely Lǚ Bùwéi 呂不韋 (292 – 235 BCE). In terms of the actual treatment described here, my interpretation is that you burn 3 cones of moxa each on the four finger nails (excluding the thumbs) on the line between the nail and the flesh, and that it is essential that you burn each cone down completely, or this method will not work.

黃帝灸法

治療神邪鬼魅,及癲狂病,言語不擇尊卑。

灸上唇裡面中央肉弦上一壯,炷如小麥子大。用鋼刀決斷更佳也。

Huángdì Jiǔ Fǎ
(The Yellow Emperor's Moxibustion Method)

To treat spectral evils and ghosts and demons, as well as conditions of *diān* insanity and *kuáng* mania, and speech that does not differentiate between high and low social status.

Burn a single cone of moxa, the size of a grain of wheat, on the inside of the upper lip, in the very center, on top of the line in the flesh. It is even better when you use a steel blade to cut it.

FORMULA NOTE

This location is known as an extra point called Xuánmìng 懸命 ("Life Suspension"), presumably because of its use in life-threatening situations. It is first mentioned in Sūn Sīmiǎo's *Bèijí qiānjīn yàofāng*, where burning 14 cones of moxa is used as a treatment for evil ghosts and hallucinatory speech. An alternate name is Guǐlù 鬼祿 ("Ghost Favor"). As in the treatment cited above, Sūn Sīmiǎo suggests that the moxibustion treatment on this point works best when it is followed by cutting through the line in the flesh with a steel blade. I am indebted to Dr. Brenda Hood for her explanation of the combination of moxibustion with bleeding in the treatment of ghost-related conditions: "The physical bleeding of a person to eliminate evil makes sense if the person is judged to be carrying some entity, especially if they consider it has afflicted the Blood level. Clinically, the majority of psycho-emotional disorders are related to dampness, blood stasis, and/or heat. Bleeding opens blockages. Moxa is Yáng in nature (invading evils are Yīn in nature), so the moxa would introduce Yáng into a system, and the bleeding would provide an outlet. In the *Nànjīng* it says to first supplement and then disperse" (personal communication).

第四十八問

大小便不通者，何也？

答曰：大腸者，傳導之官，變化出焉。傳者，傳其
不潔之物也，上與肺合。

膀胱者，州都之官，津液藏焉，氣化則能出矣。化
者，化其溲便之泄注也，內與腎合。

或臟腑不和，營衛不調，使陰陽二氣失升降之道，
致大小二腸為祕結之患。

巢氏云：熱則祕結，寒則鴨溏。熱搏於大腸，則大
便不通。熱結於小腸，則小便不通。令大小便不通
者，是大小二腸受客熱所結也。小腸受熱，化物不
出，是致膀胱不能使溲也。故便血尿血者，皆由熱
之所使也。

QUESTION FORTY-EIGHT

What is the Reason for Completely Stopped Up Defecation and Urination?

ANSWER: The large intestine occupies the office of "conveyance." Gradual and substantive change stem from it. "Conveyance" refers to the conveyance of impure substances, and it is matched with the lung above.

The bladder occupies the office of "metropolis surrounded by water." The fluids are stored inside it and are able to emerge as the result of qì transformation. "Transformation" refers to transforming the discharge of urine and feces, and it is matched with the kidney inside.

If the *zàng* and *fǔ* organs are not harmonious and *yíng* Provisioning and *wèi* Defense are not attuned, this causes the two Qì of Yīn and Yáng to lose their path of upbearing and downbearing and leads to the trouble of occlusion in the large and small intestines.

Master Chǎo said: "Heat results in occlusion, and cold results in duck slop diarrhea. When heat assaults the large intestine, defecation is stopped up. When heat binds in the small intestine, urination is stopped up. The present case of both defecation and urination being stopped up means the binding of heat that has intruded into both the large and small intestine. The small intestine contracts heat, the transformed substances [in the small intestine] fail to come out, and for this reason, the bladder is unable to induce urination. As such, blood in the feces and urine is always caused by heat.

DISCUSSION

As anybody familiar with the classical foundations of Chinese medicine should know, the explanation of the functions of the large intestine and bladder come from *Sùwèn* Chapter Eight, the "Treatise on the Secrets of the Magic Orchid" (*Línglán mìdiǎn lùn*《靈蘭秘典論》). This chapter is important as one of the foundational texts of classical medicine, so I am citing the entire section on the role of the organs as government officials here:

黃帝問曰：願聞十二藏之相使，貴賤何如？岐伯對曰：悉乎哉問也，請遂言之。

心者，君主之官也，神明出焉。

肺者，相傅之官，治節出焉。

肝者，將軍之官，謀慮出焉。

膽者，中正之官，決斷出焉。

膻中者，臣使之官，喜樂出焉。

脾胃者，倉廩之官，五味出焉。

大腸者，傳道之官，變化出焉。

小腸者，受盛之官，化物出焉。

腎者，作強之官，伎巧出焉。

三焦者，決瀆之官，水道出焉。

膀胱者，州都之官，津液藏焉，氣化則能出矣。

凡此十二官者，不得相失也。故主明則下安，以此養生則壽，歿世不殆，以為天下則大昌。

主不明則十二官危，使道閉塞而不通，形乃大傷，以此養生則殃，以為天下者，其宗大危。戒之戒之！

The Yellow Emperor said: "I would like to hear how the twelve organs employ each other and determine their hierarchy amongst each other." Qí Bó answered: "What a thorough question! Please allow me to elaborate on this:

The heart: It occupies the office of the Sovereign. Spirit luminosity stems from it.

The lung: It occupies the office of the Grand Councilor. Order and good measure stem from it.

The liver: It occupies the office of the General. Strategic planning stems from it.

The gallbladder: It occupies the office of Impartiality and Rectitude. Resolve and decision-making stem from it.

The Center of the Chest (Dànzhōng, REN-17): It occupies the office of the Servant and Messenger. Elation and joy stem from it.

The spleen and stomach: They occupy the office of the Granary. The five flavors stem from it.

The large intestine: It occupies the office of Conveyance. Gradual and substantive change stem from it.

The small intestine: It occupies the office of Receiving and Containment. The transformation of [ingested] matter stems from it.

The kidney: It occupies the office of Forceful Action. Ingenuity and acumen stem from it.

The Sānjiāo: It occupies the office of Dredging and Draining. [Free flow in] the water ways stems from it.

The bladder: It occupies the office of Metropolis Surrounded by Water. The fluids are stored inside it and are able to emerge as the result of qì transformation.

All of these twelve offices must not lose [the ability to collaborate with] each other. This being so, when the ruler is illuminated, those below are at ease. If you rely on this to nurture life, longevity results, with no danger until the end of times. If you enact this condition in all Under Heaven, great prosperity results.

When the ruler is not illuminated, the twelve offices are imperiled. This situation causes the pathways to be blocked and congested instead of flowing freely. Then the frame of the body is greatly damaged. If you rely on this to nurture life, calamity results. if you enact this condition in all Under Heaven, the ancestral temple is in grave danger. Beware! Beware!

Let us look more closely at just the explanations on the large intestine and bladder here: The phrase 傳道 chuándào has historically been read primarily in two ways: Following one interpretation, I read the term as a compound, which I have translated literally as "conveyance." Alternately, we can read 道 as "path" and explain the term in reference to 傳道之官, the officials who were sent out before an important person traveled through, whose job it was to clear the road and alert the population to get out of the way and express proper reverence to the passing dignitary. Physiologically the most straight-forward reading of this line would be as referring to food being transformed (i.e., digested) and then discharged as waste. While some clinicians also ascribe a mental dimension to the Large Intestine, related to the processing of past events and letting go, it is important to distinguish between the *zàng* organs, which are connected to the Shén, and the *fǔ* organs who are purely concerned with physical functions, especially around the processing and discharging of matter. It is also important to note that starting with this line, the internal organs are no longer described in terms of official positions but rather in terms of their function.

Next, the terms 變化 *biàn huà* and 化物 *huà wù*, as the functions of the large and small intestine respectively, look almost identical but can be read quite differently. What I have translated as "gradual and substantive change" (變化) refers to all varieties of change, both material and immaterial, or in other words transmutation, such as the life cycle of gradual maturation and then decay, or the oscillation between night and day, and metamorphosis, such as the irreversible change from the pupa to the butterfly. "Transformation of matter" (化物), on the other hand, is interpreted by most commentators as referring specifically to the digestion of food. In other words, it specifically means the processing of ingested food that is passed on to the small intestine from the stomach so that the small intestine can absorb its subtle essences and get rid of the waste. It is the small intestine's function to initially separate the clear from the turbid. While the clear is then processed into *yíng* Provisioning and *wèi* Defense Qì, the turbid is passed on to the large intestine (solids) and bladder (liquids) where they are further processed. In this sense, the small intestine is more concerned with extraction and containment, while the large intestine is charged with the task of elimination.

My translation of the role of the bladder, 州都 *zhōu dū* in Chinese, may be a surprise to some readers: It is tempting, as Unschuld has done, to follow Charles Hucker's definition of this term as "Regional Rectifier, a variant of the term Rectifier (中正 *zhōng zhèng*) used at the regional level; responsible for identifying and classifying all males considered qualified for government office." Making this explanation unlikely is the fact that the term 中正 *zhōng zhèng* is used in the *Sùwèn* passage above to refer to the office of the gallbladder. In addition, I have been unable to find any evidence of this usage before the Three Kingdoms period, or in other words AFTER the fall of the Han dynasty in 220 CE. While the *Huángdì nèijīng* certainly contains later additions -- and one could of course argue that the use of this term here is precisely one of these instances — I tend to read the text as a Hàn collection containing much pre-Hàn material. Both 州 zhōu and 都 dū are administrative terms used already in the Zhōu period. According to the *Shuōwén jiězì, zhōu* means "island" or "inhabitable land surrounded by water" in its earliest meaning, but was used to refer to an administrative unit of 2,500 households already in the late Zhou period; *dū* refers to a "city with ancestral temples" (*Shuōwén*), a fiefdom, or an administrative unit of ten towns (邑). These early definitions of both characters do seem significant to me as we contemplate the meaning of this line in terms of bladder physiology, especially the association of *zhōu* with land that is surrounded by water, a central place where waters gather. Similarly, the bladder is a place where the bodily fluids (津液 *jīnyè*) are stored, separated into clear and turbid through the action of Yáng Qì and then either steamed back up for recycling in the lung or eliminated as urine.

Qí Zhòngfǔ again refers us to his favorite source, Cháo Yuánfāng's *Zhūbìng yuánhòu lùn*, where we find a number of entries on inhibited urination, stopped urination, stopped defecation, inhibited urination and defecation, and stopped urination and defecation, grouped together in Volume Forty on women's miscellaneous conditions. To summarize, these entries discuss two basic etiological factors that can impair urination and defecation: Because of its drying action, heat, whether externally contracted or internally generated in the kidney, can impact the state of the fluids and the processing and discharge of both solid and liquid waste, when it accumulates and binds in the large and small intestine. This also seems to be the approach taken by Qí Zhòngfǔ above. As a different model, the stoppage of both urination and defecation can also be caused by blockage in the large and small intestines that is caused by "disharmony in the *zàng* and *fǔ* organs, lack of attunement between *yíng* Provisioning and *wèi* Defense, and a lack of connection between Yīn and Yáng," which Cháo identifies with the life-threatening condition 關格 *guāngé* "block and repulsion." That condition is associated with blocked urination below (and sometimes also blocked defecation) and "repulsion" above, which, most authors understand to refer to vomiting. Associated with weakness in the spleen and kidney, it is due to disharmony between Yīn and Yáng Qì so that they are blocked and bind in the abdomen, causing distention and breakdown of conveyance and transformation in the large and small intestine. Alternatively, this condition is also associated with a dual exuberance of both Yīn and Yáng Qì.

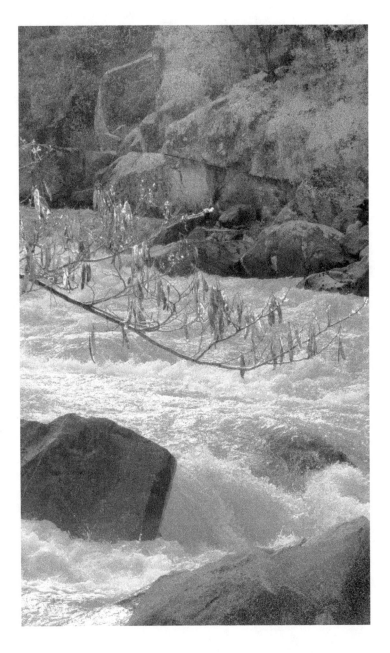

枳杏丸

治臟腑堅秘澀少。

杏仁(湯泡，去皮尖，別研)	一兩
枳殼(先研，為末)	二兩

上為細末，神麴糊為丸，桐子大，每服四十或五十丸，食前米飲薑湯下。

Zhǐ Xìng Wán
(Bitter Orange and Apricot Pit Pill)

A treatment for *zàngfǔ* hardness and constipation and rough and reduced flow.

xìngrén (soak in hot water, remove the skin and tips, and grind separately	1 *liǎng*
zhǐké (first grind it into a powder)	2 *liǎng*

Process the above into a fine powder, make a paste with shénqǔ, and form into pills the size of *wútóng* seeds. Take 40 or 50 pills per dose, downing them before meals in thin rice gruel or ginger decoction.

麻仁丸

治津液虧少，大便結秘。

麻仁(去皮)	二兩
枳實(去白，麩炒)	四兩
芍藥	四兩
大黃(炮)	四兩
濃朴	二兩
杏仁	二兩

上為末，蜜丸桐子大，米飲下二十丸，未通加至三十丸。

Márén Wán
(Hemp Seed Pill)

A treatment for a reduction in the *jīnyè* fluids and for constipation.

márén (remove the skin)	2 *liǎng*
zhǐshí (remove the white parts and stir-fry in wheat bran)	4 *liǎng*
sháoyào	4 *liǎng*
dàhuáng (blast-fry)	4 *liǎng*
nóngpò	2 *liǎng*
xìngrén	2 *liǎng*

Proceses the ingredients above into a powder and make honey pills the size of *wútóng* seeds. Down 20 pills in thin rice gruel, and if there is still no through-flow, increase the dosage to as much as 30 pills.

石韋飲子

治氣淋，小遺澀痛。

石韋 (浸，刷皮)	一兩
瞿麥	
木通	各一兩
陳皮	
茯苓	
芍藥	
桑白皮	
人參	
黃芩	各三分

上為細末，每服二錢，水一盞半，薑五片，煎七分，去滓溫服。哎咀亦得。

Shíwéi Yǐnzǐ
(Pyrrosia Drink)

A treatment for Qì strangury with rough and painful urination.

shíwéi (steep and scrub the skin)	1 *liǎng*
qúmài	
mùtōng	1 *liǎng* each
chénpí	
fúlíng	
sháoyào	
sāngbáipí	
rénshēn	
huángqín	3 *fēn* each

Process the ingredients above into a fine powder and take 2 *qián* per dose. Simmer in 1.5 cups of water with 5 slices of ginger until reduced to 70 percent. Remove the dregs and take warm. It is also possible to pound [the medicinals].

真珠丸

常觀血之流行，起自於心，聚之於脾，藏之於肝。
此三經者，皆心血所系之處也。

若三經守節，則血濡養而安和。苟一臟有傷，則血
散溢而為咎。

《指迷方》云：小便赤色，不痛不澀者，非熱非淋，
由經氣乘心，心氣散溢，血無所歸，滲入下經，故
治之多用心藥，宜服真珠丸。

真珠母(研如粉)	三分
柏子仁(研)	
當歸	各一兩
人參	
沉香	半兩
酸棗仁(炒，去皮，研)	
犀角(鎊)	
熟地(酒浸洗，蒸，乾)	一兩半
茯神(去木)	
龍齒	各半兩

上為細末，蜜丸桐子大，辰砂為衣，每服四十丸加
至五十丸。金銀薄荷湯下，日午臨臥時各一服。

Zhēnzhū Wán
(Pearl Pill)

According to the standard view, the flow of blood starts in the heart, gathers in the spleen, and is stored in the liver. These three channels are all places linked to heart blood.

If these three channels are safe-guarded and regulated, the blood is moistened and nourished, and at peace. But if even a single *zàng* organ has sustained damage, the blood scatters and spills over, with calamitous results.

The *Zhǐmífāng* states: When the urine is red in color but urination is not painful or rough, this is neither a case of heat nor of strangury, but is caused by channel Qì overwhelming the heart, so that heart Qì scatters and spills over. Having no home to return to, the blood seeps into the lower channels. For this reason, to treat this condition, we use predominantly heart medicinals. It is suitable to give Zhēnzhū Wán.

zhēnzhūmǔ (grind into powder-like consistency)	3 *fēn*
bǎizǐrén (grind)	
dāngguī	1 *liǎng* each
rénshēn	
chénxiāng	0.5 *liǎng*
suānzǎorén (stir-fry, remove the skin, and grind)	
xījiǎo (flake)	
shúdì (rinse in rice-wine, steam, and dry)	1.5 *liǎng*
fúshén (remove wood)	
lóngchǐ	0.5 *liǎng* each

Process the ingredients above into a fine powder and make honey pills the size of *wútóng* seeds. Use chénshā to coat them and take 40 to 50 pills per dose. Down in a decoction of jīnyīnhuà or bòhé. Take at noon and before going to bed, one dose each.

FORMULA NOTE

The text quoted above as *Zhǐmífāng* is called *Quánshēng zhǐmí fāng* 《全生指迷方》 (Formulas for All of Life that Point out Confusion) by its full title and was composed by Wáng Kuàng 王貺 in the early twelfth century.

My research has also found an almost literal version of this formula in a text from 1134: the *Pǔjì běnshì fāng* 《普濟本事方》 (Original Formulas for Popular Relief) by Xǔ Shūwēi 許叔微. Interestingly, that text has the following indication for the same formula, followed by practically identical instructions for preparing and taking the formula to the ones given above:

治肝經因虛，內受風邪，臥則魂散而不守，狀若驚悸。

A treatment for internal contraction of wind evil due to vacuity of the liver channel, [causing] the *hún* souls to scatter and not be safeguarded in one's sleep, and a manifestation like panic palpitations.

In terms of the exact amounts of each medicinal in the formula above, it is clear that the order of ingredients has been moved around and we are therefore uncertain of the exact amount that the formula calls for. With the help of the formula as cited in the *Pǔjì běnshì fang*, we are able to reconstruct this information: 3 *fēn* of zhēnzhūmǔ, 1.5 *liǎng* each of dāngguī and shúdì, 1 *liǎng* each of rénshēn, suānzǎorén, and bǎizǐrén, and 0.5 *liǎng* each of xījiǎo, fúshén, and lóngchǐ.

第四十九問

帶下三十六疾者，何也？

答曰：帶下者，由勞傷過度，損動經血，致令體虛受冷，風冷入於胞絡，搏其血之所成也。

諸方說帶下三十六疾者，是十二瘕，九痛，七害，五傷，三因，謂之三十六疾也。

十二瘕者，是所下之物，一者如膏，二者如青，三者如紫，四者如赤皮，五者如膿痂，六者如豆汁，七者如葵羹，八者如凝血，九者如青血，血似水，十者如米汁，十一者如月浣，十二者經度不應期也。

九痛者，一者陰中痛傷，二者陰中淋痛，三者小便刺痛，四者寒冷痛，五者月水來腹痛，六者氣滿並痛，七者汗出，陰中如蟲嚙痛，八者脅下皮膚痛，九者腰痛。

七害者，一者害食，二者害冷，三者害氣，四者害勞，五者害房，六者害妊，七者害睡。

五傷者，一者腹吼痛，二者陰中寒熱痛，三者小便急牢痛，四者藏不仁，五者子門不正引背痛。

三因（因字一本或作固），一者月水閉塞不通，其餘二固者，文闕不載。

《三因方論》云：三固者，形羸不生肌肉，斷緒不產，經水閉塞。名品雖殊，無非血病。多因經絡失於調理，產蓐不善調護，內作七情，外感六淫，陰陽勞逸，飲生冷，遂致營衛不和，新陳相干，隨經敗濁，淋露凝為瘕癖，流溢穢惡。痛害傷瘤，犯時微若秋毫，作病重如山岳。

古人所謂婦人病比男子十倍難治，而張仲景所說
三十六種疾，皆由子臟冷熱勞損，而夾帶起於陰內
也。條目混混，與諸方不同，但仲景義最玄深，非
愚淺者能解，恐其文雖異而義同也。

QUESTION FORTY-NINE

What is the Reason for the Thirty-Six Diseases "Below the Belt"?

ANSWER: "Below the belt" [conditions] are formed as the result of by taxation damage being excessive and injuriously stirring the blood in the channels. This has led to vacuity in the body and contraction of cold, and to wind and cold entering the uterine network vessels and assaulting the blood.

What the various formularies speak of as the "thirty-six diseases below the belt" is a reference to the twelve Concretions, nine pains, seven harms, five damages, and three chronic illnesses.

The twelve Concretions [refer to] the substance that is being discharged below: The first resembles [white] lard, the second resembles green-blue [very dark blood], the third resembles purple [juice], the fourth resembles red flesh, the fifth resembles scabby pus, the sixth resembles bean juice, the seventh resembles mallow broth, the eighth resembles congealed blood, the ninth resembles clear blood or blood like water, the tenth resembles rice[-rinsing] liquid, the eleventh resembles the "monthly rinse" [now early and now withheld], and the twelfth is a menstrual period that does not correspond to its proper timing.

The nine pains are: first, painful damage inside the genitals; second, strangury pain inside the genitals; third, stabbing pain with urination; fourth, cold pain; fifth, abdominal pain at the onset of menstruation; sixth, pain simultaneous with Qì fullness; seventh, discharge of fluids with pain inside the genitals that feels like gnawing insects; eighth, pain in the skin below the rib-sides; ninth, lumbar pain.

The seven harms are: first, harm from eating; second, harm from cold; third, harm from Qì; fourth, harm from taxation; fifth, harm from "bedroom matters"; sixth, harm from pregnancy; and seventh, harm from sleeping.

The five damages are: first, orifice pain; second, cold and heat pain inside the genitals; third, lower abdominal tension and hardness pain; fourth, discomfort in the *zàng* organs; and fifth, a child gate that is not straight, causing pulling back pain.

The three chronic illnesses are: first, blockages of the menstrual fluids and failure to flow through; regarding the remaining two chronic illnesses, the texts are corrupted and do not record them.

The *Sānyīn fānglùn* states: "The three chronic illnesses are emaciation of the body and inability to generate flesh, interruption of the family line and inability to give birth, and blockage of the menstrual fluids. Even though their names are different, without exception, they are all diseases of the blood. In the majority of cases, they are caused by a lack of regulation in the channels and network vessels, inadequate recuperative care after childbirth, the internal effect of the seven emotions and the external contraction of the six excesses, sexual taxation and lack of restraint, and drinking [and eating] raw and cool substances. This has led to a lack of harmony between *yíng* Provisioning and *wèi* Defense, interference between the old and the new, spoiled turbid substances along the channels, dribbling like dew, congealing and stagnating to form Concretions and Conglomerations, or spilling over as dirty and malign substances. These pains, harms, damages, and chronic illnesses may seem tiny like autumn down feathers at the time of the transgression but cause illnesses as grave as the loftiest mountains.

The ancient saying that "women's diseases are ten times more difficult to treat than men's," and Zhāng Zhòngjǐng's statement on the thirty-six types of [gynecological] illness are all due to cold and heat taxation injury in the uterus and a clandestine beginning "inside Yīn." The entries [in the various formula texts] may be confused and overlapping and the various formulas may differ. And yet, Zhāng Zhòngjǐng's meaning is extremely profound and is not something that fools and shallow minds can comprehend. In my opinion, even though these texts are different, their meaning is identical.

DISCUSSION

It is entirely appropriate that Qí Zhòngfǔ finishes off the second major section of his *Hundred Questions* with a discussion of the "thirty-six diseases below the belt" in his second-to-last entry of this section, before transitioning into reproductive conditions. For more information on the significance of the term 帶下 *dàixià* ("below the belt") and the concept of the "thirty-six diseases of below the belt," see the Preface to this book, where I have translated the relevant passages from the *Jīnguì yàolüè* and *Zhūbìng yuánhòu lùn* and briefly discussed their meaning. In its usage as a summary term for specifically gynecological conditions, it presents us here with an insightful concluding statement on the root of gynecological conditions as all being "due to cold and heat taxation injury in the uterus and a clandestine beginning 'inside Yīn.'" What exactly the mysterious phrase "inside Yīn" (陰內 *yīn nèi*) refers to in this context is not spelled out, most likely intentionally so. In medical texts and in the context of reproductive conditions in particular, Yīn tends to refer to the genitals, or in other words, the internal and external organs of the reproductive system. And that is definitely one way, and perhaps the most straight-forward way, to read this statement here, namely that the root of gynecological disorders is to be found in women's reproductive organs being affected by pathological cold or heat, usually in conjunction with wind, which were able to invade the body as the result of vacuity taxation. It is, however, also possible to read Yīn in a broader sense as referring to the Yīn aspects of the human body, thus also including associated factors like dampness, stillness, old age, obscureness and interiority, and even ghosts. Translating it literally, I leave it up to the reader to contemplate the meaning of this phrase here.

The passage above contains a number of textual corruptions like typographical errors and omitted characters. I have interpreted questionable characters and terms by referencing the lists of "thirty-six disorders below the belt" in the *Zhūbìng yuánhòu lùn* (vol. 38, section 50), *Bèijí qiānjīn yàofāng* (vol. 4, section 3), and the *Ishimpō* (vol. 21, section 24), taking both transmitted and manuscript editions into consideration. Thus I have, for example, chosen to translate the term 三因 *sān yīn* not literally as "three causes" but as "three chronic diseases" based on the fact that other lists and at least one edition of the present text has 三固 *sān gù* (lit., "three solidities") here instead. This phrase, in turn, should be read as 三痼 *sān gù*, meaning "three solidification illnesses," or in other words the three illnesses that are so solidified that they have become chronic. Similarly, I read the second type of pathological concretion, which is above called 如青 *rǔ qīng*, literally "like green-blue," as a substance that resembles very dark, greenish-blue blood, based on the fact that it is described as 青血 *qīng xùe* "green-blue blood" in the *Zhūbìng yuánhòu lùn*, but as 黑血 *hēi xùe* "black blood" in the *Bèijí qiānjīn yàofāng*. Where these texts add extra characters that clarify the meaning, I have added those in square brackets.

Some explanations for those attentive readers who are studying the Chinese source text alongside my translation of the reasons for some unusual translations: I have translated the term "sweating" (汗出 *hàn chū*) in the seventh of the "nine pains" as "discharge of fluids," because in all the other sources of this passage, the character for "sweat" (汗) is replaced with the character for "juice" (汁), with which it is easily and often confused. Similarly, I have translated the first of the five damages (腹吼痛 *fù hǒu tòng*) not literally as "pain from abdominal growling," but have chosen to interpret this as a typographical error and instead follow all other versions of this list, which have it instead as 窾孔痛 *qiàokǒng tòng*: "pain in the orifice," which we can interpret with good certainty as "pain in the vagina" in the present context. Given the similarity between the characters, it is another instance where a typographical error is the obvious answer for this discrepancy. Again based on textual comparison, I have also decided to read the term 小便 *xiǎobiàn* in the third of the five damages, in the expression 小便急牢痛 (literally, "urinary tension and hardness pain") as a typographical error for 小腹 *xiǎofù* "lower abdomen."

Among the "seven harms," there are two whose meaning is not completely clear to me: Following the pattern of all the other harms, I read 害氣 *hài qì* literally as "harmful Qì" or "harm from Qì," leaving it to the reader to decide what this could mean. I would suggest two possibilities: Most non-medical readers would understand this phrase as harmful environmental Qì, such as a sudden cold snap or pestilential wind, or in other words, any external factor that can invade the body to make the person fall ill. This meaning is often encompassed by the expression 五氣 *wǔ qì* "five Qì," which refers to wind, summer-heat, dampness, dryness, and cold. I would, however, also like to propose the possibility of reading Qì here in the sense of the emotions, especially in the sense of excessive emotions that disrupt the healthy equilibrium and calm functioning of the body. This meaning is still reflected in the modern Chinese phrase 生氣 *shēngqì* (literally, "engender Qì"), which means to "throw a fit" or "get angry." In support of that reading, I cite the famous line from *Sùwèn* Chapter Five:

人有五臟化五氣，以生喜怒悲憂恐。

Humans have five *zàng* organs, to transform the five Qì and thereby engender joy, anger, grief, worry, and fear.

The other harm that I have trouble with is the last item in this list, namely the "harm from sleeping": 害睡 *hài shuì*. Following the established pattern of all the other items in this list functioning as etiological factors rather than as the object that is being harmed, this expression should not mean "harmed sleep," in the sense of sleep disorders or disturbed sleep, but should be read literally as "harmful sleep" or "harm from sleeping."

But how could sleep have been conceived of as harmful? To answer this question in a culturally and historically sensitive manner, we must explore the ways in which the ancients thought about sleep hygiene. Clearly, there are important differences to our own ideas about sleep, starting with Zhuāngzǐ's famous statement:

古之真人，其寢不夢，其覺無憂，其食不甘，其息深深。

Oh the Perfected People of ancient times! Their sleep had no dreams, their awareness had no worries, their food had no sweetness, and their breathing was very very deep.

This same sentiment is also expressed by the Warring States philosopher Shèn Dào 慎到, who similarly said:

畫無事者夜不夢。

Those who have no affairs during the day do not dream at night.

In other words, the ideal healthy sleep in early China was one in which the person rested calmly and was not disturbed by dreams. This same sentiment is also expressed in *Língshū* Chapter Forty-Three on "Excess Evils Effusing in Dreams," where the content of dreams is used to diagnose specific states of excess or deficiency that must then be treated by draining or supplementing, respectively. What follows is my translation of the beginning of this chapter. Much of the rest of this chapter has already been translated in a slightly different version above in the discussion on the condition of "dreams of intercourse with ghosts" in Question Forty-Seven, where it is part of the last quote from the *Zhūbìng yuánhòu lùn* on the "signs of vacuity taxation and tendency to dream" (虛勞喜夢候 *xūláo xǐmèng hòu*).

黃帝曰：願聞淫邪泮衍，奈何？

岐伯曰：正邪從外襲內而未有定舍，反淫於藏，不得定處，與營衛俱行，而與魂魄飛揚，使人臥不得安而喜夢。氣淫於府，則有餘於外，不足於內；氣淫於藏，則有餘於內，不足於外。

黃帝曰：有餘不足，有形乎？。。。

The Yellow Emperor asked: "I would like to hear what one can do about excess evil spreading out."

Qí Bó answered: "Straight-forward evils invade the inside from the outside. Before taking up a fixed residence, they instead seep into the *zàng* organs. Unable to settle in a fixed location, they move together with *yíng* Provisioning and *wèi* Defense, and rise up flying with the *hún* and *pò* souls, keeping the person from finding peace in their sleep and causing a tendency to dreaming. When their Qì seeps into the *fǔ* organs, there is excess on the outside and insufficiency on the inside. When their Qì seeps into the *zàng* organs, there is excess on the inside and insufficiency on the outside."

The Yellow Emperor asked: "These excesses and insufficiencies, do they take shape?"

For the rest of this chapter, Qí Bó proceeds to list the correlations between specific dreams and the locations where evils settle in the body due to various excesses and insufficiencies, such as excess in the Yīn versus the Yáng aspect and above versus below, hunger versus starvation, excesses in each of the five zàng organs, and insufficiencies in the zàng and fǔ organs, etc.

In addition to this notion of dreaming as an expression of harmful sleep, I am indebted to Leo Lok for reminding me of Sūn Sīmiǎo's discussion of unhealthy sleeping habits in the Bèijí qiānjīn yàofāng, Volume Twenty-Seven, Chapter Two on "Dàolín Nurturing the Inner Nature." Found in this chapter and repeated in similar texts with advice on cultivating health and prolonging life is advice like not sleeping with lamps left burning, not sleeping too close to a stove, not covering the head in winter during sleep, not sleeping with the feet in an elevated position, not sleeping parallel to a long straight wall, making a habit of keeping one's mouth closed when falling asleep, not sleeping on one's belly but sleeping on the side with the knees bent and frequently (according to Sūn Sīmiǎo five times) turning sides, keeping a regular daily rhythm of rest and activity by adjusting one's times of going to bed and getting up in accordance with the seasons, avoiding loud singing or speaking before going to bed, not sleeping under window rafters, sleeping with the head facing east in spring and summer and facing west in fall and winter, not sleeping during the day, avoiding exposure to wind, etc. In addition, texts like the Yúnjí qīqiān 《雲笈七籤》 (Seven Bamboo Slips in a Cloud Satchel) from 1025 emphasized the importance of "good thoughts and a contained heart."[3]

It is noteworthy that the individual items in the various lists of "thirty-six disorders below the belt" are almost literally identical between the texts but sometimes show up in different lists. Most importantly, the list of

---

3 For more information on Daoist advice on sleeping, I refer the reader to Chén Yúnqīng 陳雲卿, et als., "Dàojiào duì wòzī de zhǔzhāng 道教對臥姿的主張" in Fóxué yǔ kēxué 2002, pp. 18-24.

"seven harms" cited by Qí Zhòngfǔ is clearly a copy of Cháo Yuánfāng's list and also identical with the one in the *Ishimpō*. Sūn Sīmiǎo's version, however, differs substantially in that he begins his "seven harms" with what is listed as the "five damages" in all the other texts, adding "a monthly rinse that is now profuse and now scanty" and "harm from vomiting." In addition he adds a different list of "five damages," namely: "first, propping fullness pain in the two rib-sides; second, heart pain stretching into the rib-sides; third, Qì binding and not flowing through; fourth, malignity diarrhea; and fifth, intractable cold before and after." In addition, he spells out the "three chronic illnesses" as "first, marked emaciation and inability to engender flesh; second, interruption of childbearing and breastfeeding; and third, blockage of the menstrual fluids." This is identical with the quotation from the *Sānyīnfāng* cited by Qí Zhòngfǔ in the section following his list of the "thirty-six disorders."

This exercise in textual research can show us how the various gynecological texts copied and interacted with each other and how texts gradually became corrupted or expanded due to an individual author's interests and skills. There are two major points that we can take away from this example: First, given the rarity of texts and of literacy among the general population still at this point in time, namely the seventh through the twelfth century, it is truly stunning how this knowledge was transmitted almost literally from one corner of the Chinese empire to the other and beyond, over a matter of centuries. Secondly, my findings show that gynecological authors, rather than creating new texts with innovative theories and treatments, continued to transmit the ancient texts with great fidelity. What makes it so difficult to trace the different layers in a single text is the fact that these authors, at least in China, saw no need to cite their sources and to differentiate clearly between old material that they were merely copying and their own innovative additions, whether in the realm of treatments or theory, even within a single paragraph or sentence. This is an important point to keep in mind when we contemplate the role of medical authors and their agency and intentions in early Chinese medical literature. It should serve as a warning against presenting any author of historical medical literature, from the mythological Yellow Emperor and the Divine Farmer to historical figures like Sūn Sīmiǎo or Qí Zhòngfǔ, as innovative physicians expressing their personal clinical experience, rather than as the transmitters and guardians of textual traditions that the historical facts reveal them to be. It is also a good reminder that the publication date of any given text cannot serve as more than a *terminus ante quem* for the content of that text. The one exception to this situation is the Japanese *Ishimpō*, probably due to the fact that the Japanese "author," or rather "compiler," saw his role more clearly as compiling what to him were extremely precious foreign texts from a distant empire with a more advanced civilization. This respect for and careful recording of his sources is one reason why this text has proven to be such a goldmine of information on early medieval Chinese medical literature for historians of Chinese medicine.

Continuing with Qí Zhòngfǔ's answer, the *Sānyīn fānglùn* cited in the second to last line is a reference to a text with the full title *Sānyīn jíyī bìngzhèng fānglùn* 《三因極一病證方論》 (Formulas and Discourse on the Disease Patterns of the Three Causes Culminating in One), which was completed by Chén Yán 陳言 in 1174. The reader should note that in the context of this title, the character 因 *yīn* does indeed refer to etiological factors, namely the six external excesses and seven internal emotions. In the original source, the quotation from this text actually uses the more correct character 瘤, which includes the disease radical, rather than the character 固, which simply means "solid" or "solidification."

Lastly, the concrete meaning of "a clandestine beginning inside Yīn" is left to the reader's imagination. I believe that Qí intentionally left his explanation vague, to leave the door open for both a narrow and a broad reading of Yīn here. In its narrowest sense, Yīn can refer to the internal reproductive organs, so this statement could mean that all gynecological conditions originate in that aspect of the female body. More broadly, though, Yīn can also include the kidney and other structures and processes associated with reproduction, or even refer to the inside of the body in general, the protected and hidden interior, the parts or aspects of the body that are not clearly discernible. And of course, Yīn here can also refer to blood when paired with Qì as its Yáng counterpart, which also makes perfect sense.

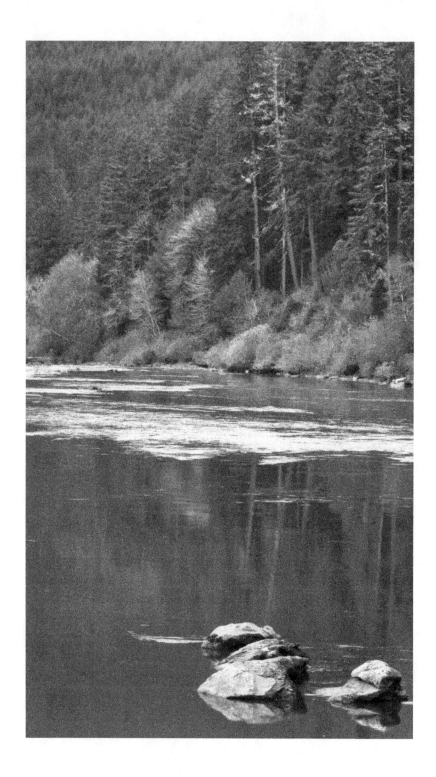

CLINICAL COMMENTARY BY SHARON WEIZENBAUM

A WORD ABOUT LEUKORRHEA

I was taught that leukorrhea was due to dampness or to dampness mixed with heat. I heard about other colors of leukorrhea but was told that basically, when a woman had leukorrhea, they needed you to help them get rid of dampness or dampness mixed with heat. Of course, as we progress in practice, many of the things we learn turn out to be much too limited for real-life patients!

The most important thing I learned about leukorrhea over time is how serious it can be and how seriously we should take it. Any time a substance is leaking out of our bodies, we are losing something precious. I had a patient once who developed leukorrhea and, much to her alarm, she watched herself age precipitously. Her hair became more brittle, the turgor of her skin diminished, and her gums receded. It was as if her life force was being drained out the bottom of her body. In fact it was! All of the exits of our body, including our pores, our bowels, our uterus, our urination, serve us. They must open regularly for us to stay alive but they also must be able to close. When you see leukorrhea, take it seriously. The zàng organs have the function of storing. Check to see if they are all able to do their job. Especially check the kidneys and spleen with the question, "are they able to absorb and consolidate the way they need to?"

Even if the leukorrhea is due to an excess, the open gates through which the excess is showing itself as leukorrhea is also still leaking essential vitality. After the excess is cleared, there will be some recuperative steps necessary.

養氣活血丹

治勞傷衝任，帶下異色。

大艾葉（炒焦，取細末）	五兩
乾薑（炮，細末）	二兩

上二件，用好醋二升半，無灰好酒二升，生薑自然汁一升，艾葉末同調於銀器內慢火熬成膏。

方入後藥末：

附子	
白芍	
白朮	
椒紅	各三兩半
川芎	
當歸	
人參	
五味子	
紫巴戟（去心，糯米炒）	各二兩

上為細末，入前藥膏子，並炒熟白麵二兩半，同和勻為劑。入杵臼內搗千下，丸如桐子大。每服五十丸，溫酒或米飲，食前任下。

Yǎng Qì Huó Xuè Dān
(Qì-Nurturing and Blood-Enlivening Elixir)

A treatment for taxation damage to the Chōngmài and Rènmài, with vaginal discharge in strange colors.

large àiyè (stir-fry until scorched, turn it into a fine powder)	5 *liǎng*
gānjiāng (blast-fry, turn into a fine powder)	2 *liǎng*

Take the two ingredients above and blend the powdered [gānjiāng and] àiyè together into 2.5 *shēng* of high-quality vinegar, 2 *shēng* of high-quality ash-free rice wine, and 1 *shēng* of pure juice [extracted] from fresh ginger. Simmer everything in a silver pot over a slow flame until it forms a paste.

A formula, for adding the medicinals below as a powder:

fùzǐ	
báisháo	
báizhú	
jiāohóng	3.5 *liǎng* each
chuanxiong	
dāngguī	
rénshēn	
wǔwèizǐ	
purple bājǐtiān (remove the core and stir-fry with glutinous rice)	2 *liǎng* each

Finely pulverize the ingredients above add to the previously made paste. Stir-fry until done with 2.5 *liǎng* of white flour and mix well to compound the medicine. Place in a mortar and pestle one thousand times. Form pills the size of *wútóng* seeds and take 50 pills per dose, in warm rice wine or thin rice gruel, before meals.

Formula Note

I have been able to trace this formula back to a slightly earlier text, the *Yáng shì jiācáng fāng*《楊氏家藏方》 (Master Yáng's Hidden Family Formulas) by Yáng Tán 楊倓 from 1178. There it is indicated for the following situation:

治產後諸虛不足，勞傷血氣，真元內弱，四肢倦乏，肌肉消瘦，及脾元虛損，或吐利自汗，或寒熱往來。

A treatment for the various kinds of vacuity and insufficiency after childbirth, with taxation damage to the blood and Qì, internal weakness of the true origin, fatigue in the four limbs, and wasting away of the flesh, as well as for vacuity detriment in the origin of the spleen, possibly with vomiting, diarrhea, and spontaneous sweating, and possibly with intermittent cold and heat.

Based on the version of the formula there, I have been able to spot missing characters and make sense of the formula instructions, marking those additions in square brackets.

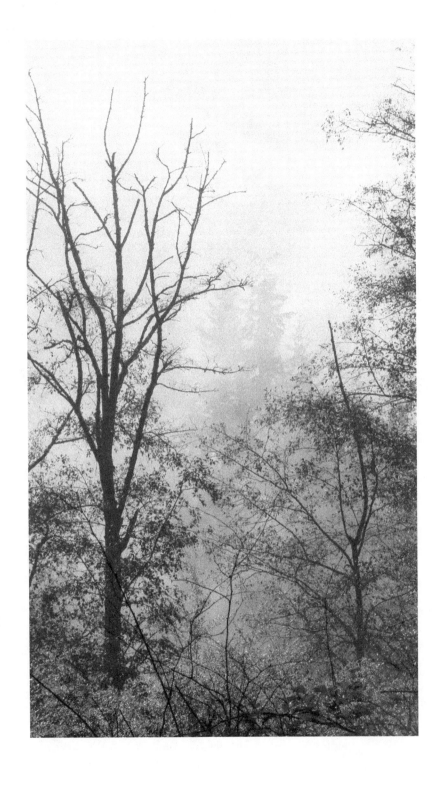

紫桂丸

補益血海，治衝任氣虛，經脈不調，或多或少，腰
疼腹冷，帶下崩漏。

禹餘糧(火煆醋淬七次)	三兩
龍骨	
艾葉(醋炒)	
牡蠣	各二兩
赤石脂	
地榆	
濃朴	
牡丹皮	
阿膠(蛤粉炒)	
當歸	各一兩
白芷	
吳茱萸(湯洗七次)	
肉桂	
附子	半兩

上為細末，麵糊丸桐子大。每服三十九，濃煎艾醋
湯空心下，常服。

Zǐ Guì Wán
(Purple Cinnamon Pill)

Supplementing and boosting the Sea of Blood, a treatment for vacuity of Qì in the Chōngmài and Rènmài, with lack of attunement in the channels, whether profusion or scantiness, lumbar pain and abdominal cold, and vaginal discharge, Landslide Collapse, and spotting.

yǔyúliáng (calcine and quench in vinegar 7 times)	3 *liǎng*
lónggǔ	
àiyè (stir-fry in vinegar)	
mǔlì	2 *liǎng* each
chìshízhī	
dìyú	
nóngpò	
mǔdānpí	
ējiāo (stir-fry with clam-shell powder)	
dāngguī	1 *liǎng* each
báizhǐ	
wúzhūyú (rinse in hot water 7 times)	
ròuguì	
fùzǐ	0.5 *liǎng*

Process the ingredients above into a fine powder and mix with flour paste into pills the size of *wútóng* seeds. Take 30 pills per dose and down them in a concentrated, simmered down decoction of àiyè and vinegar on an empty stomach. Take them constantly.

第五十問

婦人有帶下或淋漓不斷，何以別之？

答曰：產戶有三門。一曰胞門。二曰龍門。三曰玉門。衝任二脈行於中。

已產者屬胞門，未產者屬龍門，未嫁者屬玉門。

《病源》云：陰陽過度，勞傷經絡，故風冷乘虛而入胞門，損衝任之經，傷太陽少陰之氣，致令胞絡之間，穢液與血相稱兼帶而下。冷則多白，熱則多赤。久而則為淋瀝之病也。

QUESTION FIFTY

How Do You Differentiate Between the Conditions of Vaginal Discharge and Incessant Dribbling in Women?

ANSWER: The doorway of childbirth has three gates: one called Uterus Gate, a second one called Dragon Gate, and the third one called Jade Gate. The two vessels of the Chōngmài and Rènmài run through its center.

Women who have already given birth are associated with the Uterus Gate. Those who have not yet given birth are associated with the Dragon Gate. And those who are not yet married are associated with the Jade Gate.

The *Zhūbìng yuánhòu lùn* states: "Excessive sexual intercourse results in taxation damage to the channels and network vessels. Because of this, wind and cold exploit the vacuity and enter through the Uterus Gate. They injure the Chōngmài and Rènmài channels and they damage the Qì in Tàiyáng and Shàoyīn. Eventually, this causes filthy fluids in the space of the uterine network vessels to conjoin with blood and together descend as vaginal discharge. In cases of cold, [the discharge] is predominantly white; in cases of heat, it is predominantly red. If this continues for a long time, it results in the disease of dribbling.

Discussion

This entire answer is an almost literal quotation, with only some of the order changed, from the introductory essay on vaginal discharge in Cháo Yuánfāng's *Zhūbìng yuánhòulùn*, Volume Thirty-Seven, Entry Twenty-Four.

The unfortunate reality of Qí Zhòngfǔ's response is that he fails to answer his own question. It is not clear to me what the connection is between his excellent question and the explanation he provides about the three terms to use for the vagina, depending on whether women are virgins, have had intercourse but not given birth, or have given birth.

The second part of Qí's answer suggests merely that dribbling is a type of vaginal discharge that arises when the condition has become chronic, and that both of these are caused by an external invasion of wind and cold due to the vacuity and taxation damage to the channels and network vessels from excessive sexual intercourse.

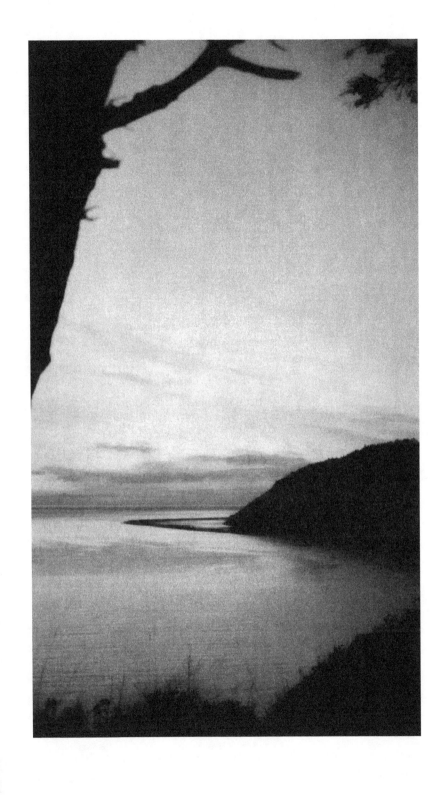

大補益當歸丸

治婦人諸虛不足。

當歸	各一兩
續斷	
乾薑	
阿膠	
甘草	
川芎	
吳朮	各一兩半
吳茱萸	
附子	
白芷	
芍藥	
官桂	
地黃	

上為細末，麵糊丸如桐子大。每服五十丸，溫酒或鹽湯下，食前。

Dà Bǔyì Dāngguī Wán
(Greatly Supplementing Chinese Angelica Pill)

A treatment for all the various forms of vacuity and insufficiency in women.

dāngguī	
xùduàn	
gānjiāng	1 *liǎng* each
ējiāo	
gāncǎo	
xiōngqióng	
báizhú from the state of Wú	
wúzhūyú	
fùzǐ	1.5 *liǎng* each
báizhǐ	
sháoyào	
guānguì	
dìhuáng	

Process the ingredients above into a fine powder and mix with flour paste into pills the size of *wútóng* seeds. Take 50 pills per dose, downing them in warm rice wine or hot salty water, before meals.

FORMULAS AND MEDICINALS
REFERENCE TABLES

GLOSSARY

BIBLIOGRAPY

INDEX

Formula Reference by Pinyin

Pinyin	Chinese	English
Bǎi Fēng Tāng	百風湯	Hundred Winds Decoction
Bǎipí Tāng	柏皮湯	Arborvitae Root Bark Decoction
Bǎizǐrén Tāng	柏子仁湯	Arborvitae Seed Decoction
Bì Yīng Sǎn	必應散	Inevitable Response Powder
Biējiǎ Wán	鱉甲丸	Turtle Shell Pill
Bǔ Yīn Wán	補陰丸	Yīn-Supplementing Pill
Chèn Tòng Sǎn	趁痛散	Pain-Alleviating Powder
Chénshā Jù Bǎo Dān	辰砂聚寶丹	Chénzhōu Cinnabar Treasures-Gathering Elixir
Chénxiāng Dǎo Qì Wán	沉香導氣丸	Agarwood Resin Qì-Conducting Pill
Chì Lóng Dān	赤龍丹	Red Dragon Elixir
Cù Jiān Sǎn	醋煎散	Vinegar-Simmered Powder
Cù Jiān Sǎn	醋煎散	Vinegar-Simmered Powder
Dà Bǔyì Dāngguī Wán	大補益當歸丸	Greatly Supplementing Chinese Angelica Pill
Dà Duàn Xià Wán	大斷下丸	Major Interrupting-Downward-Flow Pill
Dà Jiàn Zhōng Tāng	大建中湯	Major Center-Fortifying Decoction
Dà Qī Qì Tāng	大七氣湯	Major Seven Qì Decoction
Dà Shèng Yī Lì Jīn Dān	大聖一粒金丹	Great Sage Single Pill Gold Elixir
Dān Qiān Dān	丹鉛丹	Cinnabar and Lead Elixir
Dāngguī Wán	當歸丸	Chinese Angelica Pill
Dàzǎo Tāng	大棗湯	Jujube Decoction
Dìhuáng Sǎn	地黃散	Rehmannia Powder
Dìhuáng Tāng	地黃湯	Rehmannia Decoction
Dùzhòng Sǎn	杜仲散	Eucommia Powder
Èr Qì Sǎn	二氣散	Two Qì Powder

Pinyin	Chinese	English
Fúlíng Bànxià Tāng	茯苓半夏湯	Poria and Pinellia Decoction
Fúlíng Wán	茯苓丸	Poria Pill
Fúshén Sǎn	茯神散	Root Poria Powder
Guādì Sǎn	瓜蒂散	Melon Stalk Powder
Hǔ Gǔ Sǎn	虎骨散	Tiger Bone Powder
Huàn Tuǐ Wán	換腿丸	Leg-Changing Pill
Huángdì Jiǔ Fǎ	黃帝灸法	The Yellow Emperor's Moxibustion Method
Huángniú Wán	黃牛丸	Bovine Bezoar Pill
Huángqí Yǐnzi	黃芪飲子	Astragalus Drink
Huángqín Sǎn	黃芩散	Scutellaria Powder
Húmá Sǎn	胡麻散	Black Sesame Powder
Huó Xuè Dān	活血丹	Blood-Enlivening Elixir
Hǔpò Sǎn	琥珀散	Amber Powder
Jiā Wèi Lǐ Jiàn Tāng	加味理建湯	Augmented Patterning and Fortifying Decoction
Jiāng Hé Wán	薑合丸	Ginger-Encased Pill
Jiāorén Wán	椒仁丸	Sìchuán Peppercorn Pill
Jīng Jì Dān	經濟丹	Fording the River Elixir
Kǎn Lí Dān	坎離丹	Fire and Water Elixir
Kǔ Jiǔ Tāng	苦酒湯	Bitter Rice Wine Decoction
Kǔshēn Wán	苦參丸	Flavescent Sophora Pill
Lái Fù Dān	來復丹	Arriving and Returning Elixir
Lái Fù Dān	來復丹	Arriving and Returning Elixir
Lǐ Qì Tāng	理氣湯	Qì-Patterning Decoction
Lì Yàn Wán	立驗丸	Instant Efficacy Pill
Liù Shén Wán	六神散	Six Spirits Powder

Pinyin	Chinese	English
Lóngchǐ Hǔpò Sǎn	龍齒琥珀散	Dragon Tooth and Amber Powder
Márén Wán	麻仁丸	Hemp Seed Pill
Mòyào Sǎn	沒藥散	Myrrh Powder
Mùxiāng Shùn Qì Sǎn	木香順氣散	Costusroot Powder that Restores the Proper Direction of the Qì Flow
Mùxiāng Tōng Qì Wán	木香通氣丸	Costusroot Qì-Flow-Promoting Pill
Nèi Bǔ Xiōng Guī Tāng	內補芎歸湯	Internally-Supplementing Chuānxiōng and Chinese Angelica Decoction
Píng Fèi Tāng	平肺湯	Calming-the-Lung Decoction
Qín Chéngxiàng Jiǔ Fǎ	秦丞相灸法	Moxibustion Method of the Grand Counsellor of Qín
Qīng Píng Tāng	清平湯	Peace and Balance Decoction
Qū Xié Sǎn	祛邪散	Evil-Dispelling Powder
Róu Pí Tāng	柔脾湯	Spleen-Softening Decoction
Shén Jiàn Yǐnzi	神健飲子	Divine Health Drink
Shèn Shī Tāng	滲濕湯	Dampness-Percolating Decoction
Shén Zhù Wán	神助丸	Divine Assistance Pill
Shèn Zhuó Tāng	腎著湯	Kidney Clinging Decoction
Shēng Fà Yào	生髮藥	Hair-Sprouting Medicine
Shēng Méimāo	生眉毛	Making the Eyebrows Sprout
Shèxiāng Wán	麝香丸	Musk Pill
Shíhú Sǎn	石斛散	Dendrobium Powder
Shíwéi Yǐnzǐ	石韋飲子	Pyrrosia Drink
Sì Qī Tāng	四七湯	Four Seven Decoction
Sūhéxiāng Wán	蘇合香丸	Storax Pill
Táo Hóng Sǎn	桃紅散	Peach Red Powder
Tínglì Wán	葶藶丸	Lepidium Pill
Tòu Jīng Tāng	透經湯	Permeating-the-Channels Decoction

Pinyin	Chinese	English
Wàn Líng Sǎn	萬靈散	Ten-Thousandfold Magic Powder
Wǔ Xiāng Niān Tòng Wán	五香拈痛丸	Five Fragrances Pain-Plucking Pill
Xǐ Fēng Sǎn	洗風散	Washing-Away-the-Wind Powder
Xiǎo Cháihú Jiā Dìhuáng Táng	小柴胡加地黃湯	Minor Bupleurum Plus Rehmannia Decoction
Xiǎo Cháihú Jiā Dìhuáng Tāng	小柴胡加地黃湯	Minor Bupleurum Plus Rehmannia Decoction
Xiōng Qiāng Sǎn	芎羌散	Chuānxiōng and Notopterygium Powder
Yáng Bēng Jiāo Ài Tāng	陽崩膠艾湯	Yáng Landslide Collapse Donkey Hide Glue and Mugwort Decoction
Yǎng Qì Huó Xuè Dān	養氣活血丹	Qì-Nurturing and Blood-Enlivening Elixir
Yīn Bēng Gù Jīng Wán	陰崩固經丸	Yīn Landslide Collapse Menses-Securing Pill
Yīnchén Wǔ Líng Sǎn	茵陳五苓散	Virgate Wormwood and Poria Five Powder
Yù Bào Dù	玉抱肚	Jade Wrapping the Belly
Yù Zhēn Wán	玉真丸	Jade Immortal Pill
Zhēnzhū Wán	真珠丸	Pearl Pill
Zhǐ Hóng Sǎn	止紅散	Stopping-the-Red Powder
Zhǐ Xìng Wán	枳杏丸	Bitter Orange and Apricot Pit Pill
Zǐ Guì Wán	紫桂丸	Purple Cinnamon Pill
Zǐ Jīn Dān	紫金丹	Precious Gold Elixir
Zǐ Jīn Dān	紫金丹	Precious Gold Elixir
Zī Yīn Yǎng Xùe Wán	滋陰養血丸	Yin-Saturating Blood-Nourishing Pill
Zǐjīn Sǎn	紫金散	Japanese Ardisia Powder
Zǐwǎn Wán	紫菀丸	Aster Pill
Zuì Tóu Fēng Bǐngr	醉頭風餅兒	Alcoholic Head Wind Cake

Formula Reference by English

English	Pinyin	Chinese
Agarwood Resin Qì-Conducting Pill	Chénxiāng Dǎo Qì Wán	沉香導氣丸
Alcoholic Head Wind Cake	Zuì Tóu Fēng Bǐngr	醉頭風餅兒
Amber Powder	Hǔpò Sǎn	琥珀散
Arborvitae Root Bark Decoction	Bǎipí Tāng	柏皮湯
Arborvitae Seed Decoction	Bǎizǐrén Tāng	柏子仁湯
Arriving and Returning Elixir	Lái Fù Dān	來復丹
Arriving and Returning Elixir	Lái Fù Dān	來復丹
Aster Pill	Zǐwǎn Wán	紫菀丸
Astragalus Drink	Huángqí Yǐnzi	黃芪飲子
Augmented Patterning and Fortifying Decoction	Jiā Wèi Lǐ Jiàn Tāng	加味理建湯
Bitter Orange and Apricot Pit Pill	Zhǐ Xìng Wán	枳杏丸
Bitter Rice Wine Decoction	Kǔ Jiǔ Tāng	苦酒湯
Black Sesame Powder	Húmá Sǎn	胡麻散
Blood-Enlivening Elixir	Huó Xuè Dān	活血丹
Bovine Bezoar Pill	Huángniú Wán	黃牛丸
Calming-the-Lung Decoction	Píng Fèi Tāng	平肺湯
Chénzhōu Cinnabar Treasures-Gathering Elixir	Chénshā Jù Bǎo Dān	辰砂聚寶丹
Chinese Angelica Pill	Dāngguī Wán	當歸丸
Chuānxiōng and Notopterygium Powder	Xiōng Qiāng Sǎn	芎羌散
Cinnabar and Lead Elixir	Dān Qiān Dān	丹鉛丹
Costusroot Powder that Restores the Proper Direction of the Qì Flow	Mùxiāng Shùn Qì Sǎn	木香順氣散
Costusroot Qì-Flow-Promoting Pill	Mùxiāng Tōng Qì Wán	木香通氣丸
Dampness-Percolating Decoction	Shèn Shī Tāng	滲濕湯

English	Pinyin	Chinese
Dendrobium Powder	Shíhú Sǎn	石斛散
Divine Assistance Pill	Shén Zhù Wán	神助丸
Divine Health Drink	Shén Jiàn Yǐnzi	神健飲子
Dragon Tooth and Amber Powder	Lóngchǐ Hǔpò Sǎn	龍齒琥珀散
Eucommia Powder	Dùzhòng Sǎn	杜仲散
Evil-Dispelling Powder	Qū Xié Sǎn	祛邪散
Fire and Water Elixir	Kǎn Lí Dān	坎離丹
Five Fragrances Pain-Plucking Pill	Wǔ Xiāng Niān Tòng Wán	五香拈痛丸
Flavescent Sophora Pill	Kǔshēn Wán	苦參丸
Fording the River Elixir	Jīng Jì Dān	經濟丹
Four Seven Decoction	Sì Qī Tāng	四七湯
Ginger-Encased Pill	Jiāng Hé Wán	薑合丸
Great Sage Single Pill Gold Elixir	Dà Shèng Yī Lì Jīn Dān	大聖一粒金丹
Greatly Supplementing Chinese Angelica Pill	Dà Bǔyì Dāngguī Wán	大補益當歸丸
Hair-Sprouting Medicine	Shēng Fà Yào	生髮藥
Hemp Seed Pill	Márén Wán	麻仁丸
Hundred Winds Decoction	Bǎi Fēng Tāng	百風湯
Inevitable Response Powder	Bì Yīng Sǎn	必應散
Instant Efficacy Pill	Lì Yàn Wán	立驗丸
Internally-Supplementing Chuānxiōng and Chinese Angelica Decoction	Nèi Bǔ Xiōng Guī Tāng	內補芎歸湯
Jade Immortal Pill	Yù Zhēn Wán	玉真丸
Jade Wrapping the Belly	Yù Bào Dù	玉抱肚
Japanese Ardisia Powder	Zǐjīn Sǎn	紫金散
Jujube Decoction	Dàzǎo Tāng	大棗湯
Kidney Clinging Decoction	Shèn Zhuó Tāng	腎著湯

English	Pinyin	Chinese
Leg-Changing Pill	Huàn Tuǐ Wán	換腿丸
Lepidium Pill	Tínglì Wán	葶藶丸
Major Center-Fortifying Decoction	Dà Jiàn Zhōng Tāng	大建中湯
Major Interrupting-Downward-Flow Pill	Dà Duàn Xià Wán	大斷下丸
Major Seven Qì Decoction	Dà Qī Qì Tāng	大七氣湯
Making the Eyebrows Sprout	Shēng Méimāo	生眉毛
Melon Stalk Powder	Guādì Sǎn	瓜蒂散
Minor Bupleurum Plus Rehmannia Decoction	Xiǎo Cháihú Jiā Dìhuáng Táng	小柴胡加地黃湯
Minor Bupleurum Plus Rehmannia Decoction	Xiǎo Cháihú Jiā Dìhuáng Tāng	小柴胡加地黃湯
Moxibustion Method of the Grand Counsellor of Qín	Qín Chéngxiàng Jiǔ Fǎ	秦丞相灸法
Musk Pill	Shèxiāng Wán	麝香丸
Myrrh Powder	Mòyào Sǎn	沒藥散
Pain-Alleviating Powder	Chèn Tòng Sǎn	趁痛散
Peace and Balance Decoction	Qīng Píng Tāng	清平湯
Peach Red Powder	Táo Hóng Sǎn	桃紅散
Pearl Pill	Zhēnzhū Wán	真珠丸
Permeating-the-Channels Decoction	Tòu Jīng Tāng	透經湯
Poria and Pinellia Decoction	Fúlíng Bànxià Tāng	茯苓半夏湯
Poria Pill	Fúlíng Wán	茯苓丸
Precious Gold Elixir	Zǐ Jīn Dān	紫金丹
Precious Gold Elixir	Zǐ Jīn Dān	紫金丹
Purple Cinnamon Pill	Zǐ Guì Wán	紫桂丸
Pyrrosia Drink	Shíwéi Yǐnzǐ	石韋飲子
Qì-Nurturing and Blood-Enlivening Elixir	Yǎng Qì Huó Xuè Dān	養氣活血丹

English	Pinyin	Chinese
Qì-Patterning Decoction	Lǐ Qì Tāng	理氣湯
Red Dragon Elixir	Chì Lóng Dān	赤龍丹
Rehmannia Decoction	Dìhuáng Tāng	地黃湯
Rehmannia Powder	Dìhuáng Sǎn	地黃散
Root Poria Powder	Fúshén Sǎn	茯神散
Scutellaria Powder	Huángqín Sǎn	黃芩散
Sìchuán Peppercorn Pill	Jiāorén Wán	椒仁丸
Six Spirits Powder	Liù Shén Wán	六神散
Spleen-Softening Decoction	Róu Pí Tāng	柔脾湯
Stopping-the-Red Powder	Zhǐ Hóng Sǎn	止紅散
Storax Pill	Sūhéxiāng Wán	蘇合香丸
Ten-Thousandfold Magic Powder	Wàn Líng Sǎn	萬靈散
The Yellow Emperor's Moxibustion Method	Huángdì Jiǔ Fǎ	黃帝灸法
Tiger Bone Powder	Hǔ Gǔ Sǎn	虎骨散
Turtle Shell Pill	Biējiǎ Wán	鱉甲丸
Two Qì Powder	Èr Qì Sǎn	二氣散
Vinegar-Simmered Powder	Cù Jiān Sǎn	醋煎散
Vinegar-Simmered Powder	Cù Jiān Sǎn	醋煎散
Virgate Wormwood and Poria Five Powder	Yīnchén Wǔ Líng Sǎn	茵陳五苓散
Washing-Away-the-Wind Powder	Xǐ Fēng Sǎn	洗風散
Yáng Landslide Collapse Donkey Hide Glue and Mugwort Decoction	Yáng Bēng Jiāo Ài Tāng	陽崩膠艾湯
Yīn Landslide Collapse Menses-Securing Pill	Yīn Bēng Gù Jīng Wán	陰崩固經丸
Yin-Saturating Blood-Nourishing Pill	Zī Yīn Yǎng Xùe Wán	滋陰養血丸
Yīn-Supplementing Pill	Bǔ Yīn Wán	補陰丸

PINYIN	CHINESE	LATIN SOURCE	ENGLISH COMMON NAME
àiyè	艾葉	Artemisia argyi	mugwort leaf
ānxīxiāng	安息香	Benzoinum	benzoin
bādòu	巴豆	Croton tiglium	croton seed
báibiǎndòu	白扁豆	Lablab	white lablab bean
báifán	白礬	Alumen	alum
báifúlíng	白茯苓	Poria cocos	white poria
báifúshén	白茯神	Poria cocos	white root poria
báifùzǐ	白附子	Aconitum carmichaeli album	white aconite prepared lateral root
báijiāngcán	白僵蠶	Bombyx mori batryticatus	infected silkworm larva
báijílí	白蒺藜	Tribulus terrestris	goat's head bur
báiliǎn	白蘞	Ampelopsis japonica	ampelopsis root
báilónggǔ	白龍骨	Mastodon	white dragon bone
bǎipí	柏皮	Platycladus orientalis	arborvitae root bark
báisháo/ báisháoyào	白芍/白芍藥	Paeonia albiflora/ lactiflora	white peony root
báitánxiāng	白檀香	Santalum album L.	sandalwood
báizhǐ	白芷	Angelica dahurica	Dahurican angellca root
báizhú	白朮	Atractylodes macrocephala	atractylodes rhizome
bǎizǐrén	柏子仁	Platycladus orientalis	arborvitae/biota seed
bājǐtiān	巴戟天	Morinda officinalis	morinda root
bānmáo	斑貓	Mylabris	mylabris/blister beetle
bànxià	半夏	Pinellia ternata	pinellia rhizome
bèimǔ	貝母	Fritillaria verticillata var. thunbergii	fritillary bulb

PINYIN	CHINESE	LATIN SOURCE	ENGLISH COMMON NAME
bìbá	蓽茇	Piper longum	long pepper capsule and root
bìchéngqié	蓽澄茄	Piper cubeba	cubeb
biējiǎ	鱉甲	Amyda/Trionyx sinensis	turtle shell
bīnláng	檳榔	Areca catechu	betel nut
bìxiè	萆薢	Dioscorea tokoro/ hypoglauca etc.	fish poison yam
cāngzhú	蒼朮	Atractylodes lancea	atractylodes rhizome
cántuìbù	蠶蛻布	Bombyx mori	silkworm moth egg case
cǎoguǒ/ cǎoguǒzǐrén	草果/草果子仁	Amomum tsao-ko	tsaoko fruit
cǎowū/ cǎowūtóu	草烏/草烏頭	Aconitum kusnezoffii	wild aconite root
cháihú	柴胡	Bupleurum chinense	bupleurum root
chénpí	陳皮	Citrus reticulata	tangerine peel
chénshā	辰砂	mercuric sulfide	cinnabar (top quality)
chénxiāng	沉香	Aquilaria agalocha/ sinensis	agarwood resin
chēqiánzǐ	車前子	Plantago asiatica	plantain seed
chìfú/chìfúlíng	赤茯/赤茯苓	Poria cocos	red poria
chìsháo/ chìsháoyào	赤芍/赤芍藥	Paeonia rubra	red peony root
chìshízhī	赤石脂	Halloysitum	red halloysite
chìxiǎodòu	赤小豆	Vigna umbellata	red ricebean
chōngwèicǎo/ yìmǔcǎo	茺蔚草/益母草	Leonurus heterophyllus	motherwort
chuānbājǐ	川巴戟	Morinda officinalis	Sìchuān morinda root

Pinyin	Chinese	Latin Source	English Common Name
chuānjiāo/huājiāo	川椒/花椒	Zanthoxylum bungeanum	Sichuan peppercorn/prickly ash husk
chuānliànzǐ	川楝子	Melia toosendan	toosendan fruit
chuānwū/chuānwūtóu	川烏/川烏頭	Aconitum carmichaeli	aconite main root
chuānxiōng/xiōngqióng	川芎/芎藭	Ligusticum wallichii	chuānxiōng lovage rhizome
chuānxùduàn	川續斷	Dipsacus asperoides	dipsacus root
císhí	磁石	Magnetitum	magnetite
dàdòuhuángjuǎn	大豆黃卷	Glycine max	dried soybean sprout
dàfùzǐ	大附子	Aconitum carmichaeli	large aconite prepared lateral root
dàhuáng	大黃	Rheum palmatum	rhubarb root and rhizome
dǎnfán	膽礬	Chalcantitum	chalcanthite
dāngguī	當歸	Angelica sinensis/polimorpha	Chinese angelica root
dānshēn	丹參	Salvia miltiorrhiza	salvia root
dàzǎo	大棗	Zizyphus jujuba	jujube
dìhuáng	地黃	Rehmannia glutinosa	rehmannia root
dìlóng	地龍	Pheretima	earthworm
dīngxiāng	丁香	Sygyzium aromaticum	clove
dìyú	地榆	Sanguisorba officinalis	burnet root
dúhuó	獨活	AchyrAngelica pubescenbidentata	pubescent angelica rootachyranthes root
dùzhòng	杜仲	Eucommia ulmoides	eucommia bark
ējiāo	阿膠	Equus asinus	donkey hide glue
ézhú/péngézhú	莪朮/莪茂/蓬莪朮	Curcuma aeruginosa	pink and blue ginger rhizome

Pinyin	Chinese	Latin Source	English Common Name
fángfēng	防風	Ledebouriella/ Saposhnikovia divaricata	saposhnikovia root
fángkuí	防葵	Peucedanum japonicum	peucedanum root
fēngfáng	蜂房	Polistes	paper wasp nest
fénghuàpòxiāo	風化樸硝	Sodium sulfate	refined mirabilite
fěnshuāng	粉霜	mercurous chloride	refined calomel
fúlíng	茯苓	Poria cocos	poria
fúlónggān	伏龍肝	Terra flava usta	cookstove ash
fúmài/ fúxiǎomài	浮麥/浮小麥	Triticum aestivum	blighted wheat
fúshén	茯神	Poria cocos	root poria
fùzǐ	附子	Aconitum carmichaeli	aconite prepared lateral root
gāncǎo	甘草	Glycyrrhiza uralensis	licorice root
gānjiāng	乾薑	Zingiber officinale	dried ginger
gānmùguā	乾木瓜	Chaenomeles lagenaria/sinensis	dried Japanese quince
gānqī	乾漆	Rhus verniciflua/ Toxicodendron vernicifluum	lacquer
gānsuì	甘遂	Euphorbia kansui	kansui root
gānxiē	干蠍	Scorpio	dried scorpion
gǎoběn	藁本	Ligusticum sinense	Chinese lovage root and rhizome
gāoliángjiāng	高良姜	Alpinia officinarum	lesser galangal rhizome
guādì	瓜蒂	Cucumis melo	muskmelon stalk
guālóugēn	栝楼根	Trichosanthes kirilowii	trichosanthes root
guānguì	官桂	Cinnamomum cassia	quilled cinnamon bark

Pinyin	Chinese	Latin Source	English Common Name
guìxīn	桂心	Cinnamomum cassia	shaved cinnamon bark
gǔsuìbǔ	骨碎補	Drynaria fortunei/ baronii etc.N/A	drynaria rhizome
hǎitóngpí	海桐皮	Erythrina variegata	erythrina bark
hēidòu	黑豆	Glycine hispida var. nigra	black soybean
hēifùzǐ	黑附子	Aconitum carmichaeli	black aconite prepared lateral root
hēiqiānniú	黑牽牛	Pharbitis nil/ purpurea	black morning glory seed
hēlílè	訶梨勒	Terminaria chebula	myrobalan fruit
héshǒuwū	何首烏	Polygonum multiflorum/ Rheinoutria multiflora	flowery knotweed root
hēzǐpí	訶子皮	Terminaria chebula	myrobalan fruit/ chebule peel
hēzǐròu	訶子肉	Terminaria chebula	myrobalan fruit/ chebule flesh
hónghuā	紅花	Carthamus tinctorius	safflower
hòupò/ nóngpò	厚朴/濃朴	Magnolia officinalis	officinal magnolia bark
huángdān	黃丹	Minium	minium/yellow lead
huánglián	黃連	Coptis chinensis	coptis rhizome
huángqí	黃芪/黃耆	Astragalus membranaceus	astragalus/vetch root
huángqín	黃芩	Scutellaria baicalensis	scutellaria/skullcap root
huáshí	滑石	Talcum	talcum
húhuánglián	胡黃連	Picrorhiza scrophulariiflora	Picroshiza rhizome
huíxiāng/ xiǎohuíxiāng	茴香/小茴香	Foeniculum officinalis	fennel seed
hújiāo	胡椒	Piper nigrum	pepper

Pinyin	Chinese	Latin Source	English Common Name
húmá	胡麻	Sesamum indicum	black sesame
huòxiāngyè	藿香葉	Agastache rugosa (or less commonly Pogostemon cablin)	Korean mint/Chinese patchouli leaf
hǔpò	琥珀	succinum	amber
jiāngcán	僵蠶	Bombyx mori batryticatus	infected silkworm larva
jiānghuáng	薑黃	Curcuma Longa	turmeric
jiāohóng	椒紅	Zanthoxylum bungeanum	Sìchuān peppercorn peel
jiāorén	椒仁	Zanthoxylum bungeanum	Sìchuān peppercorn seed
jiégěng	桔梗	Platycodon grandiflorus	platycodon root
jīnbó	金箔	Aureum	gold leaf
jīnchāshíhú/ shíhí	金釵石斛/石斛	Dendrobium nobile	dendrobium stem
jīngjiè	荊芥	Schizonepeta tenuifolia	schizonepeta/ Japanese catnip (whole plant)
jīngjièsuì	荊芥穗	Schizonepeta tenuifolia	schizonepeta/ Japanese catnip spike
jīngsānléng	京三棱	Sparganium stoloniferum	sparganium rhizome
jīnyínbó	金銀箔	Aureum and argentum	gold and silver leaf
júhóng	橘紅	Citrus tangerina or reticulata	red tangerine peel
júpí	橘皮	Citrus tangerina or reticulata	tangerine peel
kuǎndōnghuā	款冬花	Tussilago farfara	coltsfoot flower
kǔshēn	苦參	Sophora flavescens	flavescent sophora root
liángjiāng/ gāoliángjiāng	良薑/高良姜	Alpinia officinarum	lesser galangal rhizome

Pinyin	Chinese	Latin Source	English Common Name
liánzǐcǎo	蓮子草	Althernanthera sessilis	sessile joyweed plant
língshā	靈砂	mercuric sulfide	cinnabar
liúhuáng	硫磺	sulphur	sulfur
lìzǐnèipí	栗子內皮	Castanea mollissima	chestnut endothelium
lóngchǐ	龍齒	Mastodon	dragon tooth
lónggǔ	龍骨	Mastodon	dragon bone
lóngnǎo/nǎozǐ	龍腦/腦子	Dryobalanops aromatica	borneol
lùjiǎoshuāng	鹿角霜	Cervus nippon	processed deer antler
luóbózǐ	蘿卜子	Raphanus sativus	radish seed
lùróng	鹿茸	Cervus nippon	velvet deer antler
mài/màizǐ/xiǎomài	麥/麥子/小麥	Triticum	wheat
màiméndōng/màidōng	麥門冬/麥冬	Ophiopogon japonicus	ophiopogon/Japanese hyacinth tuber
mànjīngzǐ	蔓荊子	Vitex rotundifolia	vitex fruit
márén	麻仁	Cannabis sativa	hemp seed
méngchóng	虻蟲	Tabanus bivittatus	tabanus
mòyào	沒藥	Commiphora myrrha/Balsamodendron ehrenbergianum	myrrh
mǔdānpí	牡丹皮	Paeonia suffruticosa	Tree peony/moutan root bark
mùguā	木瓜	Chaenomeles lagenaria/sinensis	Japanese quince
mǔlì	牡蠣	Ostrea rivularis	oyster shell
mǔlìfěn	牡蠣粉	Ostrea rivularis	pulverized oyster shell
mùtōng	木通	Akebia quinata or triofoliata	chocolate vine stem

Pinyin	Chinese	Latin Source	English Common Name
mùxiāng	木香	Aucklandia/ Saussurea lappa	costusroot
mùzéi	木賊	Equisetum hiemale	horsetail plant
nánmùxiāng	南木香	Aristolochia yunnanensis	Yúnnán aristolochia root
náoshā	硇砂	sal ammoniac	sal ammoniac
nǎozǐ/lóngnǎo	腦子/龍腦	Dryobalanops aromatica	borneol
niúhuáng	牛黃	Bos taurus domesticus	bovine bezoar
niúxī	牛膝	Achyranthes Bidentata	achyranthes root
nóngpò/ hòupò	濃朴/厚朴	Magnolia officinalis	officinal magnolia bark
nuòmǐ	糯米	Oryza sativa var. glutinosa	glutinous rice
pògùzhǐ	破故紙	Psoralea corylifolia	babchi
púhuáng	蒲黃	Typha angustata/ angustifolia	cattail pollen
qiānghuó	羌活	Notopterygium incisum	notopterygium root and rhizome
qiānniú	牽牛	Ipomoea or Pharbitis	morning glory seed
qiānshuāng	鉛霜	galenitum acidum	vinegar-processed galenite
qícáo	蠐螬	Holotrichia diomphalia	Korean black chafer
qīngjúpí/ qīngpí	青橘皮/青皮	Citrus tangerina or reticulata	unripe tangerine peel
qīngxiāngzǐ	青葙子	Celosia argentea	plumed cockscomb seed
qínjiāo	秦艽	Gentiana macrophylla	large gentian root
quánxiē	全蝎	Scorpio	dried whole scorpion
qúmài	瞿麥	Dianthus superbus	dianthus plant

Pinyin	Chinese	Latin Source	English Common Name
rénshēn	人参	Panax ginseng	ginseng root
ròucōngróng	肉苁蓉	Cistanche salsa	cistanche stalk
ròudòukòu	肉豆蔻	Myristica fragrans	nutmeg
ròuguì	肉桂	Cinnamomum cassia	cinnamon bark
rǔxiāng	乳香	Boswellia carterii	frankincense
sāngbáipí	桑白皮	Morus alba	mulberry root bark
sānléng/ jīngsānléng	三棱/京三棱	Sparganium stoloniferum	sparganium rhizome
sháoyào	芍药	Paeonia lactiflora/ albiflora	peony root
shārén	砂仁	Amomum villosum/ xanthioides	amomum fruit
shāshēn	沙参	Adenophora stricta/ tetraphylla	adenophora root
shēngdì/ shēngdìhuáng	生地/生地黄	Rehmannia glutinosa	fresh rehmannia root
shēngfùzǐ	生附子	Aconitum carmichaeli	raw aconite lateral root
shénqǔ	神麴	Massa medicata fermentata	medicated leaven
shèxiāng	麝香	Moschus moschiferus	musk
shíchāngpú	石菖蒲	Acorus gramineus	Japanese sweet flag rhizome
shígāo	石膏	Gypsum Fibrosum	gypsum
shíhú/ jīnchāshíhú	石斛/金钗石斛	Dendrobium nobile	dendrobium plant
shínányè	石楠葉	Photinia serrulata	photinia leaf
shíwéi	石韋	Pyrrosia lingua	pyrrosia fern leaf
shíyànzǐ	石燕子	Cyrtospirifer sinensis	spirifer fossil
shúdì/ shúdìhuáng	熟地/熟地黄	Rehmannia glutinosa	cooked rehmannia root
shuǐzhì	水蛭	Hirudo nipponica	leech

Pinyin	Chinese	Latin Source	English Common Name
shúmǐ	秫米	Panicum miliaeum	broomcorn millet
sōngzhī	松脂	Pinus	pine resin
suānshíliúpí	酸石榴皮	Punica granatum	pomegranate rind
suānzǎorén	酸棗仁	Ziziphus jujuba/spinosus	jujube seed
sūhéxiāngyóu	蘇禾香油	Liquidambar orientalis	storax oil
suōshārén	縮砂仁	Amomum villosum	Vietnamese amomum seed and fruit
tàiyīnxuánjīngshí	太陰玄精石	selenitum	selenite
táorén	桃仁	Prunus persica	peach kernel
tiānmá	天麻	Gastrodia elata	gastrodia rhizome
tiānméndōng	天門冬	Asparagus cochinsinensis	Chinese asparagus root
tiānxióng	天雄	Aconitum carmichaeli	tiānxióng aconite (processed aconite long tuber)
tiěfěn	鐵粉	ferrum	pulverized iron
tínglì	葶藶	Lepidium apetalum or Descurainia sophia	peppercress seed
tóufǎ	頭髮	Homo sapiens	human hair
tùsīzǐ	菟絲子	Cuscuta chinensis	dodder seed
wànàqí	膃肭臍	Callorhinus ursinus	seal penis and testicles
wǎncánshā	晚蠶沙	Bombyx mori	silkworm droppings
wēilíngxiān	威靈仙	Clematis chinensis/hexapetala/armandi etc.	Chinese clematis root
wǔlíngzhī	五靈脂	Trogopterus xanthipes	squirrel droppings
wǔwèizǐ	五味子	Schisandra chinensis	schisandra fruit

Pinyin	Chinese	Latin Source	English Common Name
wūxīxiè/xījiǎo	烏犀屑/犀角	Rhinoceros	rhinoceros horn shavings
wūyào	烏藥	Lindera strychnifolia/ aggregata	lindera root
wūzéigǔ	烏賊骨	Sepia	Cuttlefish bone
wúzhū/ wúzhūyú/ zhūyú	吳茱/吳茱萸/ 茱萸	Evodia rutaecarpa	unripe evodia fruit
xiāngfù/ xiāngfùzǐ	香附/香附子	Cyperus rotundus	cyperus/nut grass rhizome
xiǎomài/mài/ màizǐ	小麥/麥/麥子	Triticum	wheat
xiāoshí	硝石	potassium nitrate	niter/saltpeter
xījiǎo/wūxīxiè	犀角/烏犀屑	Rhinoceros	rhinoceros horn
xìngrén	杏仁	Prunus armeniaca	apricot seed
xìnpī	信砒	arsenicum	arsenic
xiónghuáng	雄黃	realgar	realgar
xiōngqióng/ chuānxiōng	芎藭/川芎	Ligusticum wallichii	chuānxiōng lovage rhizome
xìxiāngmò	細香墨	atramentum	fine fragrant ink
xìxīn	細辛	Asarum heteropoides	asarum plant
xuánfùhuā	旋復花	Inula brittanica or lunariaefolia	Inula flower
xuánhúsuǒ/ yánhúsuǒ	玄胡索/延胡 索	Corydalis yanhusuo	corydalis rhizome
xuānlián	宣連	Coptis teeta or japonica	Xuānchéng coptis rhizome
xuánshēn	玄參	Scrophularia ningpoensis	figwort root
xùduàn	續斷	Dipsacus asperoides	dipsacus root
xuèjié	血竭	Daemonorops draco	dragon's blood resin
xūnlùxiāng	薰陸香	Boswellia thurifera	mastic

Pinyin	Chinese	Latin Source	English Common Name
xùsuízǐ	續隨子	Euphorbia lathyris	caper spurge seed
yángqǐshí	陽起石	actinolitum	actinolite
yìyǐrén	薏苡仁	Coix lachrymae-jobi	Job's tears seed
yìzhì	益智	Alpinia oxyphylla	sharp-leaf galangal fruit
yuánhuā	芫花	Daphne genkwa	genkwa flower
yuǎnzhì	遠志	Polygala tenuifolia	polygala/snakeroot root
yùlǐrén	鬱李仁	Prunus japonica	bush cherry seed
yǔyúliáng	禹餘糧	Limonitum	limonite
zàojiǎo	皂角	Gleditsia sinensis	Chinese honey locust seed
zéxiè	澤瀉	Alisma plantago-aquatica	alisma rhizome
zhèchóng	蟄蟲	Eupolyphaga sinensis or Opisthoplatia orientalis	wingless cockroach
zhēnshā	針砂	ferrum	needle filings
zhēnzhūmǔ	真珠母	Concha margaritifera	mother-of-pearl
zhǐké/zhǐshí	枳殼/枳實	Poncirus trifoliata or Citrus aurantium	bitter orange fruit
zhīmǔ	知母	Anemarrhena asphodeloides	anemarrhena root
zhīzǐ	梔子	Gardenia jasminoides	gardenia fruit
zhūlíng	豬苓	Polyporus umbellatus	polyporus
zhūshā	朱砂	mercuric sulfide	cinnbar
zhūyú/wúzhūyú	茱萸/吳茱萸	Evodia rutaecarpa	unripe evodia fruit
zǐjīnniú	紫金牛	Ardisia japonica	marlberry fruit

MEDICINAL REFERENCE BY ENGLISH COMMON NAME

English Common Name	Pinyin	Chinese	Latin Source
achyranthes root	niúxī	牛膝	Achyranthes bidentata
aconite main root	chuānwū/ chuānwūtóu	川烏/川烏頭	Aconitum carmichaeli
aconite prepared lateral root	fùzǐ	附子	Aconitum carmichaeli
actinolite	yángqǐshí	陽起石	actinolitum
adenophora root	shāshēn	沙参	Adeonphora stricta/ tetraphylla
agarwood resin	chénxiāng	沉香	Aquilaria agalocha/ sinensis
alisma rhizome	zéxiè	澤瀉	Alisma plantago- aquatica
alum	báifán	白礬	Alumen
amber	hǔpò	琥珀	succinum
amomum fruit	shārén	砂仁	Amomum villosum/ xanthioides
ampelopsis root	báiliǎn	白蘞	Ampelopsis japonica
anemarrhena root	zhīmǔ	知母	Anemarrhena asphodeloides
apricot seed	xìngrén	杏仁	Prunus armeniaca
arborvitae root bark	bǎipí	柏皮	Platycladus orientalis
arborvitae/biota seed	bǎizǐrén	柏子仁	Platycladus orientalis
arsenic	xìnpī	信砒	arsenicum
asarum plant	xìxīn	細辛	Asarum heteropoides
astragalus/vetch root	huángqí	黃芪/黃耆	Astragalus membranaceus
atractylodes rhizome	báizhú	白朮	Atractylodes macrocephala
atractylodes rhizome	cāngzhú	蒼朮	Atractylodes lancea

English Common Name	Pinyin	Chinese	Latin Source
babchi	pògùzhǐ	破故紙	Psoralea corylifolia
benzoin	ānxīxiāng	安息香	Benzoinum
betel nut	bīnláng	檳榔	Areca catechu
bitter orange fruit	zhǐké/zhǐshí	枳殼/枳實	Poncirus trifoliata or Citrus aurantium
black aconite prepared lateral root	hēifùzǐ	黑附子	Aconitum carmichaeli
black morning glory seed	hēiqiānniú	黑牽牛	Pharbitis nil/ purpurea
black sesame	húmá	胡麻	Sesamum indicum
black soybean	hēidòu	黑豆	Glycine hispida var. nigra
blighted wheat	fúmài/ fúxiǎomài	浮麥/浮小麥	Triticum aestivum
borneol	lóngnǎo/nǎozǐ	龍腦/腦子	Dryobalanops aromatica
borneol	nǎozǐ/lóngnǎo	腦子/龍腦	Dryobalanops aromatica
bovine bezoar	niúhuáng	牛黃	Bos taurus domesticus
broomcorn millet	shǔmǐ	秫米	Panicum miliaeum
bupleurum root	cháihú	柴胡	Bupleurum chinense
burnet root	dìyú	地榆	Sanguisorba officinalis
bush cherry seed	yùlǐrén	鬱李仁	Prunus japonica
caper spurge seed	xùsuízǐ	續隨子	Euphorbia lathyris
cattail pollen	púhuáng	蒲黃	Typha angustata/ angustifolia
chalcanthite	dǎnfán	膽礬	Chalcantitum
chestnut endothelium	lìzǐnèipí	栗子內皮	Castanea mollissima

English Common Name	Pinyin	Chinese	Latin Source
Chinese angelica root	dāngguī	當歸	Angelica sinensis/polimorpha
Chinese asparagus root	tiānméndōng	天門冬	Asparagus cochinsinensis
Chinese clematis root	wēilíngxiān	威靈仙	Clematis chinensis/hexapetala/armandi etc.
Chinese honey locust seed	zàojiǎo	皂角	Gleditsia sinensis
Chinese lovage root and rhizome	gǎoběn	藁本	Ligusticum sinense
chocolate vine stem	mùtōng	木通	Akebia quinata or triofoliata
chuānxiōng lovage rhizome	chuānxiōng/xiōngqióng	川芎/芎藭	Ligusticum wallichii
chuānxiōng lovage rhizome	xiōngqióng/chuānxiōng	芎藭/川芎	Ligusticum wallichii
cinnabar	língshā	靈砂	mercuric sulfide
cinnabar (top quality)	chénshā	辰砂	mercuric sulfide
cinnamon bark	ròuguì	肉桂	Cinnamomum cassia
cinnbar	zhūshā	朱砂	mercuric sulfide
cistanche stalk	ròucōngróng	肉蓯蓉	Cistanche salsa
clove	dīngxiāng	丁香	Sygyzium aromaticum
coltsfoot flower	kuǎndōnghuā	款冬花	Tussilago farfara
cooked rehmannia root	shúdì/shúdìhuáng	熟地/熟地黃	Rehmannia glutinosa
cookstove ash	fúlónggān	伏龍肝	Terra flava usta
coptis rhizome	huánglián	黃連	Coptis chinensis
corydalis rhizome	xuánhúsuǒ/yánhúsuǒ	玄胡索/延胡索	Corydalis yanhusuo
costusroot	mùxiāng	木香	Aucklandia/Saussurea lappa

English Common Name	Pinyin	Chinese	Latin Source
croton seed	bādòu	巴豆	Croton tiglium
cubeb	bìchéngqié	蓽澄茄	Piper cubeba
Cuttlefish bone	wūzéigǔ	烏賊骨	Sepia
cyperus/nut grass rhizome	xiāngfù/ xiāngfùzǐ	香附/香附子	Cyperus rotundus
Dahurican angelica root	báizhǐ	白芷	Angelica dahurica
dendrobium plant	shíhú/ jīnchāshíhú	石斛/金釵石斛	Dendrobium nobile
dendrobium stem	jīnchāshíhú/ shíhí	金釵石斛/石斛	Dendrobium nobile
dianthus plant	qúmài	瞿麥	Dianthus superbus
dipsacus root	chuānxùduàn	川續斷	Dipsacus asperoides
dipsacus root	xùduàn	續斷	Dipsacus asperoides
dodder seed	tùsīzǐ	菟絲子	Cuscuta chinensis
donkey hide glue	ējiāo	阿膠	Equus asinus
dragon bone	lónggǔ	龍骨	Mastodon
dragon tooth	lóngchǐ	龍齒	Mastodon
dragon's blood resin	xuèjié	血竭	Daemonorops draco
dried ginger	gānjiāng	乾薑	Zingiber officinale
dried Japanese quince	gānmùguā	乾木瓜	Chaenomeles lagenaria/sinensis
dried scorpion	gānxiē	干蠍	Scorpio
dried soybean sprout	dàdòuhuángjuǎn	大豆黃卷	Glycine max
dried whole scorpion	quánxiē	全蝎	Scorpio
drynaria rhizome	gǔsuìbǔ	骨碎補	Drynaria fortunei/ baronii etc.
earthworm	dìlóng	地龍	Pheretima
erythrina bark	hǎitóngpí	海桐皮	Erythrina variegata
eucommia bark	dùzhòng	杜仲	Eucommia ulmoides

English Common Name	Pinyin	Chinese	Latin Source
fennel seed	huíxiāng/ xiǎohuíxiāng	茴香/小茴香	Foeniculum officinalis
figwort root	xuánshēn	玄參	Scrophularia ningpoensis
fine fragrant ink	xìxiāngmò	細香墨	atramentum
fish poison yam	bìxiè	萆薢	Dioscorea tokoro/ hypoglauca etc.
flavescent sophora root	kǔshēn	苦參	Sophora flavescens
flowery knotweed root	héshǒuwū	何首烏	Polygonum multiflorum/ Rheinoutria multiflora
frankincense	rǔxiāng	乳香	Boswellia carterii
fresh rehmannia root	shēngdì/ shēngdìhuáng	生地/生地黃	Rehmannia glutinosa
fritillary bulb	bèimǔ	貝母	Fritillaria verticillata var. thunbergii
gardenia fruit	zhīzǐ	梔子	Gardenia jasminoides
gastrodia rhizome	tiānmá	天麻	Gastrodia elata
genkwa flower	yuánhuā	芫花	Daphne genkwa
ginseng root	rénshēn	人參	Panax ginseng
glutinous rice	nuòmǐ	糯米	Oryza sativa var. glutinosa
goat's head bur	báijílí	白蒺藜	Tribulus terrestris
gold and silver leaf	jīnyínbó	金銀箔	Aureum and argentum
gold leaf	jīnbó	金箔	Aureum
gypsum	shígāo	石膏	Gypsum Fibrosum
hemp seed	márén	麻仁	Cannabis sativa
horsetail plant	mùzéi	木賊	Equisetum hiemale
human hair	tóufǎ	頭髮	Homo sapiens

English Common Name	Pinyin	Chinese	Latin Source
infected silkworm larva	báijiāngcán	白僵蠶	Bombyx mori batryticatus
infected silkworm larva	jiāngcán	僵蠶	Bombyx mori batryticatus
Inula flower	xuánfùhuā	旋復花	Inula brittanica or lunariaefolia
Japanese quince	mùguā	木瓜	Chaenomeles lagenaria/sinensis
Japanese sweet flag rhizome	shíchāngpú	石菖蒲	Acorus gramineus
Job's tears seed	yìyǐrén	薏苡仁	Coix lachrymae-jobi
jujube	dàzǎo	大棗	Zizyphus jujuba
jujube seed	suānzǎorén	酸棗仁	Ziziphus jujuba/spinosus
kansui root	gānsuì	甘遂	Euphorbia kansui
Korean black chafer	qícáo	蠐螬	Holotrichia diomphalia
Korean mint/Chinese patchouli leaf	huòxiāngyè	藿香葉	Agastache rugosa (or less commonly Pogostemon cablin)
lacquer	gānqī	乾漆	Rhus verniciflua/Toxicodendron vernicifluum
large aconite prepared lateral root	dàfùzǐ	大附子	Aconitum carmichaeli
large gentian root	qínjiāo	秦艽	Gentiana macrophylla
leech	shuǐzhì	水蛭	Hirudo nipponica
lesser galangal rhizome	gāoliángjiāng	高良姜	Alpinia officinarum
lesser galangal rhizome	liángjiāng/gāoliángjiāng	良薑/高良姜	Alpinia officinarum
licorice root	gāncǎo	甘草	Glycyrrhiza uralensis
limonite	yǔyúliáng	禹餘糧	Limonitum

English Common Name	Pinyin	Chinese	Latin Source
lindera root	wūyào	烏藥	Lindera strychnifolia/ aggregata
long pepper capsule and root	bìbá	蓽茇	Piper longum
magnetite	císhí	磁石	Magnetitum
marlberry fruit	zǐjīnniú	紫金牛	Ardisia japonica
mastic	xūnlùxiāng	薰陸香	Boswellia thurifera
medicated leaven	shénqǔ	神麴	Massa medicata fermentata
minium/yellow lead	huángdān	黃丹	Minium
morinda root	bājǐtiān	巴戟天	Morinda officinalis
morning glory seed	qiānniú	牽牛	Ipomoea or Pharbitis
mother-of-pearl	zhēnzhūmǔ	真珠母	Concha margaritifera
motherwort	chōngwèicǎo/ yìmǔcǎo	茺蔚草/益母草	Leonurus heterophyllus
mugwort leaf	àiyè	艾葉	Artemisia argyi
mulberry root bark	sāngbáipí	桑白皮	Morus alba
musk	shèxiāng	麝香	Moschus moschiferus
muskmelon stalk	guādì	瓜蒂	Cucumis melo
mylabris/blister beetle	bānmáo	斑貓	Mylabris
myrobalan fruit	hēlílè	訶梨勒	Terminaria chebula
myrobalan fruit/ chebule peel	hēzǐpí	訶子皮	Terminaria chebula
myrobalan fruit/ chebule flesh	hēzǐròu	訶子肉	Terminaria chebula
myrrh	mòyào	沒藥	Commiphora myrrha/ Balsamodendron ehrenbergianum
needle filings	zhēnshā	針砂	ferrum

English Common Name	Pinyin	Chinese	Latin Source
niter/saltpeter	xiāoshí	硝石	potassium nitrate
notopterygium root and rhizome	qiānghuó	羌活	Notopterygium incisum
nutmeg	ròudòukòu	肉豆蔻	Myristica fragrans
officinal magnolia bark	hòupò/ nóngpò	厚朴/濃朴	Magnolia officinalis
officinal magnolia bark	nóngpò/ hòupò	濃朴/厚朴	Magnolia officinalis
ophiopogon/ Japanese hyacinth tuber	màiméndōng/ màidōng	麥門冬/麥冬	Ophiopogon japonicus
oyster shell	mǔlì	牡蠣	Ostrea rivularis
paper wasp nest	fēngfáng	蜂房	Polistes
peach pit	táorén	桃仁	Prunus persica
peony root	sháoyào	芍藥	Paeonia lactiflora/ albiflora
pepper	hújiāo	胡椒	Piper nigrum
peppercress seed	tínglì	葶藶	Lepidium apetalum or Descurainia sophia
perilla leaf	zǐsūyè	紫蘇葉	Perilla frutescens
peucedanum root	fángkuí	防葵	Peucedanum japonicum
photinia leaf	shínányè	石楠葉	Photinia serrulata
Picroshiza rhizome	húhuánglián	胡黃連	Picrorhiza scrophulariiflora
pine resin	sōngzhī	松脂	Pinus
pinellia rhizome	bànxià	半夏	Pinellia ternata
pink and blue ginger rhizome	ézhú/ péngézhú	莪术/莪茂/蓬莪术	Curcuma aeruginosa
plantain seed	chēqiánzǐ	車前子	Plantago asiatica
platycodon root	jiégěng	桔梗	Platycodon grandiflorus

English Common Name	Pinyin	Chinese	Latin Source
plumed cockscomb seed	qīngxiāngzǐ	青葙子	Celosia argentea
polygala/snakeroot root	yuǎnzhì	遠志	Polygala tenuifolia
polyporus	zhūlíng	豬苓	Polyporus umbellatus
pomegranate rind	suānshíliúpí	酸石榴皮	Punica granatum
poria	fúlíng	茯苓	Poria cocos
processed deer antler	lùjiǎoshuāng	鹿角霜	Cervus nippon
pubescent angelica root	dúhuó	獨活	Angelica pubescens
pulverized iron	tiěfěn	鐵粉	ferrum
pulverized oyster shell	mǔlìfěn	牡蠣粉	Ostrea rivularis
pyrrosia fern leaf	shíwéi	石韋	Pyrrosia lingua
quilled cinnamon bark	guānguì	官桂	Cinnamomum cassia
radish seed	luóbózǐ	蘿卜子	Raphanus sativus
raw aconite lateral root	shēngfùzǐ	生附子	Aconitum carmichaeli
realgar	xiónghuáng	雄黃	realgar
red halloysite	chìshízhī	赤石脂	Halloysitum
red peony root	chìsháo/ chìsháoyào	赤芍/赤芍藥	Paeonia rubra
red poria	chìfú/chìfúlíng	赤茯/赤茯苓	Poria cocos
red ricebean	chìxiǎodòu	赤小豆	Vigna umbellata
red tangerine peel	júhóng	橘紅	Citrus tangerina or reticulata
refined calomel	fěnshuāng	粉霜	mercurous chloride
refined mirabilite	fénghuàpòxiāo	風化樸硝	Sodium sulfate
rehmannia root	dìhuáng	地黃	Rehmannia glutinosa
rhinoceros horn	xījiǎo/wūxīxiè	犀角/烏犀屑	Rhinoceros

English Common Name	Pinyin	Chinese	Latin Source
rhinoceros horn shavings	wūxīxiè/xījiǎo	烏犀屑/犀角	Rhinoceros
rhubarb root and rhizome	dàhuáng	大黃	Rheum palmatum
root poria	fúshén	茯神	Poria cocos
safflower	hónghuā	紅花	Carthamus tinctorius
sal ammoniac	náoshā	硇砂	sal ammoniac
salvia root	dānshēn	丹參	Salvia miltiorrhiza
sandalwood	báitánxiāng	白檀香	Santalum album L.
saposhnikovia root	fángfēng	防風	Ledebouriella/ Saposhnikovia divaricata
schisandra fruit	wǔweìzǐ	五味子	Schisandra chinensis
schizonepeta/ Japanese catnip (whole plant)	jīngjiè	荆芥	Schizonepeta tenuifolia
schizonepeta/ Japanese catnip spike	jīngjièsuì	荆芥穗	Schizonepeta tenuifolia
scutellaria/skullcap root	huángqín	黃芩	Scutellaria baicalensis
seal penis and testicles	wànàqí	膃肭臍	Callorhinus ursinus
selenite	tàiyīnxuánjīng shí	太陰玄精石	selenitum
sessile joyweed plant	liánzǐcǎo	蓮子草	Althernanthera sessilis
sharp-leaf galangal fruit	yìzhì	益智	Alpinia oxyphylla
shaved cinnamon bark	guìxīn	桂心	Cinnamomum cassia
Sìchuān morinda root	chuānbājǐ	川巴戟	Morinda officinalis
Sìchuān peppercorn peel	jiāohóng	椒紅	Zanthoxylum bungeanum
Sìchuān peppercorn seed	jiāorén	椒仁	Zanthoxylum bungeanum

ENGLISH COMMON NAME	PINYIN	CHINESE	LATIN SOURCE
Sichuan peppercorn/ prickly ash husk	chuānjiāo/ huājiāo	川椒/花椒	Zanthoxylum bungeanum
silkworm droppings	wǎncánshā	晚蠶沙	Bombyx mori
silkworm moth egg case	cántuìbù	蠶蛻布	Bombyx mori
sparganium rhizome	jīngsānléng	京三棱	Sparganium stoloniferum
sparganium rhizome	sānléng/ jīngsānléng	三棱/京三棱	Sparganium stoloniferum
spirifer fossil	shíyànzǐ	石燕子	Cyrtospirifer sinensis
squirrel droppings	wǔlíngzhī	五靈脂	Trogopterus xanthipes
storax oil	sūhéxiāngyóu	蘇禾香油	Liquidambar orientalis
sulfur	liúhuáng	硫磺	sulphur
tabanus	méngchóng	虻蟲	Tabanus bivittatus
talcum	huáshí	滑石	Talcum
tangerine peel	chénpí	陳皮	Citrus reticulata
tangerine peel	júpí	橘皮	Citrus tangerina or reticulata
Tatarinow's aster root	zǐwǎn	紫菀	Aster tataricus
tiānxiōng aconite (processed aconite long tuber)	tiānxióng	天雄	Aconitum carmichaeli
toosendan fruit	chuānliànzǐ	川楝子	Melia toosendan
Tree peony/moutan root bark	mǔdānpí	牡丹皮	Paeonia suffruticosa
trichosanthes root	guālóugēn	栝楼根	Trichosanthes kirilowii
tsaoko fruit	cǎoguǒ/ cǎoguǒzǐrén	草果/草果子仁	Amomum tsao-ko
turmeric	jiānghuáng	薑黃	Curcuma Longa
turtle shell	biējiǎ	鱉甲	Amyda/Trionyx sinensis

English Common Name	Pinyin	Chinese	Latin Source
unripe evodia fruit	wúzhū/ wúzhūyú/ zhūyú	吳茱/吳茱萸/ 茱萸	Evodia rutaecarpa
unripe evodia fruit	zhūyú/ wúzhūyú	茱萸/吳茱萸	Evodia rutaecarpa
unripe tangerine peel	qīngjúpí/ qīngpí	青橘皮/青皮	Citrus tangerina or reticulata
velvet deer antler	lùróng	鹿茸	Cervus nippon
Vietnamese amomum seed and fruit	suōshārén	縮砂仁	Amomum villosum
vinegar-processed galenite	qiānshuāng	鉛霜	galenitum acidum
vitex fruit	mànjīngzǐ	蔓荊子	Vitex rotundifolia
wheat	mài/màizǐ/ xiǎomài	麥/麥子/小麥	Triticum
wheat	xiǎomài/mài/ màizǐ	小麥/麥/麥子	Triticum
white aconite prepared lateral root	báifùzǐ	白附子	Aconitum carmichaeli album
white dragon bone	báilónggǔ	白龍骨	Mastodon
white lablab bean	báibiǎndòu	白扁豆	Lablab
white peony root	báisháo/ báisháoyào	白芍/白芍藥	Paeonia albiflora/ lactiflora
white poria	báifúlíng	白茯苓	Poria cocos
white root poria	báifúshén	白茯神	Poria cocos
wild aconite root	cǎowū/ cǎowūtóu	草烏/草烏頭	Aconitum kusnezoffii
wingless cockroach	zhèchóng	蟄蟲	Eupolyphaga sinensis or Opisthoplatia orientalis
Xuānchéng coptis rhizome	xuānlián	宣連	Coptis teeta or japonica
Yúnnán aristolochia root	nánmùxiāng	南木香	Aristolochia yunnanensis

GLOSSARY

Note: This glossary lists all deviations from Nigel Wiseman and Ye Feng's *Practical Dictionary of Chinese Medicine* found in *Channeling the Moon, Part Two,* as well as other terms that may be helpful to know, whether because the average reader with basic skills in medical Chinese terminology may not be familiar with them, because they are technical terms in gynecology, or because they are specific terms for medicinal preparation. Please note that this glossary is not intended to be a comprehensive list of TCM terminology by any means but is limited only to more specialized terms or ones that I have translated differently from Wiseman and Feng. For any terms not found in this glossary, please consult the *Practical Dictionary of Chinese Medicine.*

Actions for Medicinal and Formula Preparation

Pīnyīn	Chinese	English
bèi	焙	roast
bù jū shí	不拘時	do not restrict the timing
chǎo	炒	stir-fry
cuò	銼	grate
dǎo	搗	pestle
duàn	煅	calcine
fǔjǔ	㕮咀	pound
jiān	煎	simmer/stew
jiāng	薑	ginger-processed
jìn	浸	steep
niǎn	碾	crush with a roller
páo	炮	blast-fry
pào	泡	soak
shāo	燒	burn
suì	碎	crush
yán	研	grind
zhēng	蒸	steam
zhì	炙	mix-fry
zhǔ	煮	boil
zì	漬	drench

OTHER TERMS RELATED TO MEDICINALS AND FORMULAS

Pīnyīn	Chinese	English
dān	丹	elixir
jiān	尖	tips
jiān	煎	brew
jiǔ	酒	rice wine
ké	殼	shell
lú	蘆	shoots
miáo	苗	sprouts
mǐyǐn	米飲	thin rice gruel
mù	目	seeds
qí	臍	bottom
sǎn	散	powder
tāng	湯	decoction
wán	丸	pill
wǎn	碗	bowl
wútóng(zǐ)	梧桐子	wútóng seeds
xīn	心	core
yǐn(zǐ)	飲(子)	drink

GYNECOLOGY AND PATHOLOGY

Pīnyīn	Chinese	English
bài	敗	decay(-ed)
báidiàn	白癜	White Patch
bāo	胞	womb
bāolòu	胞漏	leaking womb
bāomén	胞門	Uterus Gate
bēng(xià)	崩(下)	Landslide Collapse (downward)
bì	閉	blockage
bì	痹	bì Impediment
biànxuè	便血	blood in the urine and feces
bùtōng	不通	lack of through-flow
chìzòng	瘛瘲	convulsion
chuāngjiè	瘡疥	scabby sores
chuánshī	傳屍	Corpse Transmission
dàixià	帶下	"below the belt," sometimes in the narrower sense as "vaginal discharge"
dàohàn	盜汗	Thief Sweating
diān	癲/顛	diān insanity
duàn	斷	interruption [of flow]
ě(xīn)	惡(心)	nausea
èlù	惡露	Malign Dew (i.e., lochia)
érzhěn(tòng)	兒枕(痛)	Child's Pillow (Pain)
èzǔ	惡阻	nausea in pregnancy
fèiwěi	肺痿	Lung Wilting
fúliáng	伏梁	Deep-Lying Beam
gǔ	蠱	gǔ toxin
guāngé	關格	block and repulsion

Pīnyīn	Chinese	English
guǐjiāo	鬼交	[dreams of] intercourse with ghosts
guǐtāi	鬼胎	ghost fetus
gǔzhēng	骨蒸	Bone Steaming
hēigǎn	黑䁓	dark discolored area
héizǐ	黑子	mole
huángdǎn	黃疸	jaundice
huǎnghū	恍惚	severe [mental] confusion
húli	狐狸	Fox [disease]
huòluàn	霍亂	Sudden Turmoil
jì	悸	palpitations
jī	積	Accumulations
jiǎ	瘕	Conglomerations
jiā	痂	scabs
jiǎoqì	腳氣	Lower-Leg Qì
jié	結	binding/to bind
jīng	驚	panic
jù	聚	Gatherings
jué	厥	Reversal
késòu	咳嗽	cough/dry cough and gurgling
kuài	塊	clot
kuáng	狂	kuáng mania
lài	癩	Lài disease
láo	勞	taxation
láozhài	癆瘵	consumption
léishòu	羸瘦	marked emaciation
lì(xià)/xiàlì	利(下)/下利	disinhibition (below)
lìfēng	癘風	pestilential wind

Pīnyīn	Chinese	English
lìjié	歷節	Joint Running
línlì	淋瀝	dribble
liú	瘤	tumors
lóngmén	龍門	Dragon Gate
lòu	漏	spotting
mào	冒	Veiling
méihé	梅核	Plum-Pit [Qì]
mèn	悶	oppression
pì	癖	Aggregations
pǐ	痞	pǐ Glomus
(quán)luá	(拳)攣	spasm
sào	瘙	eczema
shàn	疝	Mounding
tāi	胎	fetus
tiáo	調	to attune
wángxùe	亡血	blood collapse
xián	痃	Strings
xián	癇	seizure
xiāo	痟	Dissipation disease
xiāoké	消渴	Dissipation Thirst
xuàn	眩	blackout vision
xuèhǎi	血海	Sea of Blood
xuèshì	血室	Blood Chamber
xuèyùn	血運	blood dizziness
xūsǔn	虛損	vacuity detriment
yǎng	癢	itching
yǐng	癭	goiters

Pīnyīn	Chinese	English
yǐnzhěn	癮疹	dormant papules
yù	鬱	oppressive constraint
yùmén	玉門	Jade Gate
yūn	暈	dizziness
yùxuè	瘀血	static blood
zàozàng/ zàngzào	燥臟/臟躁	Visceral Agitation
zhàngnüè	瘴瘧	Miasmic Malaria
zhēng	癥	Concretions
zhòngfēng	中風	wind strike (not "stroke")
zhùwǔ	疰忤	Infixation Upset
zǐdiàn	紫癜	Purple Patch
zǐzàng/gōng	子臟/宮	uterus

OTHER TECHNICAL TERMS

Pīnyīn	Chinese	English
bó	搏	assault/battle (each other)
chéng	乘	exploit/overwhelm
fā	發	erupt/effuse
gān	干	harass
jīng	精	Essence
kè	客	intrude
kè	剋	restrain
lǐ	理	restore the correct pattern
nì	逆	counter-current [flow]
qiāng	搶	butt against
sàn	散	scatter/disperse
shèng	勝	prevail over
shùn	順	(restore) the flow in the proper direction
wèi	衛	*wèi* Defense
xiāo	消	dissipate, melt away
yíng/róng	營/榮	*yíng* Provisioning
zhì	制	control
zī	滋	saturate

Bibliography

Primary Sources

Bèijí qiānjīn yàofāng 《備急千金要方》 (Essential Formulas Worth a Thousand in Gold to Prepare for Emergencies). Sūn Sīmiǎo 孫思邈, 652.

Běncǎo gāngmù 《本草綱目》 (Classified Materia Medica). Lǐ Shízhēn 李時珍, 1596.

Chábìng zhǐnán 《察病指南》 (Guide to Scrutinizing Disease). Shī Guìtáng 施桂堂, 1241.

Chìshuǐ xuánzhū 赤水玄珠 (Dark Pearl of Red Water). Sūn Yīkuí 孫一奎, 1584.

Chǔ shì yíshū 褚氏遺書 (Posthumous Writings of Master Chǔ). Chǔ Chéng 褚澄, Southern Qí (479-502 CE).

Dàodéjīng 《道德經》 (Classic of the Way and its Virtue-Power). Attributed to Láozi, Zhōu period.

Fùrén dàquán liángfāng 《婦人大全良方》 (Compendium of Excellent Formulas for Women). Chén Zìmíng 陳自明, 1237.

Gǔjīn yītǒng dàquán 《古今醫統大全》 (Compendium of Ancient and Modern Medicine). Xú Chūnfǔ 徐春甫, 1556.

Huángdì nèijīng 《黃帝內經》 (Yellow Emperor's Inner Classic). Anon., Hàn period. Abbreviated as *Nèijīng* 《內經》 (Inner Classic).

Ishimpō 《醫心方》 (Formulas from the Heart of Medicine). Tanba no Yasuyori, 984.

Jīnguì yàolüè 《金匱要略》 (Essentials from the Golden Cabinet).
Zhāng Zhòngjǐng 張仲景, Hàn period.

Jīnguì yì 《金匱翼》 (Appendix to the *Jīnguì*). Yóu Yí 尤怡, 1768.

Jiǔzhuǎn língshā dàdān 《九轉靈砂大丹》 (Eightfold Transformation
Magical Sand Great Elixir). Unknown author, Táng to Sòng
periods.

Língshū 《靈樞》 (Magic Pivot). Anon., Hàn period. The second half
of the *Huángdì nèijīng*.

Lǚ shì chūnqiú 《呂氏春秋》 (Spring and Autumn Annals of Master
Lü). Lǚ Bùwéi 呂不韋, 239 BCE.

Mínglǐ lùn 《明理論》 (Discourse on Elucidating Principles). Short
for *Shānghán mínglǐ lùn* 《傷寒明理論》 (Discourse on Elucidating
Principles of Cold Damage). Chéng Wújǐ 成无己, 1156.

Nànjīng 《難經》 (Classic of Difficulties). Anon, Hàn period.

Neìjīng 《內經》 (Inner Classic). Anon., Hàn period. Short for
Huángdì nèijīng 《黃帝內經》 (Yellow Emperor's Inner Classic).

Nǚkē bǎiwèn 《女科百問》 (Hundred Questions on Gynecology). Qí
Zhòngfǔ 齊仲甫, 1220.

Pǔjì běnshì fāng 《普濟本事方》 (Original Formulas for Popular
Relief). Xǔ Shūwēi 許叔微, 1132.

Rúmén shìqīn 《儒門事親》 (Confucians Serving Their Parents).
Zhāng Cóngzhèng 張從正, 1228.

Shānghánlùn 《傷寒論》 (Treatise on Cold Damage). Zhāng
Zhòngjǐng 張仲景, Hàn period.

Shénnóng běncǎo jīng 《神農本草經》 (Divine Farmer's Classic of Materia Medica). Anon., Hàn period.

Shèngjì zǒnglù 《聖濟總錄》 (Encyclopedia of Sagely Benefaction). Sòng Huīzōng 宋徽宗, 1117.

Shuōwén jiězì 《說文解字》 (Explaining Characters and Analyzing Characters). Xǔ Shèn 許慎, 2nd century CE.

Sùwèn 《素問》 (Plain Questions). Anon., Hàn period. The first half of the *Huángdì nèijīng*.

Sùwèn bìngjī qìyí bǎomìng jí 《素問病機氣宜保命集》 (Collected [Comments on] Pathomechanisms, Appropriateness of Qì, and Safeguarding Life from the *Sùwèn*). Liú Wánsù 劉完素, 1186.

Tàipíng guǎngjì 《太平廣記》 (Comprehensive Records from the Tàipíng Era). Lǐ Fǎng 李昉, 978.

Tàipíng Huìmín Héjìjú fāng 《太平惠民和劑局方》 (Tàipíng Formulary from the Imperial Grace Pharmacy). Chén Chéng 陳承 et al., ed., 1078.

Wàitái mìyào 《外台秘要》 (Essential Secrets from the Outer Terrace/Palace Library). Wáng Tao 王燾, 752.

Yáng shì jiācáng fāng 《楊氏家藏方》 (Master Yáng's Hidden Family Formulas). Yáng Tán 楊倓, 1178.

Yìjīng 《易經》 (Classic of Changes). Anon., Zhōu period.

Zábìng guǎngyào 《雜病廣要》 (Comprehensive Essentials about the Various Diseases). Tanba no Genken 丹波元堅, 1853.

Zhūbìng yuánhòu lùn 《諸病源候論》 (Discourse on the Origins and Signs of the Various Diseases). Cháo Yuánfāng 巢元方, 610 CE.

Other Sources

Anon., *Zhōngyào dàcídiǎn* 《中藥大辭典》 (Great Dictionary of Chinese Materia Medica). 新文豐出版社, 1982 (originally published in 1977).

Lǐ, Jīngwěi 李經緯 et als., eds., *Zhōngyī dà cídiǎn* 《中醫大辭典》 (Great Dictionary of Chinese Medicine). 人民衛生出版社, 1980.

Smith, Hilary, *Forgotten Disease: Illnesses Transformed in Chinese Medicine* (Stanford University Press, 2017).

Unschuld, Paul U., *Huang Di Nei Jing Su Wen* (University of California Press, 2011).

Wilms, Sabine, *Humming with Elephants: The Great Treatise on the Resonant Manifestations of Yin and Yang* (Happy Goat Productions, 2018)

"The Transmission of Medical Knowledge on 'Nurturing the Fetus' in Early China." *Asian Medicine: Tradition and Modernity* 2, 2005.

The Divine Farmer's Classic of Materia Medica (Happy Goat Productions, 2017).

Venerating the Root: Sun Simiao's Bei Ji Qian Jin Yao Fang Volume 5 on Pediatrics, Parts One and Two (Happy Goat Productions, 2013 and 2015).

Wiseman, Nigel, *Practical Dictionary of Chinese Medicine* (Paradigm Publications, 2014).

Index

overwhelm 219, 241, 255, 352, 371, 435, 505, *See also* exploit/overwhelm

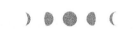

CPSIA information can be obtained
at www.ICGtesting.com
Printed in the USA
BVHW071044270820
587174BV00001B/5

9 781732 157149